TIRED
OR
TOXIC ?

A Blueprint For Health
By Sherry A. Rogers M.D.

1990

Prestige Publishing
Box 3161 3502 Brewerton Road
Syracuse, NY 13220

Library of Congress Card Catalog Number: 89-600-50

ISBN: 0-9618821-2-3

Printed in the United States

TIRED OR TOXIC ?

TABLE OF CONTENTS

Disclaimer
Dedication
About the Author
Foreword

DISCLAIMER

As with any work dealing with medicine, this attempts to teach. In the end, since there is no final test to evaluate your total comprehension of the subject, any trials should be carried out under the guidance of a qualified medical professional. This is meant to teach, not treat you.

DEDICATION

There are so many people to whom I owe thanks, that I always find this part the most difficult.

The office staff, the patients, my mentor, Dr. William J. Rea, and many more.

But one always stands above all else in my world:

TO LUSCIOUS

This book is also dedicated to the memory of......

                    FRANK MULVANA, R.N.

......who gave this world an incredible amount of healing
love and laughter.

ABOUT THE AUTHOR

Dr. Sherry A. Rogers is a fellow of the American College of Allergy and Immunology, a fellow of the American Board of Family Practice and a fellow of the American Academy of Environmental Medicine (as well as a 6 year member of the board of directors), and a diplomat of the American Board of Environmental Medicine (and on the board of directors). She also is one of the examiners for other physicians seeking fellowship and/or board status through the AAEM and ABEM, and is on the board of directors of the Pan American Allergy Society. She is also a member of the American College of Occupational Medicine.

She has written the comprehensive 650 page book on the diagnosis and treatment of environmental illness, The E.I. Syndrome, and a newly released book on how to clear the most difficult and resistant failures in the sequel You Are What You Ate.

She has published her mold research in three volumes of the Annals of Allergy, 1982, 1983, 1984, and Clinical Ecology, vol V, #3, 1987/1988, and how to diagnose chemical hypersensitivity in the Proceedings of IAQ '86, ASHRAE, The Proceedings of Indoor Air '87, West Berlin, Clinical Ecology, vol V, #4, 1987/1988, in the National Institutes of Health medical journal, Environmental Health Perspectives and in Environment International, which goes to 154 countries. These are only a few of her scientific publications.

She has authored over a dozen health magazine articles in Let's Live, Solstice, The Human Ecologist, and Bestways for example, and has been the subject of magazine articles authored by others in Prevention, Quebec Science, Solstice Science News, and Harrowsmith, as well as newspaper articles in several cities of the U.S. and Great Britain (The Yorkshire Press, etc.). She is on the medical advisory boards of Let's Live magazine and the Human Ecology Action League (Atlanta).

She has presented lay lectures on environmental medicine throughout the world, and has made television and radio appearances in over half a dozen U.S. cities (Washington, D.C., Atlanta, Buffalo, Syracuse, Phoenix, Dallas, etc.).

The services offered, besides her books, are a mold survey service for physicians and patients who want to know what types of molds are in their environments, and the formaldehyde spot test that she developed, (it gives an approximation of the level of formaldehyde in a product). She is in full time private practice seeing patients from around the world.

She teaches and lectures frequently, throughout the world. She lectures yearly in the scientific congress for the American Academy of Environmental Medicine and the international symposium, Man and His Environment in Health and Disease (American Center for Environmental Medicine, Dallas). She also teaches in training workshops for physicians as well as scientific presentations through the American Academy of Otolaryngic Allergy, and teaches in the Advanced Course for Physicians learning these new techniques (through the AAEM). She has presented courses for physicians also through the Pan American Society, Holy Name Hospital, The North American Nutrition and Preventive Medicine Association, and the International Health Foundation, as well as lectures for the Upstate Medical Center and several other hospitals.

She has presented her work in Toronto, Stockholm, West Berlin, England, and throughout six cities in China with Drs. Rea and Randolph. She has been invited by the Australian Society for Environmental Medicine to lecture for four days in that country in 1989, to present 2 papers at Indoor Air '89 in the Netherlands, and to present several papers and physician workshops for the British Society of Allergy and Environmental Medicine, 1990.

In short, she publishes original scientific research, writes books and magazine articles, teaches in the advanced courses for doctors learning all of this, and is one of the physicians who gives exams for physicians seeking certification in the field.

How did she pack so much into 46 short years? Easily. She had no choice. She had environmental illness and had to get well. Once she found the answers, she made it her business to become an expert in the field and help advance the knowledge for those who want full health.

She is me, and I invite you to read and educate yourself. For this most likely will be a major <u>turning point in your health</u> and your life; surely you will never be the same again.

For ENVIRONMENTAL ILLNESS is An Epidemic in Disguise.

FOREWORD

I am delighted to see in this book the first unparalleled and most comprehensive effort to enable the layman to learn about the era of medicine that is so new that many physicians are yet unaware of it.

This information is vitally important now as it touches everyone with nearly any symptom such as chemical sensitivity, high cholesterol, chronic fatigue, Candida-related complex, depression, Alzheimer's, high blood pressure, diabetes, heart disease, osteoporosis and more.

Having just completed a textbook for the medical profession on the same theme, I commend Dr. Sherry Rogers for this Herculean effort as I appreciate how many thousands of hours each of us has had to work independently to piece together this gigantic puzzle that explains how and why we get sick.

When I started reading this book, I was apprehensive that it might be beyond the grasp of the layman, but one has only to remember that 10 years ago words and concepts that are now commonplace, such as cholesterol, arteriosclerosis, Alzheimer's, formaldehyde, radon, PCB's, and agent orange (dioxin), were foreign. With the massive increase in environmental pollution from many angles and its resultant chemical sensitivity, terms such as xenobiotic, glutathione, xylene, toluene, toxic brain syndrome, conjugation, magnesium deficiency, chromium deficiency, and sick building syndrome will become commonplace.

The informed lay person already recognizes that as the world becomes more technological, he proportionally loses more control over his life. This book will enable him to regain control over his health as he is better able to form a team with his physician to diagnose and treat his condition. In fact, the informed layman may help educate his physician after reading this book.

A new era in medicine and living has been introduced and Dr. Rogers' book is in the forefront of educating the public on the effects of the environment on the individual.

William J. Rea, M.D.
founder, Environmental Health Center, Dallas,
thoracic and cardiovascular surgeon,
First World Professorial Chair in Environmental Medicine,
    Robens Institute, University of Surrey, England

January 3, 1990

Chapter 1: <u>A HEADACHE IS NOT A DARVON DEFICIENCY</u>

This book is not for everyone. It is only for 2 types of people: those who are sick enough, or those who are smart enough. The rest are on their own. The fact is, it is for a very select group of people, many of whom ironically enough, don't even know yet that they have anything wrong. Their family doctors cannot diagnose it, nor will the smartest medical specialists from the regional medical centers. For though there are over half a million doctors in the U.S., there are less than a few thousand physicians in the entire world who are aware of the current evolution in medicine. Furthermore, at this point in time, there are only a few hundred who have seriously begun attending courses to learn about it.

These few hundred who are developing their skills, and who come from every discipline of medicine, from internists, pediatricians, ENT, and family doctors, to immunologists and surgeons, are not in medical schools. For no medical school in the world, as of 1990, teaches this complete specialty.

Another group of physicians does not have the illness but has a superbly healthy ego so that intellectual honesty and curiosity shine through. The physician in this category is sincerely interested in the secrets of health and his patients' well being. If he or she gave you this book, your doctor is admitting that he is committed to helping you find wellness in any way he can, even if it means going against some of the now antiquated teachings he and I learned a quarter of a century ago in medical school.

With this book you will be able to determine, whether you or a loved one are an unsuspecting victim. And you will learn how to successfully treat yourselves before it is too late. You may even think that some of the symptoms that you have are already too late, but as you will learn, some of the most seemingly hopeless conditions have been helped by

the techniques in this book. Yet these conditions had previously failed to respond to the 20th century high technology medical offerings which include some of the most powerful modern medications, irradiations and surgeries.

Is Your Physician "Type E" or "Type C"?

There are no commonly used blood tests, no X-rays, no
questionnaires, no physical findings that will alert the
untrained physician to your diagnosis. And should you try
to help the physician who is unknowledgeable about the current evolution in medicine by putting the diagnosis under
his nose, you will quickly discover two types of responses:
One physician (called "type E" for egocentric) may unleash
an egocentric response upon you. Most likely you have felt
a hint of this reaction in the past when you have questioned
a diagnosis or medication. But don't take it too hard, for
you are not dealing with an open-minded individual. The
second physician (called "type C" for compassionate) will
admit he knows nothing about it but he is eager to learn so
that he can evaluate it, because he wants to help you get
well.

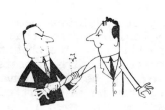

Don't try to convert every doctor involved in your
care to environmental medicine. You don't have
that much time and energy to waste. Just nurture
the ones who are type C.

For example, the kind of education we receive in medical school and internship, is an overload of material, some of which is uselessly outdated before we even graduate, the sleep deprivation, low pay, the repeated hammering and badgering by physicians, who only a few years prior were in our position; all this serves to wear us down so that we will never, ever again believe anything in medicine, no matter how logical or enticing it may appear, without the sanction, blessing and stamp of approval from the powers that be. And you'll be surprised to learn who really holds the power.

If you don't think this brain washing could happen to an intelligent, logical being, go to your doctor and complain of tiredness. If you are like the hundreds of people we saw in the last year who saw "type E" doctors, the stories are similar: nothing abnormal was found on blood tests or X-rays. The doctor proclaimed good health. The victim held his ground and politely reminded the doctor that the reason that he had come in was that he felt tired. The doctor still held his ground and reminded the victim that not only had he just completed a thorough exam, which was negative, but that his work was not to be questioned. If he

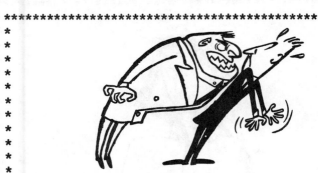

```
*********************************************************
*                                                       *
*                                                       *
*                                                       *
*                                                       *
*                                                       *
*                                                       *
*                                                       *
*                                                       *
*                                                       *
*                                                       *
*                                                       *
*      If your physician gets hostile when you try to   *
*      offer suggestions to help him solve your case,   *
*      he's more interested in protecting his ego than  *
*      your health.                                     *
*                                                       *
*********************************************************
```

4

said you were well, you were well. Luckily, many people
have "type C" doctors and they admitted that they didn't
have the answer and referred them on.

Sometimes the victim meekly tried to help doctor "type
E" by suggesting referral to a specialist, only to find to
his surprise, that this logical suggestion served to further
fuel the fires of wrath, with the unspoken message resulting; "If I don't know what you have, then no one does".
"Furthermore, as I have already expressed, if I don't know
what you have, then you don't have anything!"

Can God help us when we bestow such arrogance upon the
members of a profession who are supposed to guide us toward
health? But somehow medical school does a fantastic job in
programming us this way. And for good reason: it helps
maintain consistency, so that if you are seeing a cardiologist in California, when you move to New York you'll have
the same quality of care. So there is certainly much to be
said for not sanctioning physicians to jump wildly into
every new therapy that comes along.

```
**********************************************************
*                                                        *
*                                                        *
*                                                        *
*                                                        *
*                                                        *
*                                                        *
*                                                        *
*                                                        *
*                                                        *
*                                                        *
*                                                        *
*                                                        *
*                                                        *
*                                                        *
*                                                        *
*     If your doctor is genuinely interested in helping  *
*     you solve your case, he'll never resent any help   *
*     you can offer.                                      *
*                                                        *
**********************************************************
```

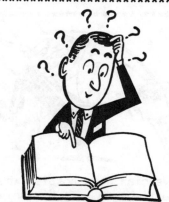

There Is No Such Thing As A Hypochondriac

The Compact Edition of the Oxford English Dictionary, Vol I, 1979, p. 1361, defines hypochondria as "a morbid state of mind, characterized by general depression, or low spirit, for which there is no real cause." And a hypochondriac as one who exhibits hypochondria.

Meanwhile, medicine borrows this name and uses it for patients who question their physician's inability to diagnose an organic disease: the hypochondriac. This term intimidates the victim sufficiently, to remove any persistence. By labeling the patient as a fake, a medical undesirable, a person who makes up symptoms to get attention, we have really put him in his place! We have not only intimidated him into a state of learning to ignore or tune out his symptoms, but we have gone one step further to assure our stance, by henceforth destroying his credibility. For once this label is applied, the next physician whom the victim of the system consults, also begins to work at a diagnosis; that is until he reads through the old records to find that Dr. X considered the patient to be a hypochondriac. Now the current doctor, if he is a "type E" can relax and breathe a sigh of relief, "No wonder I couldn't figure out what was wrong with him. There wasn't anything."

The biggest problem with this designation of hypochondriasis is that it teaches a person to ignore or tune out symptoms until they become unbearable or end-stage. The label intimidates the patient into a quiet acceptance of "half-health". Unfortunately these soft, subtle symptoms were intended by nature to serve as early warnings of worse symptoms to come if we ignore them or mask (cover them up) with medications. End-stage symptoms are much more difficult to clear, plus they eventually create permanent end-organ damage, as well as accelerate aging, and potentiate cancer.

Lately, because so many patients become infuriated by the diagnosis of hypochondriasis, a substitution has been found that saves face for the physician and simultaneously placates the patient by having a diagnosis: the chronic fatigue syndrome (also known as chronic EBV or chronic mono). More on this later.

In writing about medicine, there are generally two types of audiences that we are advised to address; one is some mythical populace that reads at an eighth grade level. The other is a pseudo-intellectual/professional level, where only referenced statements and double blind studies are allowed. I am writing for neither. I am writing for the person who wants to get well and simultaneously desires to live at optimum capacity. He just needs someone to show him how. He usually realizes his doctor will not or cannot cure him, but he has no where else to turn. If some of the following parts are too technical, as they may be, just breeze right on through. You'll be amazed how much you do absorb when you least think you can. But be gentle with yourself, for after all, you are about to learn a whole new form of medicine. So go easy on yourself if you don't grasp it all at once. For regardless, when you have finished, you'll know more about your health than many physicians at this point in time. And there will be tests you can give your doctor so you can know quickly what level of development he is at.

And when you find one who is knowledgeable or who is genuinely interested in learning, hang on to him. Not infrequently it takes 50 years for new discoveries to be thoroughly proven (because it takes that long to rewrite the medical school curriculum, get it formulated precisely in the way the powers that be want it taught, and train a new batch of physicians). Fortunately, there are countless caring, compassionate physicians who see the light and realize medicine is entering another period of evolution. They know that a headache is not a Darvon deficiency; that drugging people is not health, it's dependency. Furthermore it covers up early warning symptoms so that illness eventually progresses into something really big.

Granted some of the material may be challenging for you, but what do you expect when you are learning how to be your own doctor? You are learning a new specialty in medicine that many physicians are unaware of. If you are diligent, your efforts will pay off, as there are only two beings in the entire world who can make you truly well; God is rather busy, therefore we have to help you learn as much as possible.

Feel free to consult the glossary in the back if you are unsure of the meaning of some of these new words. It's there to help you learn faster. {Some of the more difficult chemistry will be set in these squiggle brackets, so if you're not inclined that way, you can skim those parts.}

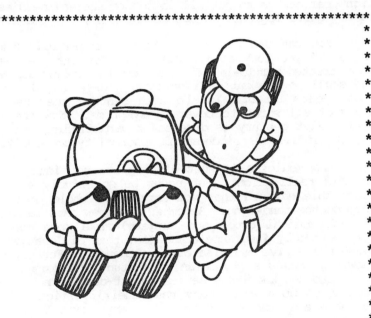

```
****************************************************
*                                                  *
*                                                  *
*                                                  *
*                                                  *
*                                                  *
*                                                  *
*                                                  *
*                                                  *
*                                                  *
*                                                  *
*                                                  *
*                                                  *
*                                                  *
*                                                  *
*                                                  *
*                                                  *
*                                                  *
*                                                  *
*                                                  *
*                                                  *
*                                                  *
* If the oil light goes on, you can always unscrew *
* the bulb, smash it with a hammer or buy a new car. *
* That's analogous to the kind of medicine insurance *
* companies pay for:  drugs, drugs and more drugs.  *
*                                                  *
****************************************************
```

You will learn how to cherish your symptoms as early warnings. For worse symptoms will appear should you chose to ignore the early warnings and merely mask them with medications. We don't have chronic pain, or high blood pressure, or asthma because the design of the world is malicious. They are early warnings; they act as a guide to tell us to alter our diet, lifestyle, or environment. They are there as a signal. They are the only warnings we have before death. It's like the car...you could just unscrew the oil light when it goes on, or you could smash it with a hammer. Both would make it go away.....but what for? The light reminds us to put oil in before the engine dies. It's really quite logical: drugs do not heal, they mask.

You can understand the current evolution of medicine better if you look at its history. For example, headaches were treated hundreds of years ago by trephining holes in the skull to let out evil spirits. Then they let out evil blood years later. In the 20th century they used potent drugs of all sorts to cover up symptoms. Now the medicine of the 21st century is directed toward finding and correcting the individual biochemical abnormality or sensitivity.

And medicine is just dipping its toe into the waters of this realization. But never be so naively enthusiastic about this new era that you expect the whole profession to jump on the bandwagon. Remember that new cars (analogous to hi-tech medical drugs and surgery) make more money (get paid better by insurance companies) than oil changes (common sense preventive medicine or maintenance). Furthermore, new knowledge means a physician must study and some prefer not to. Also new knowledge serves to out-date some of the older techniques upon which many base their prestige and income. So there are, and always will be, many "type E" dissenters. Ignorance, fear, politics (power), ego and money fuel the dissenters. While honesty, excitement, hope and facts fuel the rest.

```
****************************************************************
*    MANAGEMENT OF A HEADACHE THROUGHOUT HISTORY               *
*                                                              *
*    *    Skull trephining where holes were drilled            *
*         to let out the evil spirits                          *
*                                                              *
*    *    Phlebotomy to let out the bad blood                  *
*                                                              *
*    *    Specific drugs to calm the underlying bio-           *
*         chemical defect:                                     *
*         tranquilizers         calcium channel blockers       *
*         anti-depressants      analgesics                     *
*         vasodilators          serotonin antagonists          *
*         vasoconstrictors      serotonin agonists             *
*         beta blockers         enzyme inhibitors              *
*                                                              *
*    *    Identify and correct the underlying defect:          *
*         amino acidopathy       (e.g., taurine)               *
*         EFA deficiency         (Omega-3)                     *
*         mineral deficiency     (magnesium)                   *
*         vitamin deficiency     (B6)                          *
*         enzyme abnormality     (MAO)                         *
*         inhalant allergy       (titrated injections)         *
*         food allergy           (diet, and sometimes          *
*                                 injections as well)          *
*         psycho-social stress   (counseling, meditation*
*                                 etc.)                        *
*         Some individuals have all of the above               *
*         abnormalities                                        *
****************************************************************
```

As you learn to progressively unload yourself of unseen toxins in the following chapters, some people might even accuse you of hypochondriasis. What happens is as you get cleared out or detoxified and no longer have wall to wall symptoms, you are better able to see what turns on your symptoms. It will appear that things are bothering you that never did before, when in actuality, you were so overloaded before you could not tell what bothered you.

A word about references. Due to the glut of references available, I tried to limit the numbers used, while still demonstrating the massive amount of data that exists. Suffice it to say, all of this has backup in the literature and a key reference that will site all the scientific evidence is in press (<u>Chemical Sensitivity</u>, Rea, 1990). Also for the interested physician, the courses and publications of the American Academy of Environmental Medicine (Appendix) provide much data. Thanks to the wonderful world of computer assisted searches, we have more data than we can collate. For to include thousands of individual references would be to make this a volume that you would need a backhoe loader to help you carry to the beach.

Furthermore, the dissenter who insists on references for every single sentence, is not the one for whom this is written. It is for the person who wants to get healthy. I love it; I have yet to meet a dissenter who has ever successfully recognized and treated the type of patient we are addressing. Upon questioning, he is totally ignorant of the entire discipline of environmental medicine, and all the available references. Furthermore, he would never dream of searching further references for years as many of us have done. And even when you put them under his nose, he still refuses to acknowledge them. He has been brainwashed that a headache is a Darvon deficiency and no one is going to convince him otherwise. Besides it's an infinitely quicker, and therefore financially more rewarding way to get rid of the patient and on to the next one. And for sure the patient will return, for you've hooked him. Prescription drugs have become his lifeline to a symptom-masked day.

This work is for the person who is honestly not functioning with all oars in the water. For the person who is going through life at half mast, who thinks he feels fine because he has learned through the years to tune out so much. He has learned to rationalize that he is just getting older, that he works too hard, that he has stress and that is why he doesn't awaken feeling vivacious, playful and energetic every day. It is for the person who has periodic physicals and is told that he is perfectly healthy, and yet he feels dreadful a great deal of the time. He is hooked on all sorts of stimulants and relaxants to help him ignore the messages coming from the body. He uses coffee, candy bars and soda to get him up, and alcohol and tranquilizers to get him down. It is for the person who never quite feels well, who has chronic tiredness or exhaustion or fatigue, but who deep down wants to have unbounded energy and enthusiasm for life.

Most people who think they are tired, are actually toxic. And with the principles, herein, you will learn how you got toxic, how to diagnose it, and how to detoxify your body and bring yourself to levels of wellness that you have never experienced before. The body is not only capable of healing a number of things, but of regenerating to undreamed of levels of wellness, if only given a chance. It is a miraculous, God-given piece of machinery that has been more carefully engineered than any computer or modern day device, and it is all yours for the taking.

If you choose, you can feel as exhilarated everyday as you do on a vacation. But first you must possess greater knowledge. We invite you to come join with us and learn how to make your body and mind all that they are capable of being. And all through your own efforts. Nothing will be done to you by anyone other than yourself. For only you possess all the necessary qualities of a true healer.

So come along and learn whether you are really pooped or poisoned, tired or toxic.

Chapter 2:   EVERY CATASTROPHE IS A BLESSING IN DISGUISE

Remember in the 70's when people foam insulated their homes with urea foam formaldehyde insulation (U.F.F.I.)? They flocked to our offices with numerous complaints. We quickly learned that the commonest symptoms from urea foam formaldehyde insulation fumes were depression, fatigue, poor memory and thought process, headache and flushing, dizziness, burning eyes and throat, laryngitis, dermatitis, bronchitis, cough, asthma, palpitations, arthritis, hemorrhaging, and much more.

This was like rubbing Aladdin's lamp, because now we could think back to patients of the past who had had depression, fatigue, headache, and dizziness, that we were unable to help. It was quite possible that these people were also suffering from formaldehyde induced symptoms. But when we questioned them, many of them had not had a foam insulated home.

Fortunately studies began emerging to show us that recently urea foam insulated homes were not the only source of formaldehyde; they were just a dramatic teaching example provided by having had sudden exposure to massive amounts of formaldehyde. We learned that houses with urea foam formaldehyde insulation, in one study, had a mean formaldehyde level of 0.12 ppm (parts per million), while a regular house without U.F.F.I. had a mean level of 0.03 ppm. But an energy efficient home had levels of 0.10 ppm which nearly rivaled one with formaldehyde. This is because the tightening kept in the formaldehydes that outgassed from many other products. A trailer or mobile home was dreadful at 0.40 ppm, and a shopping mall was 1.50 ppm. And so it was that we learned many places had even higher levels of formaldehyde than a recently foam insulated home.

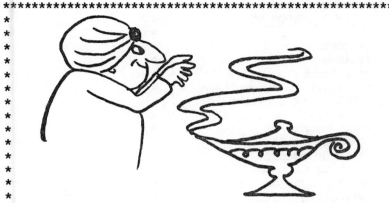

```
************************************************************
*                                                        *
*                                                        *
*                                                        *
*                                                        *
*                                                        *
*                                                        *
*                                                        *
*                                                        *
*                                                        *
*                                                        *
*                                                        *
*                                                        *
*                                                        *
*                                                        *
*     The formaldehyde insulation catastrophe was like   *
*     rubbing Aladdin's lamp.  It taught us that the      *
*     bizarre symptoms that some people had were due to   *
*     other chemicals.                                    *
*                                                        *
************************************************************
```

The disturbing fact is that OSHA or the Safety and Health Administration (which is part of the U.S. Department of Labor) in 1971 set the standard for formaldehyde in an 8-hour work day as 3 ppm. In 1976 the National Institute for Occupational Safety and Health recommended 1 ppm, and in 1981 recommended formaldehyde be handled as a potential occupational carcinogen (cause of cancer).

```
************************************
*     COMMONEST SYMPTOMS OF        *
*     U.F.F.I. EXPOSURE            *
*                                  *
*     depression                   *
*     fatigue                      *
*     poor memory                  *
*     inability to concentrate     *
*     can't think straight         *
*     "like thinking in a fog"     *
*     feel unreal                  *
*     headache                     *
*     dizzy or spacey              *
*     flushing of face             *
*     burning eyes or throat       *
*     laryngitis                   *
*     chronic cough, asthma        *
*     arthritis                    *
*     rashes                       *
*     heart palpitations           *
*     and much more.......         *
************************************
```

But OSHA, which is responsible for establishing regulations held fast to 3 ppm (Cox, JE, OSHA reconsidering formaldehyde, ASHRAE Journal, p. 10, Sept. 1985). This is in spite of known symptomatic responses (Kane, LE, Alarie, T, Sensory irritation to formaldehyde and acrolein during single and repeated exposures in mice, Am. Ind. Hyg. Assoc. J., 38:509, 1977):

Symptoms	Concentration ppm	Exposure Time min.
eye irritation	0.01	5
able to smell it	0.05	1
runny nose	0.05	5
sore throat	0.5	5
cough	0.8	5
headache, disoriented	0.8-1.0	10-30

```
**************************************************
*   COMMON FORMALDEHYDE VALUES                   *
*                                                *
*   normal house                0.03 ppm         *
*   house with UFFI             0.12             *
*   energy-efficient home       0.10             *
*   mobile home                 0.40             *
*   office building             0.44             *
*   hospital                    0.55             *
*   shopping mall               1.50             *
*   permanent press fabrics     0.70             *
*   paper products              1.00             *
*   biology lab                 8.50             *
**************************************************
```

It makes one wonder how sick you would have to become. And in 1985 OSHA, the government regulatory body whose role it is to protect us still clung to 3 ppm, in spite of publications affirming damage to genetic material which could initiate cancer (Graefstrom, RC, Fornore, AJ, Autrup, H, Lechner, JF, Harris, CC, Formaldehyde damage to DNA and inhibition of DNA repair in human bronchial cells, Science, 220, 216-217, 1982).   And, of course, other researchers confirmed adverse health effects at exposures of 0.12-1.6 ppm (Main, DM, Hogan, TJ, Health effect of low-level exposure to formaldehyde, J. Occup. Med., 25, 896-900, 1983).

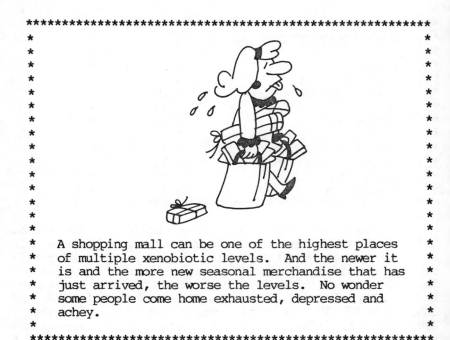

```
*************************************************************
*                                                           *
*                                                           *
*                                                           *
*                                                           *
*                                                           *
*                                                           *
*                                                           *
*                                                           *
*                                                           *
*                                                           *
*                                                           *
*                                                           *
*                                                           *
*                                                           *
*                                                           *
*   A shopping mall can be one of the highest places        *
*   of multiple xenobiotic levels.  And the newer it        *
*   is and the more new seasonal merchandise that has       *
*   just arrived, the worse the levels.  No wonder          *
*   some people come home exhausted, depressed and          *
*   achey.                                                  *
*                                                           *
*************************************************************
```

ENTER: A New Era In Medicine

Yet still there were people expressing these cerebral (brain) symptoms, but the formaldehyde levels of their buildings were not particularly high. They measured the inside air levels through local environmental testing laboratories and checked the household contents with the formaldehyde spot test (see Appendix) and they were OK. That was when the tight building syndrome, which was actually described by Dr. Theron Randolph (Chicago) over 25 years ago, became popularized (Randolph, TG, Human Ecology and Susceptibility To The Chemical Environment, Charles C. Thomas Publ., Springfield IL, 1962). We learned that formaldehyde was only one of many culprits that could cause these symptoms in a tightened building. Trichloroethylene, hexanes, toluene, xylene, benzene, phenol, phthalates, styrene, and many other hydrocarbons, could likewise cause these symptoms (Bardana E, Formaldehyde, Immunology and Allergy Practice, 2:3, 11-23, 1980).

For example, chemical analysis of the outgassing of a common carpet revealed that benzene, formaldehyde, methacrylate, tetrachloroethylene, toluene, xylene, methylnaphthalene, phthalates, and styrene were among the chemicals that outgassed in a 20th century home or office. The head space analysis of vinyl floor tile, for example, (Proceedings of Indoor Air, Stockholm, 1984) showed similar chemicals of trichloroethane, toluene, hexanol, cyclohexanone, benzaldehyde, phenol, benzyl chloride and more.

```
**********************************************************
*                                                        *
*      COMMON CAUSES OF THE TIGHT BUILDING SYNDROME      *
*                                                        *
*      formaldehyde          ozone                       *
*      toluene               carbon monoxide             *
*      xylene                carbon dioxide              *
*      trichloroethylene     dust                        *
*      perchloroethylene     alkanes                     *
*      hexanes               other hydrocarbons          *
*      nitrous oxides                                    *
*      Bardana, Immunol. & Allergy Practice, 1986        *
**********************************************************
```

If we looked at the air analysis of a normal hospital, we saw all those chemicals and many more. In fact it looked like the hospital was one of the most unhealthy places to be. If you looked at just the cleaning supplies that are commonly used by the janitorial service, they contained toluene, phenol, formaldehyde, xylene, butane, and methylene chloride.

```
*****************************************************************
*   COMMON CARPET CHEMICALS                                    *
*                                                              *
*   formaldehyde  benzene                methyl naphthalene    *
*   toluene       methacrylate           pthalates             *
*   xylene        tetrachloroethylene    styrene               *
*****************************************************************
```

```
*************************************************************
*   HEAD SPACE ANALYSIS                              *
*   OF VINYL FLOOR TILE                              *
*                                                    *
*   toluene          benzyl chloride                 *
*   phenol           benzol chloride                 *
*   trichloroethane  benzyl butyl ether              *
*   benzaldehyde     decanol                         *
*   butanol          1 (2-butoxy ethoxy)             *
*                       ethanol                      *
*   hexanol          2-butanone                      *
*   cyclohexanone                                    *
*************************************************************
```

And so environmentally induced symptoms, or the tight building syndrome, or environmentally-induced illness, or environmental illness (for short) was seen to be the product of two major culprits: (1) the addition of many new 20th century chemicals and products which outgas these chemicals daily to our home and office environments, and (2) the tightening of offices and homes to conserve energy which further served to concentrate, or keep inside the building, the outgassing of chemicals. And when people ran out of chemicals, they would have huge trucks of carcinogenic lawn pesticides delivered to their front doors!

Clearly new construction is a major trigger. In an EPA (Environmental Protection Agency) study, the total hydrocarbons in a new office were 1100 ng/L, compared with 130 ng/L in an old office. Furthermore, there are many intelligent alternatives, such as tacking down carpet

```
*******************************
*      GASES IN HOSPITAL AIR   *
*                              *
*      acetone                 *
*      acrolein                *
*      ammonia compounds       *
*      benzene                 *
*      carbon dioxide          *
*      chlorine                *
*      ethylene oxide          *
*      formaldehyde            *
*      halogenated hydrocarbons*
*      other hydrocarbons      *
*      hydrogen cyanide        *
*      mercury                 *
*      methane                 *
*      nitrogen compounds      *
*      nitrogen oxides         *
*      nitrous oxides          *
*      ozone                   *
*      pesticides              *
*      phenols                 *
*      phosphates              *
*      potassium hydroxide     *
*      sodium hydroxide        *
*      styrene                 *
*      sulfur compounds        *
*      toluene                 *
*      xylene                  *
*      many others             *
*                              *
*      Indoor Air,             *
*      Stockholm, 1984         *
*******************************
```

```
***********************
* COMMERCIAL CLEANING  *
* SOLUTIONS OFTEN      *
* CONTAIN              *
*                      *
* toluene              *
* phenol               *
* formaldehyde         *
* xylene               *
* butane               *
* methylene chloride   *
***********************
```

```
***********************
*    EXHALED BREATH    *
*    ANALYSIS OF 355   *
*    URBAN RESIDENTS   *
*    IN NEW JERSEY     *
*                      *
*    chloroform        *
*    trichloroethane   *
*    benzene           *
*    styrene           *
*    0-xylene          *
*    carbon tetra-     *
*        chloride      *
*    xylene            *
*    dichlorobenzene   *
*    ethyl benzene     *
*    trichloroethylene *
*    tetrachloroethylene*
***********************
```

instead of using polluting adhesives. Gluing a carpet has been the demise of many an office setting and its inhabitants, and in light of modern knowledge is just plain ridiculous. Carpet adhesive in the same EPA study had an emission rate of 234 mcg/m2h while the carpet itself had 36 mcg/m2h. (Project summary, Indoor air quality in public buildings: Volume II, Sheldon, L, et al, EPA, Environmental Monitoring

Systems, Research Triangle Park, NC, 27711, EPA/ 600/56-88/0096 Sept. 1988).

Along with adhesives for carpet and moldings being a source of several toxic chemicals, chip board (particle board) is a common source of formaldehyde and its symptoms in new construction or renovation. (Andersen, I, et al, Indoor air pollution due to chipboard used as a construction material, Atmospheric Environ., 9, 1121-1127, 1975). Headache and fatigue were the predominant formaldehyde-induced symptoms in many studies. (Main, DM, et al, Health effects of low-level exposure to formaldehyde, J. Occup. Med., 125:12, 896-900, Dec. 1983).

And as you can begin to appreciate from these minuscule samplings of the volumes of research data, the implications to man are endless. A new nursing home had 93 ng/L hydrocarbons while an old one had 12. Poor Granny may have been thought of as senile when she really had hydro-carbon brain fog. The mother of one of my patients moved into a new residence when her husband died. In a short time, she became "senile", so it was decided to get her into a nursing home. Between moving out of her new apartment and into the home she had to stay with her daughter. And lo and behold, she got normal again. What about the other people in renovated offices, schools, institutions, and homes who are not aware that they are among those who have brain functions that are adversely affected by 20th century chemicals?

A study of the exhaled breath analysis of 355 urban residents in New Jersey (Indoor Air, Stockholm, 1984), revealed such chemicals as chloroform, trichloroethane, benzene, styrene, xylene, carbon tetrachloride, and much more. These chemicals were actually coming out of their lungs, and out of their blood streams, because they were normal constituents of their everyday air.

In short, evidence began accumulating from researchers all over the world that these new 20th century chemicals were actually in our bodies. It was then only a short time

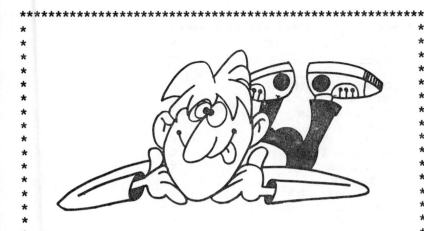

```
**********************************************************
*                                                        *
*                                                        *
*                                                        *
*                                                        *
*                                                        *
*                                                        *
*                                                        *
*                                                        *
*                                                        *
*                                                        *
*                                                        *
*                                                        *
*                                                        *
*                                                        *
*   The commonest symptoms of chemical sensitivity were  *
*   feeling dopey, dizzy, spacey, and unable to          *
*   concentrate.                                         *
*                                                        *
**********************************************************
```

before we learned that once inside the body, the fate of these chemicals was to break all the rules of medicine. Take, for example, the common copy machine found in most all offices. Trichloroethylene is just one of many chemicals found in these machines that outgasses into the office air. Since everything that is in the air gets into your blood stream (that is how you die from odorless carbon monoxide), trichloroethylene (TCE) is in nearly everyone's bloodstream. It is also a solvent; it is used in correcting fluid for typing errors; it is a common ingredient in dry cleaning and rug shampooing chemicals; it is in floor polishes, and it is an old anesthetic (so you know it easily crosses the blood brain barrier and preferentially causes brain function loss). The symptoms that TCE causes are confusion, poor attention, undue fatigue, poor reaction time, peripheral neuropathy (numbness and tingling), poor coordination, head-ache, dizziness, poor decision making, muscle cramps and much more (Feldman, <u>American Journal of Industrial Medicine</u>, 1980).

```
***********************************
*       COMMON SYMPTOMS OF        *
*       TRICHLOROETHYLENE         *
*                                 *
*       poor concentration        *
*       poor coordination         *
*       undue fatigue             *
*       drowsiness                *
*       poor reaction time        *
*       numbness & tingling       *
*       confusion                 *
*       headache                  *
*       dizziness                 *
*       poor decision-making      *
*       muscle cramps             *
*       _____           *
*       Feldman, American J.      *
*       Indust. Med. (1980)       *
***********************************


*******************************************
*       PRODUCTS CONTAINING               *
*       TRICHLOROETHYLENE                 *
*                                         *
*       solvent in machines & oils        *
*       dry cleaning fluid on clothes     *
*       carpet shampoo                    *
*       floor polish                      *
*       copy machines                     *
*       furniture glues                   *
*       typewriter corrective solution    *
*       an much more......                *
*******************************************
```

```
***********************************************************
*                                                         *
*              CHEMICAL SENSITIVITY                       *
*                                                         *
*      * discovered in 1951 by Dr. Theron Randolph        *
*      * rediscovered 30 years later and evolved:         *
*           U.F.F.I. taught us the symptoms               *
*           U.F.F.I. was not the only source of HCHO      *
*           Formaldehyde is not the only chemical         *
*           Evidence of levels                            *
*           Brain primary target organ                    *
*                                                         *
***********************************************************
```

Quick Stop Summary

So there tends to be a recurring theme running through all of these analyses:

(1) Chemicals like benzene (a known cause of leukemia) and benzene derivatives like toluene, phenol and xylene as well as other hydrocarbons, like formaldehyde, trichloroethylene, and styrene (from plastics) tend to be in most homes and offices to varying degrees.

(2) Because these are all lipid-soluble chemicals (they easily pass into lipid cell membranes) they pass easily into the blood stream when they are inhaled.

(3) Once in the body, they pass easily into the brain (the most lipid organ of the body). So the commonest symptoms are brain symptoms: depression, inability to think straight, exhaustion, dizziness and headache.

```
***************************************************************
*                                                             *
*              BRAIN IS THE PRIMARY TARGET ORGAN              *
*                                                             *
*        (1) It is a lipid substance that solvents readily    *
*                penetrate                                    *
*        (2) Dysfunctional detoxication creates chloral       *
*                hydrate                                      *
*        (3) Detox bottleneck raises aldehyde levels          *
*                                                             *
***************************************************************
```

Furthermore, analysis of coronary artery plaques (the arteriosclerotic patches in blood vessels in the heart) demonstrated that organochloride pesticides, chlorinated benzene pesticides, plasticizers, BHT (a toluene that is a common food additive), and many other hydrocarbons were actually deposited or incorporated into these areas. Clearly the body, once being exposed to these, in attempts to get rid of them, often was unable to dispose of them and so sequestered or stored them in places of ongoing inflammation and damage, such as arteriosclerotic (cholesterol) plaques within arteries.

```
*********************************************
*    CORONARY PLAQUE ANALYSIS SHOWS         *
*                                           *
*    organo chloride pesticides             *
*    chlorinated benzene pesticides         *
*    plasticizers (phthalates)              *
*    BHT (toluene)                          *
*    aromatic hydrocarbons                  *
*    alkanes                                *
*********************************************
```

And so the victims of formaldehyde insulation taught us a great deal about the symptoms of chronic unrecognized exposures to formaldehyde and other 20th century chemicals. At the same time scientists were quietly learning about the effects of silent polyvinyl chloride poisoning as they studied astronauts who felt unwell in space flight simulators (for they were literally encased in plastic cocoons). Similarly the alcoholics and drug addicts gave us an opportunity to learn how the body attempts to get rid of foreign chemicals. Other catastrophes, like Bhopal, Minimata Bay, agent orange in Vietnam, Chernobyl and other accidents also provided us with invaluable lessons in environmental medicine that would have otherwise taken us decades more to discover.

Diagnosing Chemical Sensitivity

Fortunately there is a technique to diagnose chemical hypersensitivity right in the physician's office. It is called provocation-neutralization. And it is based on a homeopathic principle which has been substantiated by the excellent research of Dr. Jacques Benveniste of Paris, France (Nature, 1988).

For every substance that causes a response in a person, there is a dose that provokes symptoms and a dose that neutralizes, or turns them off. This is a time-honored observation and has many examples in the body. Everything in nature has a good or optimal dose. On either side of this optimal or peak response is the adverse effect. The further to the left or right of the best response one goes, the closer one comes to the ultimate adverse response, death. For example, water is necessary for life. But too little and we die. Or, too much and we also die. The same goes for food and oxygen. Look at thyroid, a hormone that regulates metabolism. Too little and we are tired, fat and constipated. Too much thyroid and we are nervous, thin, and have diarrhea. But the optimal, or good dose, makes us feel well. Every vitamin, mineral, amino acid and essential fatty acid, every medicine, yes, everything causes a good and a bad response. Essentially, it all hinges on the dose.

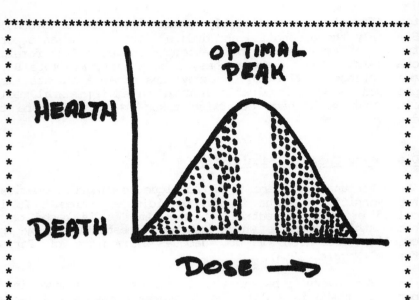

```
***********************************************************
*                                                         *
*                                                         *
*                                                         *
*                                                         *
*                                                         *
*                                                         *
*                                                         *
*                                                         *
*                                                         *
*                                                         *
*                                                         *
*                                                         *
*                                                         *
*                                                         *
*                                                         *
*                                                         *
*                                                         *
*                                                         *
*                                                         *
*                                                         *
*   Principle of Provocation-Neutralization Testing:      *
*   Every substance, including air, food, water and       *
*   even thyroid hormone, has an optimal or best dose     *
*   for the body.  The further one strays from this       *
*   optimal or best dose, the more adverse the effect     *
*   becomes.  Ultimately, too little is just as fatal     *
*   as too much.                                          *
*                                                         *
***********************************************************
```

And so it is with chemicals tested with the provocation-neutralization technique. Doses on either side of optimal can mimic the symptoms that the chemical produces in the body while an optimal dose clears them. Basically there is a dose of a chemical that will turn on a person's symptoms, if they are sensitive to this chemical, and then another dose that will turn them off. The doses used are minuscule and much less than the total dose that a person inhales in any one day. We even proved this technique by doing it in horses with asthma, and indeed we could turn on their asthma and coughing, and turn it off. It has been filmed and published (<u>Clinical Ecology</u>, vol. 5, #4, 1987/1988). We also published the techniques for physicians who want to learn how to do it in the prestigious U.S. government's National Institutes of Health journal, <u>Environmental Health Perspectives</u> (vol. 76, pg 195-198, 1987).

Besides our 2 publications (<u>Environmental Health Perspectives</u> and <u>Clinical Ecology</u>) on provocation- neutralization, there are many others. Here are just the top five I picked up from a pile of many others on my desk.

1. Scadding, GK; Brostoff, J; Low dose sublingual therapy in allergic rhinitis due to house dust mites. <u>Clin. Allergy</u> 1986; 16:483-491.

2. Rea, WJ; Podell, RN; Williams, M; Fenyses, I; Sprague, DE; Johnson, AR; Elimination of oral food challenge reaction by injection of food extracts. <u>Arch. Otolaryngol.</u> 1984; 110:248-252.

3. Boris, M; Weindorg, S; Schiff, M; Low dose antigen therapy attenuates asthma. <u>Otolaryngol. Head Neck Surg.</u>, June 1988, Vol. 98, No. 6.

4. William P. King, MD, Wallace A. Rubin, MD, Richard G. Fadal, MD, Walter A. Ward, MD, Richard J. Trevino, MD, William B. Pierce, MD, J. Alan Stewart, MD and John H. Boyles, Jr., MD - Provocation-neutralization: A two-part study Part I. The intracutaneous provocative food test: A multi-center comparison study. <u>Otolaryngol. Head Neck Surg.</u>, September 1988, Vol. 99, No. 3, pp. 263-272.

5. William P. King, MD, Richard Fadal, MD, Walter Ward, MD, Richard Trevino, MD, William Pierce, MD, J. Alan Stewart, MD and John H. Boyles, Jr., MD - Provocation-neutralization: A two-part study Part II. Subcutaneous neutralization therapy: A multi-center study. <u>Otolaryngol. Head Neck Surg.</u> September, 1988, Vol. 99, No. 3, pp. 272-278.

Let's look at how it is used in the office: Charles was a 39 year old engineer who presented to the office with a history of severe arthritis for a year and a half. He knew that when he was at home his arthritis was even worse, but if he was out of town on a consulting job, his arthritis actually improved a little. He consulted specialists in internal medicine and rheumatology but found the drugs they prescribed to be of little help. Besides, he was too smart to be suckered into thinking that he had an arthritis drug deficiency and should be taking this for the rest of his life in order to enjoy health.

We measured his serum formic acid (a metabolite of formaldehyde in his blood), and found that after a weekend at home it was 10, but after a day at work it was 6. Normal is less than 5. A monitor for formaldehyde in his home showed that the level was .06 ppm, which is too high for someone who is chemically sensitive, preferred being 0.02 ppm.

With the provocation testing, we injected an extremely small dose of formaldehyde {0.01 cc of a #3 dilution}, and actually caused ringing in the ears, a warm feeling, sweaty palms, and achey joints. "This is just how I've been feeling, especially at home," he said.

Then when we neutralized it {with a 0.05 cc of a #5 dilution}, his symptoms were terminated. When he was tested, he was not told what he was being tested to and he was given several tests of placebos (normal saline or salt water). In this way, we were able to be sure that he was not faking a response. We would even change the order of the tests and retest him on another day. Every time the normal saline control failed to provoke a reaction, but the formaldehyde duplicated his symptoms. Then the "good" or optimal dose turned them off.

It was clear that the particle board subflooring in his brand new home was the source of the formaldehyde. WHEN HE MOVED, HIS ARTHRITIS DISAPPEARED.

Another young man was a 42 year old dentist who had had headache, nausea, hand and leg tremor (not good symptoms for a dentist, you might note), depression, inability to concentrate, dizziness, chest pain, and shortness of breath. He had consulted a family doctor, internist, pulmonologist, allergist, gastroenterologist, and industrial hygienist. His symptoms were worsening, he had no diagnosis, no hope for recovery, and was incapacitated.

Testing him to the chemicals, single blind, in the office, revealed that normal saline placebos did nothing. Then when we tested to formaldehyde, we duplicated his head-ache, dizziness and nausea. When we put on the neutralizing dose his symptoms cleared. We could do the same thing with toluene and xylene. Again we inserted salt water placebos throughout the tests and nothing happened. HE WAS SO CHEMI-CALLY SENSITIVE THAT UNTIL HE WAS ABLE TO MOVE, HE HAD TO SLEEP IN HIS GARAGE, and use oxygen delivered through stain-less steel tubing and a ceramic mask, in order to operate on his patients.

Formaldehyde hypersensitivity can occur at any time, and neither of these men had had a foam insulated home that triggered it. That's why the catastrophe of formaldehyde insulation was so useful. It taught us the symptoms so that now we merely had the task of locating the source. It led to the discovery that many household products, cleansers, foam cushions, formaldehyde containing adhesives in furni-ture, carpets, paints, permanent press clothes, particle board and other construction materials, mattresses and hun-dreds of daily products (right down to shampoo, toothpaste, and ice cream) often contain formaldehyde. Often, once the sensitivity to formaldehyde begins, it leads to a snowball effect where the victim starts becoming sensitive, as the dentist did, to many other chemicals. And, then he exhibits a resetting of the thermostat where he gradually begins to become more and more sensitive to chemicals that before caused minimal or no reaction.

We have on video (a double blind study of) one woman whose rheumatoid arthritis, pain, stiffness, and limitation of motion can be neutralized within minutes with the correct dose of phenol. Her rheumatoid arthritis began within a few years of much home renovation and the addition of a new bedroom. Phenol levels in the inside air become elevated from the outgassing of new construction and when new furnishings are brought into a home. Within minutes of testing her to phenol, we unexpectedly hit her neutralizing dose. She was suddenly able to get in and out of a chair and actually skip and wave her arms. This is a lady whose professor husband had to comb her hair and brush her teeth for her before they came. This study was repeated many times in a double blind fashion and even filmed. (Double blind means that in addition to a single blind test where the patient doesn't know what's being tested, here the nurse doing the tests did not even know what she was testing. The nurse is merely given a number of test doses to sequentially administer, one every ten minutes, and instructed to record the responses.)

Although the gradual worsening of people who become chemically sensitized is bad enough, it turns out that for many victims, it is only the beginning of their problems. Once the immune system is triggered, and breaks down, sensitivities rapidly spread. The average victim becomes sensitive to pollens, dust, and molds, foods, chemicals, Candida, and much more. Furthermore they often have a host of nutritional (vitamin and mineral) deficiencies that lead to a malfunctioning or an ailing detoxication system; so that now they develop a toxic build up of foreign chemicals in the blood stream, as they are not able to metabolize and dispose of them as other people do. This all serves to give them increasingly more symptoms with time, as they baffle more and more physicians.

Look at the dentist. By the time he came for diagnosis, he could no longer even go into his home for any time longer than to shower. He had become so supersensitive that the home chemicals that had previously posed no problem had become intolerable. If he stayed in his home for half an hour his symptoms would recur.

```
***********************************************************
*                                                         *
*      COMMON SOURCES OF FORMALDEHYDE                      *
*                                                          *
*      construction materials:                            *
*                adhesives, paints, paving,               *
*                particle board, ceiling tile,            *
*                floor tile, plaster board                *
*      permanent press, easy-wear, no-iron, or            *
*                color-fast fabrics                        *
*      spray starch                                        *
*      shampoo, conditioner, tooth paste                  *
*      cosmetics                                           *
*      mattresses, couches, foam cushions                  *
*      commercial and home cleaning supplies               *
*      carpet and carpet pads                              *
*      paper products                                      *
*      shopping malls, fabric stores                       *
*      plastics                                            *
*      dyes                                                *
*      cigarettes                                          *
*      auto and industrial exhaust                         *
*      air fresheners                                      *
*                                                          *
*      _____               *
*      Rogers, S. The E.I. Syndrome, Prestige             *
*      Publishing, Syracuse, NY                            *
***********************************************************
```

The classic patient who has developed chemical sensitivity has been to over a dozen specialists, has no diagnosis, and is eventually referred to a psychiatrist. Some patients have come into the office with an over six foot long pharmacy print out of just the medications prescribed to them in the preceding year by well-meaning physicians in an attempt to help them with their symptoms. Eventually, most have been told that their symptoms are all in their heads. And, indeed, this is partly true, because the typical hydrocarbon, such as trichloroethylene, is metabolized via many possible routes to a number of chemicals. One path the chemical may pass through in order for the body to get rid of it is called the ALDEHYDE PATHWAY. When the aldehyde pathway, for example, becomes over burdened through inhaling many other chemicals, or through an undiscovered vitamin or mineral deficiency that is crucial in that pathway, the body then shunts the chemistry to produce chloral hydrate, the old "Mickey Finn" or "knockout drops". So, indeed, these people have a very good reason for the spacey, dizzy, inability to think and concentrate symptoms that they complain of. They actually produce the old "Mickey Finn" chemical in their brains.

We have an epidemic in disguise, and what a joke this has been on mankind. For here we have a group of people who are seriously ill, and often barely able to function. Their major target organ is the brain, and so they are not only depressed and irritable, but they cannot think well to function in performing their duties to make a living for their families. They go to well-meaning physicians, who have no knowledge of this area of medicine, and are told that their symptoms are probably hypochondriacal, and that they should take a tranquilizer and learn to relax in the evening. Meanwhile, the prescribed drugs only serve to further overload a malfunctioning detoxication system and accelerate the downhill course. They get no sympathy from physicians, relatives, friends or employees because medicine, in order to save face, bestows the implied label of hypochondriac on conditions it does not understand, and for which it does not yet have blood tests and X-rays for diagnosis. Meanwhile the sick have only one direction in which to go: they get sicker.

Chapter 3:   INTRODUCTION TO THE DETOXICATION SYSTEM

You have heard of the respiratory system. Diseases of it range from colds to pneumonia, asthma, emphysema and more.

You have heard of the cardiovascular system. Its problems include hypertension, heart attacks, and phlebitis.

You have heard of the gastrointestinal system. Problems with this include ulcers, hiatus hernias, gall stones, hepatitis and colitis.

You have heard of the genitourinary system, with kidney, prostate, bladder, uterus, and ovarian problems.

You have heard of the musculoskeletal system, with arthritis, fibrocytis, ruptured discs, torn tendons and broken bones.

You have heard of the endocrine system with malfunctions of the glands like the thyroid, pituitary, and adrenal, for example.

You have heard of the nervous system with diseases ranging from migraines to strokes, Parkinsonism to multiple sclerosis, and manic depression to schizophrenia.

And until this decade, you probably were not aware of the immune system. It governs allergies, auto immune diseases, like thyroiditis, rheumatoid arthritis, lupus, and extends to the deadly diseases of AIDS and cancer.

But you and thousands of physicians are unacquainted with a system whose importance is ushering in an evolution in medicine. Knowledge of this system antiquates our current classification system of diseases and opens up the era of ultimate wellness. Simultaneously it begins to bring to a close the era of drugs and surgery to merely suppress symptoms.

We are now able, instead, to find the actual cause of symptoms and banish them in healthful ways. Gone is the outdated idea that a headache is a Darvon deficiency. For indeed that is how we have handled symptoms since the era of drugs began early in this century. Antiquated is the idea that every unexplainable symptom is due to "a bug", "a virus", or "all in your head". Mysterious viral infections and hypochondriasis have ineffectively dominated the diagnostic picture long enough.

So what is this system? None other than the DETOXICATION SYSTEM. It exists in every cell of the body, and its existence before this century has been virtually unknown. But with the advent of drugs, scientists became curious as to how the body got rid of these. As a result much of the biochemistry has been worked out in the last couple of decades. Then the space program scientists started studying how the astronauts metabolized, or detoxified, or got rid of all the outgassing plastic (polyvinyl chloride) fumes that permeated their blood streams while inside the shuttles. At the same time other scientists started studying how the body defends itself against all sorts of poisons, including pesticides and all of the hydrocarbons of the 20th century.

Xenobiotics Will Become A Household Word

Hydrocarbons are merely chemical compounds with hydrogen and carbon. But many of the ones we are exposed to daily are synthesized or made from coal and petroleum. Different names for these petro chemical derivatives include, VOC's (volatile organic hydrocarbons), aliphatic and aromatic hydrocarbons, and pesticides. These are the commonest categories of foreign chemicals that get into the blood through air, water, and food. A term that lumps all of these foreign chemicals together, and means simply that --- foreign chemicals --- is XENOBIOTICS (pronounced as though it began with a "Z" as with Xerox).

```
************************************************************
*                                                          *
*                                                          *
*                                                          *
*                                                          *
*                                                          *
*                                                          *
*                                                          *
*                                                          *
*                                                          *
*                                                          *
*                                                          *
*                                                          *
*                                                          *
*                                                          *
*                                                          *
*                                                          *
*                                                          *
*                                                          *
*                                                          *
*                                                          *
*     The detoxication system is like the janitorial      *
*     service of the body.  It keeps it clean so accumu-   *
*     lated chemicals do not destroy the machinery.  For   *
*     when the machinery is damaged, we have serious       *
*     disease.                                             *
*                                                          *
************************************************************
```

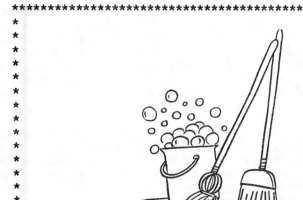

Unfortunately, much of the information about xenobiotic or foreign chemical metabolism (detoxication) has not yet filtered into the medical school curriculum, so most doctors are unaware of its importance and mechanisms. This is a major roadblock to entering the next era of medicine, for to be ignorant of the nutritional biochemical intricacies of the detoxication system, is to be left practicing the medicine of the past. Usually once a physician comprehends how this system works, he is never again content to treat by the old "diagnose and drug 'em" method. For in knowledge lies power, and herein lies the power to clear previously impossible and incurable conditions.

Because we are polluting our world at an unprecedented rate, there are skips and jumps in our knowledge. So xenobiotics like PCB's, agent orange, DDT, dioxin, diazinon, benzene, and formaldehyde become household words while the medical world, for the most part, continues business as usual as though these didn't exist ---- or at least as though they had no bearing on our current symptoms and complaints.

You might wonder why we have a detoxication system to begin with. Somebody up there must have known that we were going to be foolish enough to try to poison ourselves someday. Sure there are natural poisons, such as mycotoxins from molds and cyanides from cassava root and fruit seeds, but this detoxication system is turning out to be a heavy duty piece of machinery, capable (in some people) of Herculean biotransformation of twentieth century, dangerously toxic, man made substances.

Nearly everything entering the body must be processed or metabolized or chemically changed or altered in some way so that the body can do what it wants with it. Most of the foreign chemicals or xenobiotics get detoxified or metabolized into safer, less toxic forms so they can be safely excreted without further poisoning or damaging the organ of excretion. Sometimes, however, the body detoxication pathways are overloaded or damaged by previous chemicals and an even more potent chemical is created. For some chemicals the body appears to have no way to detoxify them or in trying to do so, actually makes a more toxic chemical. So instead of detoxifying, the body is actually toxifying. Since this activation of chemicals is not making them less toxic, many biochemists prefer (and rightly so) the term biotransformation for the name of the process handling foreign chemicals. We're sticking with detoxication (as scores of the world's most knowledgeable toxicologic biochemists have), however. (It's easier to say "detox" than "biotransform").

```
***********************************************************
*                                                         *
*                                                         *
*                                                         *
*                                                         *
*                                                         *
*                                                         *
*                                                         *
*                                                         *
*                                                         *
*                                                         *
*                                                         *
*                                                         *
*                                                         *
*                                                         *
*                                                         *
*                                                         *
*                                                         *
*                                                         *
*   Some physicians are still tied up totally in the      *
*   drug era.  For without knowledge of the detoxica-     *
*   tion pathway and chemical sensitivity, they are       *
*   unable to find the cause of most medical problems.    *
*                                                         *
***********************************************************
```

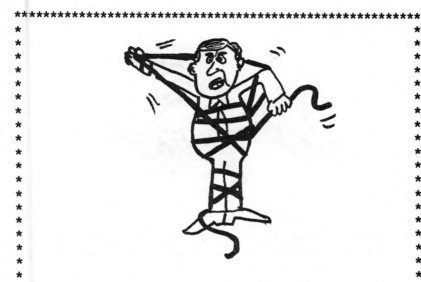

Basically chemicals get into the body by three major routes. They are in the air and you breathe them. The capillary system of the lung absorbs them and within seconds they are in the blood stream. Actually, a part of everything around you is in your blood stream, for everything is continually undergoing oxidation (aging, rusting, breaking down, deterioration, dehydrogenation). As it does so, molecules of it are mixed with the air and it is able to be breathed. This is why you can smell a lemon on the table from six feet away, because molecules are in the air and floating away from their original source. Likewise, you don't have to be able to smell something for it to be in your blood stream. Deadly, yet odorless, carbon monoxide has never been smelled by anyone.

```
***********************************************************
*                                                         *
*                                                         *
*                                                         *
*                                                         *
*                                                         *
*                                                         *
*                                                         *
*                                                         *
*                                                         *
*                                                         *
*                                                         *
*                                                         *
*                                                         *
*                                                         *
*                                                         *
*    Everything you can smell is in your blood stream.    *
*    And what's worse is that so also are the gasses you  *
*    cannot smell.                                        *
*                                                         *
***********************************************************
```

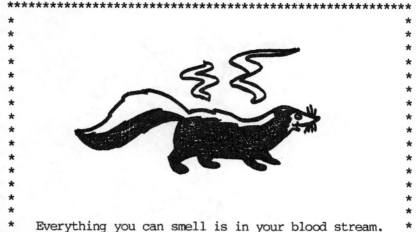

The next commonest way for a foreign chemical or xenobiotic to reach the blood stream is by eating it or drinking
it.   Many do this with pesticides, mycotoxins, dyes, additives, and hundreds of other chemicals daily.   The chemicals
get absorbed into the blood stream right along with the
food.

The third commonest way is by absorption through the
skin.   Skin absorption is so good that more and more prescription medicines are being manufactured in a patch form
(nitroglycerin, estrogen, and motion sickness medications).
If I put a sunscreen on my body, within minutes I can taste
it and it feels like it is coming out of my tongue.   Most
people are not this sensitive, for a number of reasons, but
many are and are not aware of it because they are too overloaded from other sources.   But if you take any drug, we can
measure the levels of it in your blood, or just as easily in
your saliva within a short time after absorption.   This is
because once inside the body, chemicals permeate the entire
body, and saliva is one of many detox routes.

People who slather creams, colognes and oils on their skin don't realize that it is just like eating it, for it reaches the blood stream as though they had eaten it. That is why with industrial and farming accidental spills of chemicals and pesticides on workers, the first and most immediate treatment must be to thoroughly wash the chemical off the skin. For every wasted second means that more of it is absorbed. A person could actually die just as easily from having certain chemicals and pesticides on his skin as he can had he swallowed the poison directly.

Once in the blood stream, the body wants to do two things with poisons or foreign chemicals (xenobiotics). First it usually wants to make them less poisonous. Then it has to figure out a way to excrete or get rid of them. You see if you send an inhaled, ingested, or absorbed poison directly to the kidney for excretion, for example, without first changing it to a less toxic form, it will damage the kidney as it passes through into the urine. So it is wiser to first change this chemical to a less destructive substance before sending it to the kidney. This is often carried out in Phase I of detoxication.

Phase I detoxication occurs in the wavey set of membranes inside the cell called the endoplasmic reticulum (ER). There are three types of reactions to choose from --- oxidation, reduction and/or hydrolysis. These are fancy names for merely removing an electron ("burning it off"), adding an electron or removing hydrogen from the original or parent compound. Sometimes this is all that needs to be done, and the changed compound or metabolite is ready for safe excretion. Sometimes several of these reactions occur.

But what if the kidneys get too overloaded? Nature has provided a back up. Outside of the endoplasmic reticulum, but still inside the cell (called the cytoplasm or cytosol), is Phase II of the detoxication system. In this

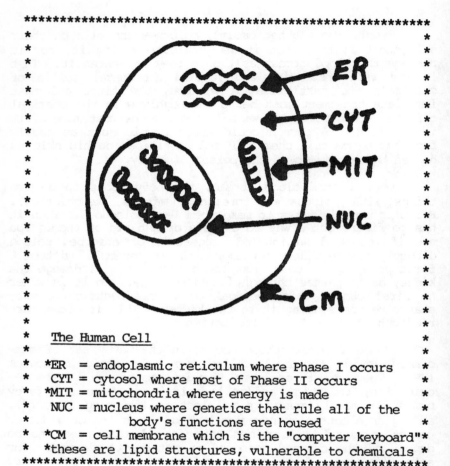

The Human Cell

*ER = endoplasmic reticulum where Phase I occurs
CYT = cytosol where most of Phase II occurs
*MIT = mitochondria where energy is made
NUC = nucleus where genetics that rule all of the
        body's functions are housed
*CM = cell membrane which is the "computer keyboard"
*these are lipid structures, vulnerable to chemicals

step a large protein or amino acid (a part of a protein) is
hooked on to the metabolite (the oxidized or changed chemical) making it bigger, more electrically charged and hence,
more polar. In this form, it is more readily soluble in
water and can be more easily excreted through the bile and
pass into the stool. This spares the kidney of having to do
all the work and provides a mechanism to get rid of more
toxic and difficult compounds for which Phase I alone is not

sufficient. The Phase II process is called conjugation, which merely means coupling (attaching) with another molecule. Conjugates can be excreted in the urine or bile.

Here is an easy way to conceptualize Phase II conjugation: Imagine a poultry farmer has a fire in his barn and there is a stampede of chickens flocking to the one door of the barn. The farmer wants to save his prize layer so he picks her up in his arms and runs with her out the door to save her. This is analogous to molecular conjugation (Phase II). A substance made by the body (like glutathione) attaches onto the foreign chemical making it much easier for it to be whisked our the door (safely into the bile and gut).

Glutathione (GSH) is a tripeptide, which means 3 amino acids go into its construction {glutamic acid, cysteine, and glycine}. It is the major conjugator in phase II to help the body detox foreign chemicals, medications, radiation and even it's own hormones (Muster, A, Anderson, ME, Glutathione, Am. Rev. Biochem., 52: 711-760, 1983). It also functions directly or indirectly in many other important body reactions regarding making new genetic material, enzymes and hormones. So it becomes readily apparent that if it is compromised because of loss in bile or urine from chemical exposure or overload, many other seemingly unrelated functions of the body will also be affected.

You know how important glutathione (GSH) is in cleaning up chemicals in the body and getting rid of them before they do harm. Since the formation of GSH is dependent on the amino acid cysteine, increasing the levels of this helps many people detox better. There's even a more efficacious derivative of it, N-acetyl cysteine that has even prevented tumors (De Flora, S, et al, Inhibition of urethan-induced lung tumors in mice by dietary N-acetylcysteine, Cancer Letters, 32, 235-241, 1986).

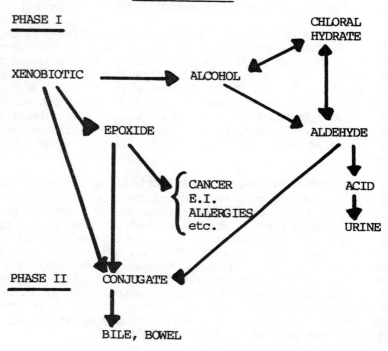

RUDIMENTARY SCHEMATIC OF
DETOX PATHWAYS

Actually things are a bit more complicated than it would appear, however, for any one chemical. For once a chemical reaches the blood stream it has about a dozen choices of which metabolites or compounds it can be changed into and like us, sometimes the body goofs and actually changes the xenobiotic into a more, not less, toxic compound. Instead of detoxication, toxication occurs. That is why, as stated, many scientists correctly prefer the term biotransformation (meaning simply, changing the form of a chemical through the chemistry of the body) to detoxication (which implies that we always make a substance less toxic, when in fact we sometimes do not).

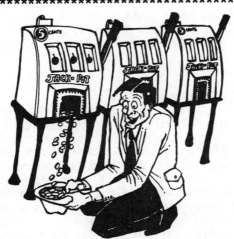

If you find a physician who knows the phases of detox, you've hit the jackpot. Keep him or her, because he is fascinated with the biochemistry of wellness.

So if there are a dozen or so possible pathways for a chemical to take to become biotransformed or detoxified, how does the body decide which path to take? It depends on many factors. When a chemical reaction occurs, such as in Phase I, it does so with the aid of specialized proteins called enzymes. And when I say specialized, you have no idea how specialized these can be. There are many of them that only facilitate one type of reaction and won't have anything to do with any other types of reactions, even if the body is in dire trouble. So if the body is overloaded with a particular poison, if that enzyme does not play a specialized role in breaking down that poison, it just sits idly by and becomes a spectator of destruction.

Furthermore, many enzymes need a particular vitamin or mineral present in order to work. These enzymes become paralyzed or inactive if that vitamin or mineral is not present.

Why The Sick Get Sicker

Many of the detoxication processes require energy {for example, the 3 principle transferases (conjugators) are called UDPGA, PAPS, and GSH. These reactions all require ATP which is the body's packaged energy source. Remember these squiggle brackets will contain more technical information that not everyone will need, so do not worry if you do not understand it}. So when you use energy to detoxify chemicals, you are putting an increased demand or burden on the body. But what is far more disturbing is that as a person's detox system gets overloaded with unseen, odorless chemicals, eventually there is no room at the "Inn". The body cannot process them for a while. So, they float around in the blood and aimlessly destroy things. For instance, they can start to eat holes in the mitochondrial lipid membrane inside the cell where energy (in the form of ATP) is manufactured. So now, even if the system eventually catches up and is able to detox these chemicals, they may have damaged the energy generating mechanisms and/or other pivotal detox enzymes so that detox is impaired. Now you can begin to see how the sick get sicker. And to give a medicine could be the deadly straw to this overloaded camel.

Some people because of genetics or heredity, already lack certain specific enzymes. That is one reason why some people are very ill from medicines and anesthetics that are otherwise harmless to the majority of the population. And in this century especially, sometimes a particular enzymatic pathway is temporarily blocked or overloaded because it is already too busy dealing with some other chemical that got there first. Sometimes this damage is permanent, rather than temporary.

So in summary, the choice of pathways depends on the heredity or individual genetics of each person, the availability of specific vitamins and minerals in the detox paths which enable them to function, the unseen overload or burden from other chemicals, and the unseen previous damage from other chemicals.

```
**************************************************
*       Which Pathway A Xenobiotic Takes To Get   *
*       Detoxified Depends Upon.............       *
*                                                  *
*    * GENETICS                                    *
*              (What enzymes are available)        *
*                                                  *
*    * NUTRIENT LEVELS                             *
*              (What vitamins, minerals, amino     *
*              acids and essential fatty acids     *
*              are available)                      *
*                                                  *
*    * TOTAL LOAD                                  *
*              (How many other chemicals are       *
*              competing)                          *
*                                                  *
*    * DETOX DAMAGE                                *
*              From Former Chemicals               *
*              (What pathways that have been       *
*              damaged)                            *
**************************************************
```

In A Nutshell

You don't have to be a biochemist to understand this. In a nutshell, many chemicals found in our 20th century air, outgas from many sources. Trichloroethylene is in most people's blood streams because of carpets, adhesives, copy machines, machine oils, and even dry cleaning fluid.

Depending on how healthy the detox pathway is in an individual, it can attach to DNA (genetic material) and cause cancer, chemical sensitivities, birth defects, new disease, or accelerate aging. Or it can attach to the kidney so that now the person starts losing proteins and minerals. This in turn causes other diseases (they are caused by the deficiencies created). Or it can attach to the liver and make it less able to handle chemicals. It can attach to glutathione (GSH) and the body gets rid of it. Unfortunately for every molecule of xenobiotic (bad chemical) the body gets rid of, it also permanently looses a molecule of GSH. So a heavy exposure puts a big drain on the detox system and can eventually deplete it. Or the chemical can hook into and damage the pathways where the chemicals are being degraded.

If there is a backlog of chemicals because the body is overwhelmed, chloral hydrate can be formed and brain fog results. There are many other possibilities but you get the picture. There is exponential worsening. It's worse than a chain reaction or automobile accident with a massive pile-up of cars.

For in this case, when a chemical gets bogged down and cannot get through the overloaded detox system, not only does it float in the blood stream and cause symptoms, but so do all the subsequent chemicals to which the person is exposed. And these chemicals can actually damage (sometimes irreversibly) other detox enzymes. So now the entire system just keeps becoming progressively more damaged with each exposure. And new damage results in new symptoms and target organs. The poor victim feels as though he has joined the disease-of-the-month club, for he keeps continually "falling apart".

Biochemical Bottlenecks In Detoxication

You know that tingly feeling of joy you get when you learn something new that will be very relevant to your life (like how to fix that computer glitch)? Well believe it or not, you're going to get that feeling many times throughout this book as your level of understanding grows. So right now, you're going to have to trust me and stride through some bio (body) - chemistry (biochemistry: how the body works). Try to resist thinking "What on earth am I doing reading this stuff?" You will be rewarded in the end, but the pathway to this happy end is through this field.

So let's look a little closer at the detoxication scheme to learn where some of these vitamins and minerals fit in. Superficially there are some biochemical bottlenecks through which a majority of detoxication reactions pass. If there is an overload in and of these pathways, we are in serious trouble. In understanding how this operates, one automatically understands the biochemistry of the person who is "allergic to", or sensitive or hypersensitive to chemicals. We call this chemical sensitivity or E.I. (environmentally-induced illness or environmental illness for short). Once the mechanism for understanding the process is in place, we are then equipped to better help this person heal himself.

In Phase I there are two bottlenecks. Many foreign chemicals are first metabolized into alcohols which then must be metabolized from an alcohol stage into an aldehyde. From the aldehyde stage a chemical can become transformed into an acid and safely excreted in this acidic form through the urine.

Each conversion step which then transforms our original toxin to a different chemical or metabolite is usually made possible through enzymes. These are specialized proteins that sometimes contain or require as co-factors specific minerals and/or vitamins.

For example, the enzyme to get from the alcohol form to the aldehyde is <u>alcohol dehydrogenase</u> and must have a specific amount of zinc in it to function. One of the enzymes to get the aldehyde into an acid is aldehyde oxidase, and this needs molybdenum and iron to function. The problem is that voluminous studies by researchers around the world and even some by the U.S. government itself admit that the average U.S. diet does not supply 100% of many of these pivotal minerals. In fact, many studies have shown that one-third or more of the people were low in a particular nutrient. For example, in one study 13% of randomly selected patients had normal zinc levels and 68% ingested less than two-thirds of the RDA for zinc (Elsborg, L, The intake of vitamins and minerals by the elderly at home, <u>Int. J. Vit. Nutr. Res.</u>, 53:321-329, 1983). When you apply some statistics to the over 40 nutrients at once, you realize quickly that probably at least one in every three people is deficient in at least one nutrient. And this is what we see in private practice. The problem is that this puts these unsuspecting victims of processed foods at a distinct disadvantage in terms of detoxifying chemicals. And it makes them more vulnerable to becoming chemically sensitized when compared with someone who has a full deck of nutrients.

What's even more worrisome is this. If either enzyme is malfunctioning for lack of its mineral, for example, then the body can shift the chemistry to another pathway to form chloral hydrate. Remember, it's the chemical that was called "Mickey Finn" or "knock out" drops, and that is exactly what some people act like when they are exposed to certain chemicals that overload their detoxication systems from plastics, glues, carpets, dry cleaning fluid and much more that is found in the everyday environment (Hepatotoxicity of vinyl chloride and 1,1-dichloroethylene, Reynolds, ES, et al, <u>Am J. Pathol.</u>, 81:1, 219-231, Oct. 1975). This happens especially if they are deficient in zinc or molybdenum, since these are key minerals in the alcohol and aldehyde conversion enzymes. The result of either of these deficiencies is the potential synthesis of chloral hydrate in the brain, producing the classic symptoms: spacey, dizzy, dopey, unable to concentrate, depressed for no reason, tired, impotent, and/or a peculiar numbness or tingling in parts of the body.

This can all happen merely because a person is unknowingly deficient in zinc or molybdenum or other minerals that are also crucial in these pathways. It can also happen if one of these pathways is already too overloaded and busy trying to metabolize chemicals from another source.

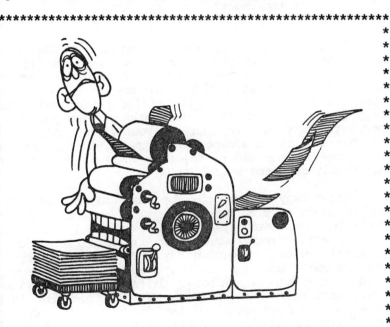

If you get foggy-headed at work from the copy machine, for example, chances are you have a nutrient (vitamin or mineral) deficiency and chemical overload from other areas of your life.

```
****************************************************************
*   CLUES TO SUSPECTING YOU ARE CHEMICALLY SENSITIVE          *
*                                                              *
*   You smell things much better than most people             *
*   You can't tolerate alcohol well                           *
*   Perfumes and strong cleansers bother you                  *
*   You are worse in certain stores                           *
*   There are many medications you cannot take                *
*   Vitamins often make you worse                             *
*   Your reaction time is poorer in city traffic than         *
*           in the country                                    *
****************************************************************
```

So if your detox pathways are working as fast as they can in metabolizing the phenols, xylene, and trichloro-ethylene from your new carpet and furniture, plus the alcohol you drink every night, you may be the only one who becomes a space cadet when the office is painted. You get brain fog and just can't think straight. You get moody and short with people. You increase your errors while decreasing your ability to accept criticism. This may lead you to drink more at the end of the day. How do you ever escape this deadly downward spiral?

Right away you see that because you are never degrading the exact same number and types of chemicals at any one moment in time, that this explains, very aptly, why a chemically sensitive person can react so fiercely one day, and not nearly as bad on another day. Or how, for example, one week you could have a particular symptom to an exposure, and the next week have a completely different symptom. You have merely used different pathways. It does not mean that you are a full fledged hypochondriac, or going off your rocker. But if one is totally ignorant of the biochemistry of detoxication, the victim appears to be a down and out malingerer, and in need of urgent psychiatric help. Clearly any prescribed medication can further overload this already ailing system, for it provides it with one more chemical that it must waste its precious detoxication energy and nutrients on.

```
**************************************************************
*                                                            *
*                                                            *
*                                                            *
*                                                            *
*                                                            *
*                                                            *
*                                                            *
*                                                            *
*                                                            *
*                                                            *
*                                                            *
*                                                            *
*                                                            *
*                                                            *
*                                                            *
*                                                            *
*                                                            *
*   If one day you're happy, and another day you're          *
*   dopey and spacey, chances are you're not tired,          *
*   you're toxic.  On the toxic days your detox system       *
*   is merely overloaded.  Let's find out why and            *
*   correct it.                                              *
*                                                            *
**************************************************************
```

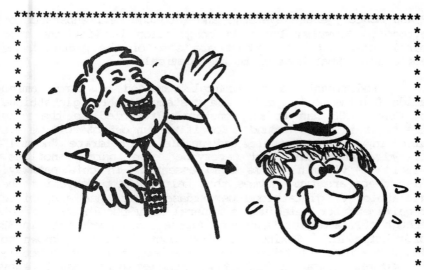

If the <u>aldehyde</u> pathway is blocked (due to say an un-diagnosed molybdenum deficiency, or over exposure to form-<u>aldehyde</u> in a new carpet or clothing, or drinking too much alcohol, or the aldehyde enzymes are damaged by a pesticide exposure), then the aldehyde backlog or build up occurs. What are the symptoms of that? Facial flushing, disorienta-tion, inability to think straight, easily confused, palpita-tions or cardiac arrhythmia, spaciness, poor equilibrium ---many of the same symptoms of a chemical exposure for someone who is chemically sensitive. And as you will learn later on, the solution is not just to take large doses of zinc or molybdenum, for in fact this could make you worse.

Now let's jump out of the endoplasmic reticulum (ER), home of Phase I detoxication {also known as the cytochrome

P-450 monooxygenase system}, and into the cell substance or cytosol. Remember Phase II conjugation is (for the most part) occurring here. What are some of the proteins and amino acids that hook on to the chemicals?

Predominant is a chemical composed of three amino acids (glutamine, glycine, and cysteine) called glutathione or GSH. GSH has to be constantly recycled so there is plenty of it to go around. For if we run out of this we are also in serious trouble and unable to tolerate "normal" everyday chemicals that everyone else barely notices. Niacin or vitamin B3 is also essential in this pathway. Also there are two enzymes that help to keep recycling the glutathione: glutathione peroxidase (which has a specific requirement for selenium, a mineral many people do not get enough of), and glutathione reductase (this needs vitamin B2 or riboflavin). Taking the birth control pill is known to lower the level of riboflavin in the body and in some people it becomes seriously depleted. This explains, easily, why some women developed severe chemical hypersensitivity after they began the birth control pill.

PAPS is an abbreviation for another chemical {3'-phosphoadenosine, 5'-phosphosulfate} that conjugates in Phase II, and it also requires the amino acid cysteine. Glucuronic acid is another conjugator and it requires zinc.

Also, there are amino acids like glycine and cysteine that are capable of conjugating chemicals all by themselves. {Meanwhile you can begin to appreciate that the sulfur containing amino acid cysteine is going to be important since it is already used in 3 ways during 3 Phase II detox: in glutathione or GSH, PAPS, and alone as an amino acid conjugator}.

It is interesting that most of the Phase II conjugations, like glutathione, PAPS and cysteine, all have sulfhydryl groups in them. This means that sulfur is very important in the diet to help the body detox chemicals. No wonder studies show that inbred strains of laboratory animals have less cancer when eating a high sulfur diet of

```
************************************************************
*                                                          *
*          Oxidation Reactions Catalyzed by                *
*     The Cytochrome P-450-containing Monooxygenases        *
*                                                          *
*   hydroxylation              addition of hydroxyl        *
*                              group (-OH)                 *
*                                                          *
*   epoxidation                addition of oxygen,         *
*                              makes it highly reactive    *
*                              and toxic                   *
*                                                          *
*   N-, O-, or S- dealkylation add H to N, O, or S         *
*                                                          *
*   deamination                remove -NH3 group           *
*                                                          *
*   N-hydroxylation            add -OH group to N          *
*                                                          *
*   sulfoxidation              add =O to sulfur            *
*                                                          *
*   desulfuration              remove sulfur               *
*                                                          *
*   dehalogenation             add =O and remove halide    *
*                                                          *
*   _____          *
*                                                          *
*           Reductive Biotransformation By                 *
*             The Cytochrome P-450 System                  *
*                                                          *
*   azo reduction              split N=N bond              *
*                                                          *
*   aromatic nitro reduction   NO2 becomes NH2             *
*                                                          *
*   reductive dehalogenation   halide replaced by H        *
*                                                          *
*   _____          *
*                                                          *
*   (Sipes, G, Gandolfi, AJ, Biotransformation of          *
*   toxicants, 64- 98, Cassarett's and Doull's             *
*   Toxicology, 1986, see appendix).                       *
*                                                          *
************************************************************
```

5 Major Phase II Conjugation Reactions	Example	Preferred Route of Excretion
acylation	amino acids like glycine to form urinary metabolite hippuric acid	kidney
acetylation	addition of Acetyl CoA to form mercapturic acid	kidney
methylation	addition of methyl group	
glucuronidation	addition of sugar group	kidney (bile if M.W. > 350)
sulfonation	conjugation with PAPS, conjugation with GSH	kidney bile

(Tucker, GT, Drug metabolism, Br. J. Anaesth., 51, 603-618, 1979; Spies, G, Gandolfi, AJ, Biotransformation of toxicants, 64-98, Casarett's and Doull's Toxicology, 1986, see appendix).

Brassaciae or cruciferous vegetables (the cauliflower, cabbage, Brussel sprouts family of vegetables), and onions. These all contain extra sulfur.

Many other vitamins, minerals, amino acids, and essential fatty acids are involved in the smooth function of the detoxication system. For example, magnesium is in nearly 300 enzymes and is a necessary co-factor for many of these reactions. This thumbnail sketch merely serves to introduce you to some of the more common biochemical bottlenecks, and get you oriented. You are doing great. The diagrams will help you visualize and summarize the highlights.

So what happens when the biochemical bottlenecks of Phase I become overloaded? Several things, all of which create symptoms and eventual disease, leading to end organ failure and death. First, as the major alcohol and aldehyde paths slow down, chemistry can be shifted to other metabolites called epoxides. These epoxides are highly reactive and unstable products, capable of initiating the changes that eventually lead to cancer, accelerated aging, allergies, E.I., immunosuppression (AIDS), mutagenesis (dangerous and undesired changes in one's genetics enabling them to get cancer), and teratogenesis (birth defects) (page 42).

Remember, many people can be exposed to a potentially carcinogenic (cancer causing substance), but only a few get the cancer. It certainly has a great deal to do with how often their chemistry is pushed to epoxides (called epoxidation). Now you can begin to see that two factors would tend to do this: (1) overload of the detox paths with other chemicals, and (2) missing vitamins and minerals in the pathways so that metabolites get shifted to epoxides.

Look at the dozen children in Woburn, Massachusetts who developed leukemia when the town's water supply was contaminated with trichloroethylene. Now you can begin to understand why it is so difficult to incriminate particular

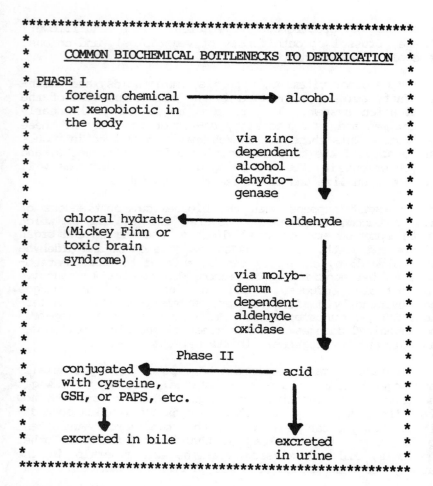

```
****************************************************
*                                                  *
*     COMMON BIOCHEMICAL BOTTLENECKS TO DETOXICATION *
*                                                  *
* PHASE I                                          *
*     foreign chemical  ─────────▶ alcohol         *
*     or xenobiotic in                             *
*     the body                                     *
*                          via zinc                *
*                          dependent               *
*                          alcohol                 *
*                          dehydro-                *
*                          genase                  *
*                                   ▼              *
*     chloral hydrate  ◀──────── aldehyde          *
*     (Mickey Finn or                              *
*     toxic brain                                  *
*     syndrome)                                    *
*                          via molyb-              *
*                          denum                   *
*                          dependent               *
*                          aldehyde                *
*                          oxidase                 *
*                                   ▼              *
*               Phase II                           *
*     conjugated  ◀──────────── acid               *
*     with cysteine,                               *
*     GSH, or PAPS, etc.                           *
*         ▼                          ▼             *
*     excreted in bile          excreted           *
*                               in urine           *
****************************************************
```

chemicals as agents of disease. They are not the sole factors, but only one of many contributing factors. The predilection for children is easy to understand because their immune systems are immature. Wouldn't it have been interesting to know the heredity, however (how many of these children's family histories had cancer or E.I.), and to know their diets (how many ate predominantly sugar coated breakfast cereals, hot dogs, and canned school cafeteria spaghetti for lunch, and pizza for dinner, all of which easily lead to zinc, molybdenum, selenium, and magnesium deficiencies), and how many had compromised detoxication pathways (spent time gluing model planes, lived in a brand new house or trailer, had new carpeting, new foam filled fire retardant and pesticided-by-law mattresses, and polyester sheets with scented fabric softener, or were regularly exposed to natural gas or pesticides in the school or home)?

Also when regular first-pass pathways are not optimally functional, chemicals get shuttled from auxiliary path to path in search of one that can accommodate them. In doing so, one of the first things that can happen is that they may interfere with the detoxication of other chemicals so that chemicals which normally do not have any trouble getting detoxified (and hence cause no build up, and cause no symptoms) are suddenly triggering symptoms. This is exactly what is seen in the victim of chemical sensitivity. All of his life he is unaffected by toluene, for example, and suddenly he starts reacting to carpets, cleansers, pesticides and plastics. Everyone is sure he is loony! Everyone that is, who is ignorant of the biochemistry of detoxication.

```
*********************************************************
*                                                       *
*                                                       *
*                                                       *
*                                                       *
*                                                       *
*                                                       *
*                                                       *
*                                                       *
*                                                       *
*                                                       *
*                                                       *
*                                                       *
*                                                       *
*                                                       *
*   I know this chemistry has been a real pain for you. *
*   I also know you don't understand it all.  You're    *
*   not supposed to yet.  So do not worry.  It will all *
*   make sense in the end.  Just keep reading and you   *
*   will be amazed at how much you know at the end..... *
*   .... enough to get yourself really well, possibly   *
*   for the first time in your life, and for the rest   *
*   of your life!                                       *
*                                                       *
*********************************************************
```

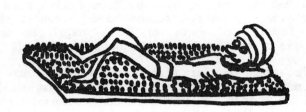

Orphaned Chemicals Raise Havoc With Membranes

These orphaned chemicals that keep charging around the body looking for a pathway that can detoxify them, can create a great deal of damage during their search. Don't forget the whole purpose of the detoxication system is to make these chemicals less toxic and get rid of them as quickly as possible. But when all the pathways are blocked, these nasty critters do the worst things possible; they poison and damage enzymes so that some day even when the body is no longer over burdened by chemicals, it does not regain normal function. And how often have we seen this? You put a chemically sensitive person in the cleanest environment you can, and he still does not recover --- not until a significant amount of healing has taken place. You will learn how to bring this about for yourself.

Worse yet, these orphaned chemicals also damage actual membranes of the cell. For one, the outside membrane of the cell must not have any holes in it, or the cell's contents leak out and the cell dies. Long before death occurs, however, other chemicals can leak in through these holes and damage the genetics and other regulatory proteins. This creates new and baffling symptoms for the physician who is totally untrained in environmental medicine. For he is prone to using his only tool (drugs) which only further compromise the system. The end result? THE SICK GET SICKER.

Bear in mind, once these chemicals have leaked inside the cell, they can attach to other membrane structures, like the mitochondria, where energy is manufactured, and the endoplasmic reticulum where Phase I of detoxication takes place. But if the person complains of exhaustion to a physician unknowledgeable in environmental medicine, some of the common diagnoses they come in with are chronic mono, EBV, or chronic yuppie fatigue syndrome: diagnoses that have no universally agreed upon pathogenic diagnostic criteria and for which there is no treatment.

```
*********************************************************
*                    DETOXICATION                      *
*                                                       *
*      Inhaled, ingested, or absorbed xenobiotics       *
*                (foreign chemicals):                   *
*                      ↓                                *
*                Phase I detoxication                   *
*                                                       *
*      ──────────────────────────►  excreted in urine  *
*                      ↓                                *
*                Phase II detoxication                  *
*                                                       *
*      ──────────────────────────►  excreted in urine or*
*                                   in bile to gut      *
*                                                       *
*      Any of these pathways can be blocked or damaged by: *
*         *    vitamin deficiency                       *
*         *    mineral deficiency                       *
*         *    amino acid deficiency                    *
*         *    fatty acid deficiency                    *
*                                                       *
*         *    foreign chemicals for which the body has no *
*                 mechanism for detoxifying             *
*         *    newly formed metabolites (breakdown products) *
*                 of xenobiotics                        *
*         *    detox enzymes poisoned by heavy metals (like *
*                 mercury, aluminum, cadmium)           *
*         *    detox pathways just plain overloaded from *
*                 everyday chemicals in the environment *
*         *    poor genetics (lack of specific detox enzymes) *
*********************************************************
```

```
************************************************************
*                                                          *
*    HOW THE SICK GET SICKER                               *
*                                                          *
*    Chemicals back up in the bloodstream when the detox   *
*    system is ailing.                                     *
*                                                          *
*    This Can Result In:                                   *
*    *    chemicals stored in fat, brain and other lipid   *
*              tissues like regulatory membranes           *
*    *    chemicals float freely and poison or damage      *
*              enzymes and other parts of the detox        *
*              system                                      *
*    *    chemicals recycle in detox path and overload     *
*              it so new chemicals cannot be               *
*              metabolized                                 *
*    *    formation of metabolites that are more           *
*              dangerous than the parent compound, like    *
*              free radicals that eat holes in regula-     *
*              tory membranes (nucleus, mitochondria,      *
*              endoplasmic reticulum, and cell body        *
*              membranes)                                  *
*    *    chemicals and their metabolites get shuttled     *
*              into new pathways that produce new          *
*              symptoms (chloral hydrate's toxic brain     *
*              symptoms)                                    *
*    *    backlogged chemicals poison or damage parts of   *
*              the energy systems (mitochondrial en-       *
*              zymes and membranes) that run detox         *
*    *    backlogged chemicals damage the endocrine,       *
*              nervous and immune systems, so any          *
*              symptom imaginable results                  *
************************************************************
```

```
**************************************************
*                                                *
*      Symptoms Are Not Diagnostic               *
*            And Can Mimic One Another            *
*                                                *
*      pollen & dust sensitivity                 *
*      house dust & animal dander sensitivity    *
*      mold sensitivity                          *
*      food sensitivity                          *
*      chemical (pesticides, hydrocarbons)       *
*      nutritional deficiencies                  *
*      Candida/intestinal microbes               *
*      toxicity (mercury, lead, cadmium)         *
*      stress                                    *
*                                                *
**************************************************
```

The cell membrane, or covering of the outside of the cell, is sort of like a computer key board: the lipid structure from which directions for wellness, or for allergies and inflammation (like arthritis, colitis, etc.) originate. So you can see that chemical damage to a membrane has far reaching effects. The enzyme you already heard about, glutathione peroxidase, is one of many that are important (along with vitamin E) in helping these membranes maintain their strength and integrity against the onslaught of chemicals. Since glutathione must have selenium to function, you can now see why selenium and vitamin E are important in protecting membranes. They keep orphaned chemicals from destroying membranes: the process that raises havoc and creates many diseases. But don't run out and corner the market in selenium, yet. Going beyond 400 mcg a day of this mineral can cause your hair and nails to fall out, for one. Let's get you more informed before you start helping yourself.

All of this enables us to progressively and more clearly visualize how a malfunctioning, or dysfunctional detoxication system gets backlogged, and how these backlogged chemicals, with all escape routes blocked, bounce around, damaging vulnerable cell membranes. If the damage is in the membranes of the mitochondria, where energy is made, you get a resultant, unexplained exhaustion. If the chemicals damage membranes of the endoplasmic reticulum, where Phase I of detoxication occurs, you get a further compromised detoxication process so that now you begin reacting to, or not tolerating things that never bothered you before. And if chemicals damage the cell envelope or outside cell membranes, the result can be many symptoms like increased chemical vulnerability, allergies, and inflammatory and auto-immune conditions, like arthritis, colitis, asthma and much more. For all these membranes are made from specialized fats or lipids, very sensitive to chemicals.

Eventually, with enough overload to your detox system and resultant membrane damage, it will seem like every time you turn around you seem to have developed another ailment. You're afraid to tell your doctor since he hasn't figured out the causes of the first three complaints yet, and now you have additional ones.

The average American diet is notoriously high in sugar. When sugar is refined, many of its precious minerals like chromium and magnesium are significantly reduced. When one ingests refined (white table) sugar (as opposed to raw sugar cane), he gets very little minerals like chromium. The problem is, although minerals are required to metabolize the sugar, the body actually loses chromium in the urine when sugar is ingested, so it becomes a doubly depleting substance (Hombridge, KM, Chromium nutrition in man, *Amer. J. Clin. Nutr.* 27: 505-514, May 1974; and Boyle, E, Mondschein, B, Dash, H, Chromium depletion in the pathogenesis of diabetes and arteriosclerosis, *South. Med. J.*, 70, 12, 1449-1453, Dec. 1977).

You can quickly appreciate how someone that consumes a lot of sugar gets mineral deficiencies. Then, when the office is painted or new carpet is installed at home, he is the only one to start with these cerebral toxic brain symptoms. If that were not enough, the DOMINO EFFECT or avalanche of new symptoms begins to occur as the backlog of chemicals from the ailing and overloaded detox system actually begins to poison the very detox enzymes themselves.

It is not enough that the chemicals can cause brain-fog and other bizarre symptoms, but these chemicals go the ultimate mile and begin to damage the very system that we depend upon to clear them from our bodies.

Clearly, when chemicals enter the blood, there are only three paths available. They can be detoxified, so the body can get rid of them. They can be stored in the fat and vital tissues until the body can figure out how to get rid of them. Or the body can actually use them, and incorporate them into enzymes or tissues. The latter turns out to be to the detriment of the host. For example, cadmium and lead from industrial and auto exhaust, can accumulate in kidneys and cause hypertension.

And, as mentioned, some chemicals are not made less toxic, but actually more toxic. An example of this is methanol (wood alcohol), which is oxidized to become formaldehyde in the body, and it is well-known that this build up of formaldehyde (from drinking wood alcohol) can cause blindness.

Suicide Inhibitors Of The Detox Pathway

Clearly not all xenobiotics are detoxified, but some are actually made more toxic. Some metabolites (the products that the inhaled and ingested chemicals were turned into in the body) become so toxic by this change that they poison the detox system. We call this suicide inhibition. For put it another way, the body has turned these chemicals into ones that turn off a portion of the detox pathway, or can even poison or kill it forever.

You recall that in the liver cell, the endoplasmic reticulum (ER), is where Phase I of detoxication occurs through the cytochrome P-450 system. The ER constitutes 15% of the total cell volume; the surface area of the ER is 8 1/2 times that of the mitochondria (energy manufacturer) and 37 1/2 times that of the cell membrane (Kulkarni, AP, Hodgson, E, Metabolism of insecticide by mixed function oxidase systems, Pharmoc. Ther., 8, 379-475, 1977).

More importantly, is the fact that common indoor chemicals like trichloroethylene (copy machines, carpet adhesives, dry cleaning fluid) and vinyl chloride (plastics in notebooks, toys, computers, furnishings) can be metabolized to suicide inhibitors of cytochrome P-450 (<u>Casarett's and Doull's Toxicology</u>). This is an extremely important mechanism in creating overload and resultant chemical sensitivity in the vulnerable person.

Now one can appreciate how a normal person can become chemically sensitive after even one exposure to a renovated environment, for example. And once that detox system is functioning suboptimally, subsequent (previously unnoticed) exposures progressively inhibit the detox system.

Clearly many other common indoor chemicals are also suicide inhibitors of the very detox enzymes that are one major source of protection from the 20th century man-made environment. Combine this with the biochemical bottle necks, and it has spelled disaster for many of us as we became highly chemically sensitive. But the problem does not end there, for the system is now primed for a massive cave-in from triggers barely noticed by others. For example, chloral hydrate can inhibit aldehyde dehydrogenase, as can magnesium deficiency, many drugs, alcohol, acetaldehyde and aldehyde buildup, and mercury from pesticides, dental amalgams (fillings), and exhaust fumes from industry and burning at toxic dumps, and much more. (Weiner, H, Flynn, TG, <u>Enzymology and Molecular Biology of Carbonyl Metabolism: Aldehyde Dehydrogenase, Aldo-Keto Reductase, and Alcohol Dehydrogenase</u>, Alan R. Liss, Inc., NY, 1987).

Don't let these foreign words frustrate you. I know you don't understand all of this, but you will get the general picture. The tough stuff is there more for your security so that no one can try to undermine your progress toward wellness by telling you there's no evidence.

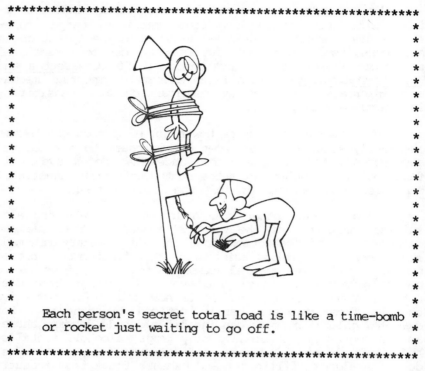

```
*********************************************************
*                                                       *
*                                                       *
*                                                       *
*                                                       *
*                                                       *
*                                                       *
*                                                       *
*                                                       *
*                                                       *
*                                                       *
*                                                       *
*                                                       *
*                                                       *
*                                                       *
*                                                       *
*                                                       *
*                                                       *
*                                                       *
*        Each person's secret total load is like a time-bomb *
*        or rocket just waiting to go off.              *
*                                                       *
*********************************************************
```

Each person's secret total load is like a time-bomb or rocket just waiting to go off.

It has been extremely naive of man, who has polluted the outside air so badly that he changes the weather global-ly and wipes out entire forests and destroys precious monu-ments with acid rain, to think that this has no bearing on human beings. To go one step further he has concentrated even worse chemicals indoors, while still claiming they are harmless and that there is no evidence.

The individual's ability to recover or snowball and become progressively worse is dependent upon many factors, as you are about to discover, but especially one's genetics, nutrient status of the detox system, and total environmental body burden or load. In essence, in terms of developing chemical sensitivity we are all like soldiers walking through a field of land mines: no one knows when his number will come up. But we can teach you how to survive when it does and how to avoid many of the land mines.

Lastly, many of these chemicals, aside from the devastation they can wreak in initiating chemical sensitivity, can cause cancer by damaging the genetic material. In fact even though many of us recover remarkably, we are still more vulnerable to chemicals than we were before and this is more likely a genetic change as well.

Vinyl chloride from plastics (1), benzene from gasoline and room deodorizers (2), and many more chemicals have been incriminated. The damage to genetics comes from the chemicals themselves, their metabolites, the free radicals they generate and even the chemicals that result from the free radical destruction of the membranes {malondialdehyde, a breakdown product of lipid peroxidation reacts with DNA causing it to lose template activity, cross-link and have single strand breaks} (3).

(References from above paragraph)

(1)   (Ward, AM, et al, Immunological mechanisms in the pathogenesis of vinyl chloride disease, **Brit. Med. J.,** 1, 936-938, 1976).

(2)   (Graestrom, RC, et al, Formaldehyde damage to DNA and inhibition of DNA repair in human bronchial cells, **Science,** 220, 216-218, April 8, 1983).

(3)   (O'Brien, PJ, Free-radical-mediated DNA binding, **Environ. Health Persp.,** 64, 219-323, 1985).

Clearly, of the known cancer causing agents (viruses, ultraviolet and ionizing radiations, and chemicals), chemicals are of major importance. But it is a multi-staged process. That's why everyone who smokes does not get lung cancer. The sneakier compounds to prove cause and effect relationship are the ones that do not cause cancer directly by themselves, but are strong promoters or initiators. Hence our best protection is to keep our total load to a minimum (Miller, EC, et al, Mechanisms of chemical carcinogenesis, **Cancer,** 47:5, 1055-1064, March, 1987).

Clearly new rules in medicine are emerging as we enter the era of molecular medicine; and two of the most important rules to keep in mind are:
1. The total environmental load.
2. The biochemical individuality of each person.

Give your brain a rest now. It must be churning fiercely, for you have done a miraculous job. You have just burst the bonds of obsolete medical concepts and taken a giant step into the medicine of the 21st century. You will never be the same again. It will be difficult for anyone to

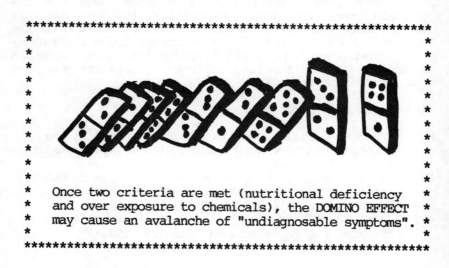

Once two criteria are met (nutritional deficiency and over exposure to chemicals), the DOMINO EFFECT may cause an avalanche of "undiagnosable symptoms".

foist a drug on you for lack of anything better to do. And your fertile brain will be always seeking ways to unload and maintain the health of your precious detox system, for you now appreciate that it is ever so vital to your total mental and physical well-being. And when you find that physician who shares this approach to your health, treasure him or her.

Chapter 4 :   A MEDICAL RENAISSANCE CHANGES THE RULES OF
MEDICINE

There is a blossoming renaissance in medicine, and out
of half a million U.S. physicians, only a small army of less
than two thousand is yet aware of it. As has been true
throughout the history of science and medicine, new truths
threaten old egos, upon which much financial, as well as
psychological security rests.

For example, Semmelweiss merely suggested to his colleagues that invisible germs were carried on their hands.
If only physicians would wash their hands after doing autopsies, before running down the hall to deliver the babies,
perhaps nine out of ten women would not die of childbirth
fever. This simple request, that we now take for granted,
met with derision, animosity, jealousy, hostility and anger.
How could one man be any smarter than they were? But when
it became common knowledge about town that his patients
lived longer, his gynecology practice boomed. Since this
cut into the business of his fellow colleagues, they got
hostile, bad-mouthed him, and they ostracized him.

Human nature being what it is, once you've chosen
camps and decided to arbitrarily denigrate something it's
very difficult to humble yourself and dig in to try to learn
what it's really about. Their jealousy stifled any scientific curiosity. They just sought any excuse to get rid of
this embarrassing thorn in their sides. After all if you
don't kill 90% of your patients, it sets you apart from the
pack: and when you deviate from the pack in medicine as a
physician, you're automatically labeled a quack.   (And
you've already learned that when you deviate from the pack
as a patient in terms of being able to suppress your symptoms with drugs, you're called a hypochondriac.)   Anyway,
they kicked him out of the medical society. He died of
suicide, penniless. You probably naively think, as I did,
that this no longer goes on in medicine today.   (Chapter
10).

Medical growth, renaissance or evolution is initially resisted by relabeling it as "medical controversy". Growth, renaissance or evolution, requires change of basic concepts and patterns, and many wish to cling to the old and familiar for the duration of their practice lives. After all, old physicians do not want to go back to school, medical school curriculums would need a total revamping, insurance data bases would require a drastic restructuring, personnel would have to be retrained; so let's not rush into this. The present system is working. Why rock the boat?

```
**************************************
*                                    *
* ANYONE WHO IS NOT UP ON A SUBJECT  *
* IS USUALLY DOWN ON IT.             *
*                                    *
**************************************
```

The reason is obvious: Many people look awful, feel awful, and are aging too rapidly. And they are products of obsolete medical concepts that are not adequate for diagnosing and treating disease in the 21st century.

Fortunately in spite of this outmoded mind set, we now have drugless methods to bring relief to patients with long-standing asthma, eczema, migraine, depression, panic disorder, chronic mononucleosis, "Yuppie Fatigue Syndrome", chronic cystitis, chronic vaginitis, lupus, sarcoid, dizziness, sinusitis, rheumatoid arthritis, learning disorders, spastic colon, schizophrenia and undiagnosable symptoms of just feeling terrible, spacey, dizzy, exhausted, unable to concentrate or poor memory, and nearly any symptom you can think of. And this is just the beginning. For rather than drugging a symptom or surgically cutting it out, we now can find the individual biochemical glitches and environmental triggers for most symptoms.

```
***************************************************************
*                                                             *
*     Current Outdated And Obsolete Medical Concepts          *
*                       Include:                              *
*                                                             *
*     *   All symptoms are bad and should be treated with     *
*         potent drugs.  By this logic, a headache must       *
*         be a Darvon deficiency.                             *
*     *   All patients with a singular disease and            *
*         similar symptoms such as all patients with          *
*         arthritis, or all patients with asthma, colitis,    *
*         or schizophrenia must have the same cause and       *
*         consequently the same treatment.                    *
*     *   Chronic exhaustion, depression, and spaciness       *
*         are symptoms of hypochondria.                       *
*     *   Nobody needs vitamins in the United States if       *
*         they eat regular food.                              *
*     *   Cookbook medicine is mass applicable and provides*
*         an adequate data base for insurance reimburse-      *
*         ment.  Those who fall through the cracks of         *
*         this system do not merit treatment or reimburse-   *
*         ment or are treated by quacks.  Therefore reim-     *
*         bursement for their services is denied.             *
*                                                             *
***************************************************************
```

The Brain Is The First To Be Affected

One key to understanding the medicine of the 21st century is to appreciate biochemical individuality. For contrary to current medical views, all patients with rheumatoid arthritis, for example, are not the same, do not look the same, do not smell the same, do not taste the same, do not eat the same, do not live the same, and do not have the same cause for their similar symptoms and therefore will not respond to the same treatment. That is why the singular magic bullet has not been found, and extremely potent drugs to annihilate symptoms are the only currently universally used methods. For example, many now pain-free rheumatoid patients have told me their rheumatologists turned colors when they happily went back to announce they no longer needed medications. They were surprised that the doctor did not share their joy at having discovered that a variety of foods had caused their arthritis pain. This is difficult for me to understand when even the scientific literature supports it. My only conclusion is that they did not want to be bothered with learning how to teach these people to go on the diagnostic diet, to see if hidden food sensitivity might apply to a particular person.

The twenty five year old speciality of environmental medicine (begun as the Society for Clinical Ecology) recognizes that the majority of people who have no diagnosis or who have been told "You have to learn to live with it", "It's all in your head", or "You must take these medicines the rest of your life", really have environmentally-induced illness or, for short, Environmental Illness or E.I. For anyone who has freed rheumatoid arthritis patients, for example, of their pain knows that if you have a room full of 100 patients with rheumatoid arthritis, no two will have the exact same set of causes. They are each biochemically unique. Not all have food sensitivity as one of their triggers either.

Only by identifying the hidden and unsuspected causes of symptoms for each individual can health be restored.

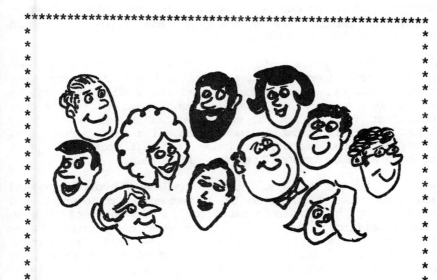

We don't all look different just to make life interesting. We _are_ different biochemically too.

Case Examples:

1)   A retired 62 year old industrial arts teacher had such painful arthritis he could not shake hands. He was also tired all the time. After finding that wheat, chocolate, beef and a few other foods cause his pain and swelling, he took up mountain climbing.

2)   A restaurant manager, 34 years old, was diagnosed as having "sarcoid or systemic lupus" by a prestigious medical center. Only dangerous doses of prednisone allowed her to function for the last five years. She was off all medications and totally clear of symptoms (arthritis, depression, dermatitis, colitis, exhaustion) and feeling actually more

energetic than she had ever been within one month of identifying and treating the causes. She has remained well and
without medication for four years.

3) For two years a 52 year old engineer consulted over
half a dozen specialists, and had had all the tests they
could think of. They were stumped for a diagnosis and he
was unable to work. All medications made him feel worse.
But after identifying the environmental causes of his body
aches, tremors, numbness, chest pain, dizziness, exhaustion,
depression, and heart arrhythmias, he continues to be able
to keep himself symptom free for eight years.

4) An 8 year old was labeled hopelessly hyperactive and
was prescribed high doses of amphetamines to control his
behavior by the pediatric neurologist. In spite of this he
poured boiling water on this three year old sister, threw
the iron at his father and his grades were all F's. Within
three months of identifying the causes of his symptoms, he
was off all medications and receiving A's and B's.

5) A 33 year old man had ten years of chronic diarrhea
and thick scaley dermatitis from head to toe. He also had
violent mood swings. He consulted specialists at four different medical centers in a large city, and used thousands
of dollars worth of treatments. After identifying the
causes he was clear for the first time in ten years within
two weeks of treatment.

6) A 7 year old girl had guttate psoriasis. The pediatrician and dermatologist recommended a lifetime of steroid
creams (which could cause the skin to look prematurely
wrinkled and atrophic or thin by the time she reached her
twenties). By finding the cause, she was clear in one month
and has remained that way for four years, with no drugs.

In these cases you saw many different target organs:
the joints, the nose (chronic sinusitis), the lungs
(asthma), the bowel (colitis), skin (eczema, psoriasis),
nervous system (with numbness and tingling or hyperactivity,
or mood swings), the heart vessels (with arrhythmia), but
there is almost always additional involvement of the common-

est target organ, the brain. Frequently, most of these people are initially too intimidated and embarrassed to mention how exhausted they are. Instead they concentrate on the more visible symptoms that can be more readily verified. Medicine, unfortunately, delegates brain symptoms (exhaustion, depression, schizophrenia, feeling unreal, spacey, confused, unable to concentrate, poor memory, panic attacks, manic episodes, mood swings, attention deficit disorder, learning disorder and hyperactivity) to the psychiatrists.

In all cases the causes of the symptoms were found so that drugs, which had been at best only partially effective anyway, were no longer needed.

The Name Of The Game Is The Name

Why is there a need for a new specialty of Environmental Medicine? The reason is to bridge the excellent acute care medicine that we have in this country with the medicine that is now necessary in the 21st century.

After all, if you have an auto accident today, you will most likely get first rate, state of the art care. We excel in acute care medicine in this century. But look at what happens when we treat degenerative or chronic conditions.

A typical example I hear daily goes like this: "What have you done to get rid of your headaches before you came here, Mrs. Jones?"

"I saw my family doctor who referred me to a neurologist. He ordered a CAT scan of my head and did many other tests as well."

"And what did he tell you?"

"He told me I have migraines and would have to take these drugs the rest of my life."

So in essence, she complained of headaches and he renamed it as migraines, then gave the unspoken message that it reflects a deficiency of medication, because that is how it was treated. It appears that the name of the game in medicine is merely to relabel or put a name on a condition, then drug it. In other words, the name of the game is the name.

```
***********************************************************
*                                                         *
*                                                         *
*                                                         *
*                                                         *
*                                                         *
*                                                         *
*                                                         *
*                                                         *
*                                                         *
*                                                         *
*                                                         *
*                                                         *
*                                                         *
*   As soon as your symptoms can be compartmentalized,   *
*   then the specialist for that problem is consulted.    *
*   Meanwhile the whole person is not dealt with.         *
*                                                         *
***********************************************************
```

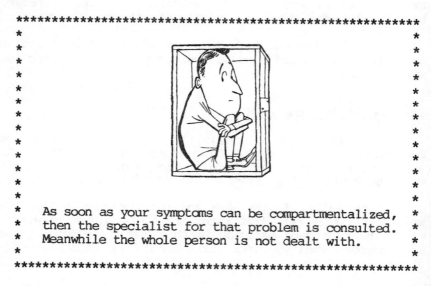

It goes on all day in many ways: "What have you done in attempt to get rid of your stomach problems before you came here Mr. Smith?"

"I saw my family doctor who referred me to a gastroenterologist. He scheduled many bowel X-rays after which he looked into the bowel with a long scope. He told me I have a spastic colon and would have to take these pills to control it."

And so it goes with referral to the target organ specialist; the disease is merely relabeled. It's as though the name of the game is to find the name. Having done so, the rest is easy: drug it or cut it out and throw it away.

Is there something wrong this this system? Absolutely! It gives many blatantly erroneous messages to the patient.

It suggests that:

(1) The diagnosis or the name of the condition is paramount to getting well. This justifies hundreds, and often thousands, of dollars of tests. If he's experienced, most of the time the physician knows beforehand when the results are going to be negative. He is seldom surprised. But if he doesn't carry through with the tests anyway, like the brain scan (or newer nuclear magnetic resonance imaging scan) of hundreds of dollars, then he destroys his presumed reason for being and might be sued for malpractice. Clearly the name of the condition is often merely a simplistic restating of, or translation of, the symptoms in medically acceptable (to physicians and insurance companies) jargon.

(2) Symptoms reflect a deficiency of some expensive synthetic prescription drug, for that indeed is how the majority are treated.

(3) Meanwhile, the patient can eat, drink, and smoke what he wants and live any way he chooses. For these activities have little bearing on his wellness. Only recently has this started to break down as people are slowly (much too slowly) shown how to reduce their cholesterols with diet change (although many of the current suggestions are still antiquated and actually harmful, see Chapter 7).

```
***************************************************
*    OUTMODED                                     *
*       *   concept of hypochondria               *
*       *   intricate diagnostic categories       *
*       *   need to routinely drug all            *
*           symptoms                              *
*       *   cook-book medical treatment           *
*       *   lack of patient responsibility        *
*           for health                            *
***************************************************
```

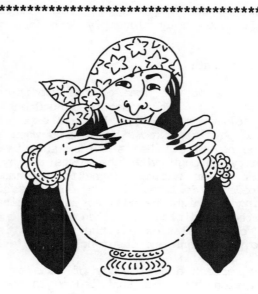

```
**********************************************************
*                                                        *
*                                                        *
*                                                        *
*                                                        *
*                                                        *
*                                                        *
*                                                        *
*                                                        *
*                                                        *
*                                                        *
*                                                        *
*                                                        *
*                                                        *
*                                                        *
*                                                        *
*                                                        *
*                                                        *
*                                                        *
*                                                        *
*                                                        *
*     There ought to be a happy medium between acute     *
*     care and molecular/environmental/preventive        *
*     medicine in this country pretty soon.  For example,*
*     there are simple things that people can do to begin *
*     to rule out hidden food allergies as a cause.      *
*                                                        *
**********************************************************
```

What's worse is that these disease names usually represent the beginning of end-stage degeneration of a particular target organ. They are the only way the body has of telling us the adaptive mechanisms are failing, because symptoms have been ignored and covered up too long with medications. So when we suppress the symptoms with medications, there is only one thing that can happen. We get symptoms in another target organ. But because the symptom doesn't appear related to the first problem, and because medicine is fragmented with specialties where each doctor only wants to concern himself with one target organ, no one recognizes the dangerous warnings. Drug therapy forces a switch in target organ. For you are still eating or breathing something that the body is alarmed about.

If we didn't have nutritionally inferior diets and an environmental chemical overload, we could continue to ignore the detox system.

Obsolete Rules Of Medicine

1) health is the absence of disease
2) symptoms are bad and should be suppressed
3) drugs and surgery are the way to health
4) all patients with similar symptoms have the same cause
5) no one needs vitamins or minerals
6) most diseases have singular causes
7) diseases can be treated by specialists who see one organ
8) small harmless doses of everyday chemicals from our food, air and water do not bioaccumulate

---

As The World Changes, New Rules Of Medicine Became Necessary

Let's look at some of my new rules of 21st century medicine:

I.   **Man is exposed to more chemicals than ever before** in the history of the world. (These include a plethora of chemical products that outgas volatile hydrocarbons. Furthermore he has used pesticides in plastics, fabrics, mattresses, foods, and more; he regularly ingests contaminated food, air, water, and prescription medicines). The 21st century has therefore created new problems that change many of the rules of medicine. Although the following facts may be new to many physicians, there is voluminous evidence in the biochemical literature for nearly everything that is presented (and this evidence is avail- able in a variety of instructional courses for physicians through the American Academy of Environmental Medicine, as just one example). Buildings constructed and furnished with materials that outgas these new chemicals are tightened to conserve energy; and outdoor air, mainly due to vehicular, toxic waste incinerators, and industrial exhausts is also getting progressively polluted. These chemicals react in a multitude of previously unseen ways in the environment and in our bodies.

A.   Because many of these chemicals are hydrocarbons, they are lipid soluble and the brain is the primary target organ. Lipids, or specialized fats in all cell membranes are more abundant in the brain and nervous system than anywhere else in the body. As most modern chemicals are solvents, this means they prefer and can penetrate lipids most easily. Therefore the first organ to become symptomatic is the brain. It is well documented in the scientific literature that these chemicals produce symptoms for which there are no blood tests, no x-rays.

B.   This damaged detoxication system can be permanently or temporarily malfunctioning and a variety of pathways can be intermittently affected producing a complex and fluctuating array of symptoms. Because the detoxication system in many

```
**********************************************************
*                                                        *
*                                                        *
*                                                        *
*                                                        *
*                                                        *
*                                                        *
*                                                        *
*                                                        *
*                                                        *
*                                                        *
*                                                        *
*                                                        *
*                                                        *
*     Medicine often gives the message, eat, drink and   *
*     be merry, for we have a pill for every symptom.    *
*                                                        *
**********************************************************
```

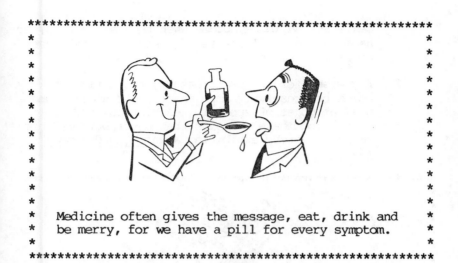

Medicine often gives the message, eat, drink and be merry, for we have a pill for every symptom.

victims is already overloaded by other chemicals (and its malfunction is further compounded by inferior nutrition, from eating processed foods), many people do not clear these extra xenobiotics (foreign chemicals) when they are moved into "clean air" and eat "clean (organic) food". Many have a permanently damaged xenobiotic detoxication system. On the way to becoming permanently damaged, the following phenomena occur:

1. The <u>spreading phenomenon</u> occurs when a patient starts reacting to a variety of inhalants, foods, chemicals and molds that never before bothered him. This occurs when key detoxication pathways finally become overloaded and break down, such as alcohol dehydrogenase or aldehyde dehydrogenase. Because these are common final pathways, for not only inhaled and ingested xenobiotics, but also normal body metabolites (like brain hormones and neurotransmitters). Symptoms can easily become triggered by many seemingly unrelated entities. So by being poisoned by a pesticide exposure or an over abundance of everyday room chemicals, they

can start having symptoms when they eat a food, or
have an emotional stress, for example, that never
bothered them before.

2. Likewise, for the same reasons, the patient be-
    comes progressively more reactive to smaller and
    smaller doses of specific xenobiotics, and to
    foods, chemicals or molds that never bothered him
    before, thereby exhibiting a <u>heightened sensi-
    tivity</u>.

****
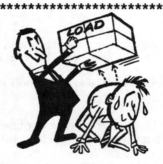

As causes of symptoms are discovered, there is a
gradual unloading until that wellness can occur.
****

It's easy to see how this occurs. Suppose each
day you're exposed to formaldehyde from your new
carpet at home. The detox path is able to handle
this so you are not aware of a problem. Suddenly
they paint at work and the xylene becomes the
straw that breaks the camel's back. You not only
get spacey and unable to concentrate at work, but
you start having a flare-up of your old back pain
at home. Meanwhile you no longer tolerate
shopping malls and get very depressed in them
within an hour. And every time you eat anything
with wheat (bread, beer, whiskey, donuts, pasta)
you become very depressed. The end result is that

it is as though you have gone off your rocker, when in actuality you have reset your thermostat to a lower level of reactivity. But to someone who is ignorant of the biochemistry of detoxication, it appears that you are a bonafide hypochondriac.

3. Symptoms fluctuate, seemingly unpredictably, since the total load (dose of each individual offender and total combined load of all offenders) presented to the individual is never exactly the same at any two moments in time. The day you get stuck in traffic on the way to the office, the newly carpeted office makes you spacey. The days when you take the bypass and miss all the exhaust, the office doesn't bother you.

4. There is tremendous individual biochemical variation in target organ. No two people have the exact same symptoms and triggers. As Gray's Anatomy shows, there is even great physical variation; for example, there are many shapes and positions that a stomach can have. And the biochemistry of each individual is infinitely more variable. One person can get leukemia from chronic exposure to benzene in gasoline, while in someone else it can cause peripheral nerve damage with numbness and tingling. In another it will cause headache. Just look at the variability in symptoms we saw among genetically related family members when they had urea formaldehyde foam insulated their home. One was spacey, one was nauseated, one had headache or arthritis and two were unaffected. If this is what happens with people with similar genetics, imagine the variation in response in a factory or office.

5. Because of this biochemical individuality there is likewise tremendous individual variation in susceptibility to chemicals.

6. There has been (ala the 1983 Nobel laureate Dr.

Barbara McClintock) a genetic change in some
individuals. This can occur for a variety of
reasons. Suppose you were deficient in a key
nutrient like zinc, which is crucial in DNA
(genetic) repair enzymes {zinc is pivotal in DNA
polymerase}. When some foreign chemicals (xenobiotics) are metabolized, they form dangerous
substances called adducts that attach to our
genetic material, DNA. If the repair enzyme {zinc
dependent DNA polymerase} is deficient (for lack
of zinc), we cannot repair this damage. This
explains why many of us seem to have actually
become chemically sensitive overnight.

7. Nearly all materials are continually oxidizing and
   small amounts of them are continually being given
   off or released into the air. These osmols
   penetrate the blood stream and the blood/brain
   barrier, irrespective of whether an odor is
   perceptible (one can die of carbon monoxide
   poisoning while never smelling it). Hence people
   with a "reset" thermostat react at much lower
   levels than "normal" people, when no one else is
   even able to perceive an odor. Often because of
   heightened sensitivity (almost like a traffic jam
   in the over burdened, poorly functioning liver of
   the victim) this chemical accumulates in the blood
   stream of the effected person. Eventually he may
   even smell the chemical while others still cannot.
   This creates further frustration and undermines
   the credibility of the victim. For example, when
   I'm around someone with perfume or aftershave, I
   can taste it coming out on my tongue, while they
   can't even smell it after they've had it on a few
   hours.

8. The damaged detoxification system has far reaching
   effects on much more than the immune system. It
   extends to all systems since they are irrevocably,
   biologically entwined. For if the liver is
   traffic-jammed and unable to further breakdown or
   metabolize a chemical, the chemical ends up aim-

lessly floating around in the body bathing the cells of every system. These cells, wherever they are, inevitably suffer and become damaged. These damaged cells could be in the nervous system and result in depression, or they could be in the endocrine system and injure the function of the ovaries with resultant infertility (as many pesticides do). They could be in the pancreas and result in diabetes or pancreatitis (Acute pancreatitis following continuous exposure to organophosphate insecticide, Internal Medicine World Report, March 1-14, 1989). All bets are off as to how each person will respond.

Obviously when symptoms occur in the endocrine system, musculo-skeletal system, neurologic system, or energy metabolism system, etc. seemingly unrelated symptoms, as infertility, muscular/skeletal pains, weakness, exhaustion or even gastro/intestinal disturbances can occur on top of the already existing troublesome symptoms. This gets very discouraging and these people often feel like they have a new disease every week. For indeed, when the detox system is not understood, the sick get continually sicker.

9. The environment for one individual is never the same at any two moments in time and is constantly changing. Hence, symptoms will unpredictably change, and even things that once caused reactions may not cause a reaction on another day because the total load is never the same. For example, the office paint will bother someone more after a night of alcoholic drinks or a night in a smokey, pesticided bowling alley, than if he had stayed home and played baseball with the kids outdoors in fresh air. The detox system needs time each day to catch up.

10. Chronic exposure to deleterious substances often leads to the induction of enzymes to help the body adapt to this offender. After a while the trigger

is not perceived as being directly related to
symptoms because of <u>adaptation</u> (a rise in enzymes
that help to degrade this chemical) has occurred.
This phenomenon <u>is called masking</u>. But once the
trigger is removed for a specific period of time,
the compensatory rise in enzymes no is longer
stimulated and the enzyme level returns to normal.
For example, your first cigarette may make you
sick, but after years, you can easily smoke 2
packs a day. Then quit for 6 months. During this
time your adaptive or masking enzymes will drop
back to normal levels. Suddenly smoke 2 packs
again in one day and you'll probably be sick. The
same principles apply for man's adaptation to
everyday chemicals in air, food and water.

```
*************************************************************
*                                                           *
*                                                           *
*                                                           *
*                                                           *
*                                                           *
*                                                           *
*                                                           *
*                                                           *
*                                                           *
*                                                           *
*                                                           *
*                                                           *
*                                                           *
*                                                           *
*                                                           *
*                                                           *
*   All bets are off as to what symptoms you might          *
*   have once the detox system breaks down and starts       *
*   to back up and damage other systems like the nerv-      *
*   ous, endocrine and immune systems.                      *
*                                                           *
*************************************************************
```

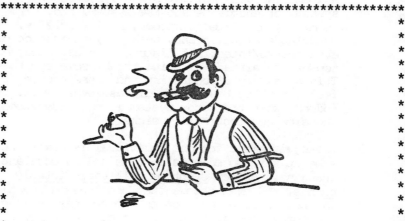

Obviously all this adaptation or masking requires
energy and extra nutrients. And there is a limit

as to how much adaptive reserve each of us has.

The most insidious part of this is when some new chemical is added to all of this (new carpet, recent construction or new furniture) and the system breaks down. You can see how the person

****
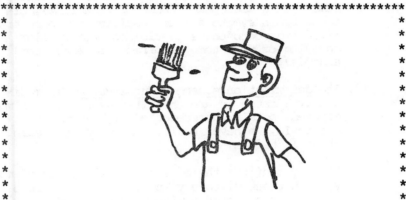

Total load: If you paint inside your house during the time they put in new carpets at work, you're more likely to be the one who becomes chemically sensitive.

****

who has been steadily having 2 packs of cigarettes a day with no problem cannot understand why he should stop smoking when it was the new carpet that made him sick. He doesn't see that when the detox system fails, it starts failing for many other chemicals that it was previously able to handle. So once you start reacting to anything you'll heal much faster if you can reduce the unseen overload to your system in as many sensible ways as possible. The trick is to understand what things that you take for granted that are readily overloading you and will continue to overload you.

11. There is steady bioaccumulation throughout life. Many inhaled and ingested chemicals cannot be totally disposed of. They accumulate in minuscule, unnoticeable amounts until there is sudden breakdown of the system; suddenly we see a person with cancer (from benzene inhaled from gasoline fumes) or a neuropathy (numb or weak limb), or toxic brain symptoms like inability to concentrate (from organophosphate pesticides from regular spraying of your home or office for ants, for example).

12. The detoxication scheme is undervalued in medicine. Because we are the first generation of man exposed to this unprecedented high level of chemicals, we never really had a need to learn about it before.

(a) History confirms there is frequently a lag of many years between discovery and incorporation into medical practice of a widely based non-drug related therapy. But it is especially difficult to study something when the lag time between exposure and malignancy, for example, might be twenty years or more.

(b) Individuality of biochemical response, target organ response and total load vary tremendously. For example, some people lack specific enzymes to detoxify certain chemicals. That is why some cannot take certain drugs. Biotransformation or detoxication of benzene is inhibited, for example, by the presence of toluene. You will recall the target organ for benzene (a known cause of leukemia) is the bone marrow. So if two rubber tire makers are both exposed to benzene, the one to get leukemia will more likely be the one whose wife paints the inside of his house every 2 years (and who gets higher toluene exposure).

The precise target organ will be dependent upon

the individual's biochemistry and the total load
of other chemicals vying for metabolism at the
same time. Since toluene inhibits the breakdown
of benzene, it makes it more likely that it will
cause leukemia.

****

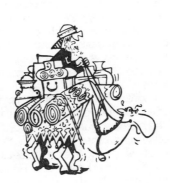

If you are not as well as you'd like to be, start
by assessing your total load and see what could be
over-burdening your detox system.

****

(c) Human xenobiotic responses cannot be adequately
studied in animals: the rat has six times the
level of some detoxication enzymes, like hepatic
glutathione S-transferase as compared with man
Sulfo-transferases like glutathione S-transferase,
have a high affinity for phenolics. So that means
a rat wouldn't be harmed by common phenol-
containing dentifrices and household cleaning
products as easily as man would. Rats thrive in
filth and rarely get infected; the rat does not
have a folate system and cannot get formaldehyde
toxicity as readily as man does, and the rat does

not produce offspring with phocomelia (offspring born without limbs) with thalidomide, like man did either.

(d) There's another principle of environmental medicine that must be understood before one can comprehend a person's symptoms. That is bipolarity. When you first get exposed to a particular food or chemical that causes a reaction, you may react by being very hyper, wild, up, or anxious as with an overdose of coffee or alcohol. The same phenomenon can occur with a sensitivity to sugar, chocolate, soda, or wheat, for example. The person gets "wired" initially with these if he is sensitive. This is his reaction. Often these people are super salesmen or the life of the party, so this is not considered an undesirable quality, much less a symptom. However, when the reaction runs down, he swings the other way and gets utterly exhausted or depressed. If, however, he recognizes the connection with his allergies, that he feels good when he has sugar or wheat, when he wears down he gives himself another fix to get "up" again.

You can readily appreciate how if this were a wheat or sugar reaction that wore off every 3 or 4 hours, how this would be a one-way street to rapid weight gain and obesity (or hypoglycemia, Candida overgrowth, and irritable bowel), especially if it were not recognized and treated. Worse yet, with the passage of months and years, the nutrients in the reaction pathways get depleted and the person no longer gets "up" (the stimulatory phase). He just stays chronically down (the depressive phase). But he is now so hooked on the food that he can't get off. If he misses a meal he gets a headache or irritable or some other symptom. Everyone learns that he has to have his "fix" (that 4 p.m. coffee or nightly martini) or else! So he's seemingly locked into feeling lousy and getting progressively more over

weight while he continues to exhaust his adaptive
detox enzymes.

And to make this weight gain even worse, sometimes
an overload of a xenobiotic will poison some of
the metabolic enzymes or endocrine glands
(thyroid) that are needed to get the weight back
off.

C.   Part of these problems is genetic, but part of it is
related to the degree of <u>nutritional depletion</u> that the individual has. This varies because of the following factors:

1.   <u>Food processing removes a large percentage of
     vitamins and minerals</u> from foods. It changes
     fatty acids from beneficial to harmful types that
     accelerate aging and degenerative disease (Chapter
     7). Irradiation of food destroys a significant
     level of vitamins also. Changing tastes (where
     people are hooked on sweets, salts, and fats),
     depleted soils (we feed the world!), and increased
     medication prescriptions (these use up vitamins
     and minerals) also further compromise one's
     nutrient status.

     Furthermore, abnormal levels of certain bowel
     flora like yeasts grow in the intestines after
     antibiotics. This leads to inflammation of the
     gut wall which then poorly absorbs nutrients.
     At the same time, (antibiotics kill the good
     protective bacteria in the gut that help make some
     vitamins and detoxify chemicals).

     Additionally, with our current level of chemical
     pollution in the bloodstream (remember all those
     chemicals the New Jersey residents had in their
     blood?), these chemicals damage parts of vitamins
     and their enzymes and block mineral-containing
     enzymes, putting an even greater stress on the
     nutrient system. As well, the chemical overload
     can shunt biotransformation processes to other
     pathways that are not normally subject to deple-

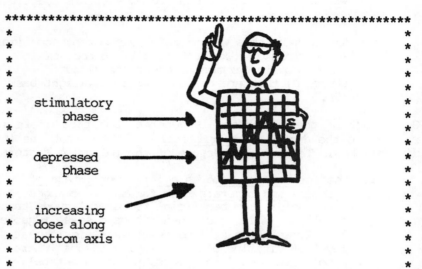

```
****************************************************
*                                                  *
*                                                  *
*                                                  *
*                                                  *
*                                                  *
*   stimulatory                                    *
*      phase                                       *
*                                                  *
*                                                  *
*   depressed                                      *
*      phase                                       *
*                                                  *
*                                                  *
*   increasing                                     *
*   dose along                                     *
*   bottom axis                                    *
*                                                  *
*                                                  *
*   Bipolarity:  As the dose increases, you pass out *
*   of the depressed phase into the stimulatory phase *
*   as more adaptive enzymes are induced.  But if the *
*   dose keeps increasing, you deplete all enzyme  *
*   reserves and fall into the depressed phase.    *
*                                                  *
****************************************************
```

tion. With an extra unexpected load in a pathway, further nutrients can get depleted.

And lastly, biochemical individuality and the stress of chronic disease also have a great role to play in the final nutrient status of each person. Stress causes over-synthesis of stress hormones that require extra nutrients for their eventual metabolism.

So food processing has a seriously silent and epidemic effect on our lives. For example, vitamin E has been removed from most grocery store oils and flours. Exposures to various pesticides

and chemicals can cause brain symptoms which
actually mimic Alzheimer's. The brain is more
vulnerable to attack by these when vitamin E is
not standing guard at the cell membrane. Vitamin
E is necessary to prevent Alzheimer's.

2. To compound our problem of declining nutrient
status in this century, <u>nutritional depletion is
not readily recognized</u> because of many reasons (1)
there is no interest in it because it is a non-
prescription item, so the physician has no power
over its use and (2) pharmaceutical companies
cannot patent the products to make a profit.

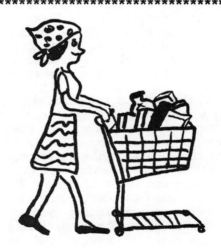

Many foods in a bag, box, jar, can, or wrapper
have had substantial amounts of key detox nutrients
removed in processing.

Therefore, there is little interest in nutritional

therapies nor is there money for research.

It is believed by many who never check nutrient levels in their patients, nor read nutritional biochemistry and medical journals, that because the U.S. is so affluent, a deficiency is not likely. Another reason for the failure to appreciate the extent of nutritional deficiencies is that many nutrients' (vitamin, mineral, amino acid, and essential fatty acid) levels are not readily available in commercial laboratories, nor are the functional assays. Furthermore, just to be able to know which test to order requires sophisticated biochemical knowledge that many physicians do not yet possess. And some physicians are still stuck with prehistoric thinking and persist in looking for a single disease or syndrome as a hallmark of a specific nutrient deficiency. They ignore the fact that a deficiency of B12, for example, can cause fatigue in one person and numbness in another.

In reality a single deficiency (because it is important in a variety of enzymes) can manifest as a variety of symptoms. For example, zinc is in over 90 enzymes, magnesium is in over 300. How can there be a single deficiency syndrome? I can show you 30 people who were deficient in magnesium and each one had a different symptom that was cleared when the deficiency was corrected. Likewise one particular symptom can be cleared by different nutrients in different people. Vitamin B6 can clear depression, PMS, carpel tunnel syndrome, exhaustion, pernicious vomiting of pregnancy, and much more. This can befuddle the physician who is unknowledgeable about nutritional biochemistry.

3. There are many examples of serious errors currently being perpetuated in medicine due to lack of knowledge in nutritional biochemistry. These current medical errors include the manage-

ment of hypercholesterolemia with margarines and corn oil, the prophylaxis of osteoporosis with estrogen and calcium, the treatment of hypertension with drugs, and the failure to recognize magnesium deficiency or Candida related complex (both of which can masquerade as nearly any symptom one can think of. See Chapter 7).

****

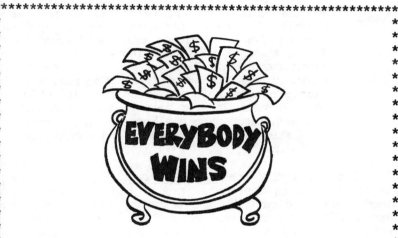

21st century molecular medicine is very cost effective and will save millions of dollars for a health care system that is in shakey financial shape. For instance, identifying a magnesium deficiency and changing the diet has relieved many individuals of over $100 in blood pressure medicine a month.

****

4. Every day you are wearing down and losing some of your detox nutrients. When you detox a molecule of pesticide, for example, from school, or a molecule of nicotine from your cigarettes, or a molecule of acetominophen (Tylenol) for your headache, you are using up glutathione. Remember that's the molecule analogous to the chicken

farmer grabbing up his prize hen. This carries
the chemical into the bile ducts of the liver and
into the intestine for excretion. It is lost
forever. And so is the cysteine (probably the
most important detox amino acid) and other
nutrients.

If your diet can keep up with the chemical demands
and losses of this century, fine. If not, as
cysteine is lost faster than it can be synthesized
from methionine (another amino acid found in the
diet), then you will have increasing inability to
detox chemicals. Plus you will have less taurine
(that is made from cysteine). The result of low
taurine can be seizures, recurrent infections,
heart disease, poorer detoxication of chemicals,
and much more. You see how one tiny example
snowballs (Taurine, Huxtable and Babeau, see
Appendix).

II.   Clearly there are two different types of medicine.
The first type is the acute form of medicine where x-rays,
blood tests, medications, and surgery, form the mainstay of
current diagnosis and treatment. This type of medicine concentrates on illness and disease. The second form of medicine concentrates on wellness and prevention.

A.   Acute care medicine, which has very little to do with
wellness and prevention, is dramatic, often highly technical, usually independent of patient involvement and intel-
lect, and expensive. I call this hi-tech medicine. It is
indispensable in its own right.

B.   The second form of medicine deals with wellness and
prevention and focuses on patient education and responsibility. It is not hi-tech medicine; it is not as expensive, nor as mystical. When illness becomes chronic, more
patient education and responsibility is needed. I call this
intelligent medicine.

1.   Benefits are not possible without the patient
being involved and sharing a large part of the

responsibility.

2. This entails a vast amount of educating of the patient, and consequently dilutes some of the physician control and mystique.

3. Patients learn to listen to (and not block out because of fear of being intimidated by a label of hypochondriasis) and appreciate body symptoms as early warnings. For example a headache is not seen as a Darvon deficiency, but a reason to

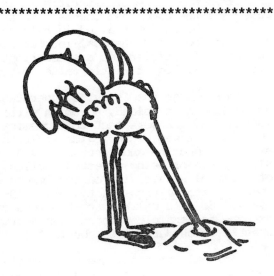

```
************************************************************
*                                                          *
*                                                          *
*                                                          *
*                                                          *
*                                                          *
*                                                          *
*                                                          *
*                                                          *
*                                                          *
*                                                          *
*                                                          *
*                                                          *
*                                                          *
*                                                          *
*                                                          *
*                                                          *
*                                                          *
*                                                          *
*        This is what it's like to practice medicine in    *
*    this era without knowledge of nutritional biochem-    *
*    istry.                                                 *
*                                                          *
************************************************************
```

review what you are eating and breathing and what

biochemical abnormalities you may have.

4. There is no need for organ limited specialists, because the treatment is not going to be limited to drugs to mask symptoms. For example, arthritis pain is not going to be covered up by non-steroidal anti-inflammatory drugs, but rather dietary and xenobiotic (foreign chemical) triggers will be sought. Therefore, it becomes inconsequential if the arthritis is named or labeled rheumatoid, lupus, or degenerative. Because the underlying cause is sought, the label is often meaningless. Who cares what type of arthritis it is? It's the cause not the name that counts. So a rheumatologist who is not trained in helping you figure out what foods and chemical intolerances and what nutritional deficiencies are contributing to your symptoms will be of little value to you.

You know enough chemistry to understand that just as no man is an island, no organ within man is an island. By the mere fact that chemicals are in the blood stream, it's logical that the immune system, endocrine and central nervous systems are all capable of being affected (Kollen, LD, Effect of chemical sensitivity on the immune system, Immunol. and Allerg. Pract., 7:10, 13-25, Oct., 1985). So it's unlikely that anyone can help your asthma, for example without also addressing your spastic colon, arthritis, brain fog and cystitis.

5. Conventional lab tests are not heavily relied upon because they detect only end-stage degeneration. For example, significant loss of liver function must occur before damaged enzymes are seen on regular blood tests. Only when end-stage degeneration (chronic disease) or seriously decompensated (acute breakdown) stages occur are these tests positive.

6. This is not a cookbook form of medicine where one symptom is pathognomonic (specifically diagnostic)

for one disease that is treated with one drug. For example, twenty arthritis patients will all have different foods and chemicals as the triggers of their symptoms. And some will also have an unsuspected magnesium deficiency as the cause for their relentless muscle spasm. Likewise, one trigger, such as formaldehyde, can cause twenty different symptoms in twenty different people.

7. Intelligent medicine requires in depth knowledge of nutritional biochemistry and the biochemistry of detoxication on the part of the physician. Because this form of medicine is in its infancy, we can't yet always find all the causes in everyone. But the track record has been so overwhelmingly good, that it's worth evaluating in the person who wants to avoid drugs. For those who won't, or can't make the necessary changes, they have the optional choice of falling back on drugs.

III. Often issues that are confusing to physicians new to the discipline or point of view of environmental medicine, need explaining. Some of the key issues follow:

A. The bizarre psychiatric symptoms that fluctuate wildly: alcohol and aldehyde metabolism (or breakdown) are two of the common pathways through which chemicals pass to become detoxified. In other words, these are the two biochemical bottlenecks of Phase I detoxication. Acetaldehyde is a potently destructive chemical to important regulatory membranes, proteins, enzymes, and purines. So acetaldehyde must be quickly gotten rid of or metabolized by the body. It must not be allowed to accumulate because it is so damaging.

But it's fairly easy for the aldehyde path to become overloaded. Breathing plastic fumes, formaldehyde-coated paper, carpet and fabric fumes, trichloroethylene from newly shampooed carpets or dry cleaned clothes, aldehydes from auto exhaust can all raise the blood level of aldehydes. So can being highly stressed, since most brain hormones or neurotransmitters also metabolize to aldehydes. Unfortun-

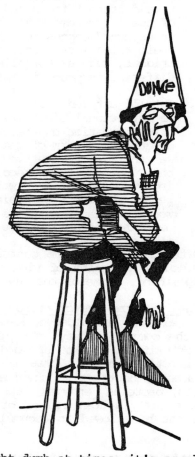

```
****************************************************
*                                                  *
*                                                  *
*                                                  *
*                                                  *
*                                                  *
*                                                  *
*                                                  *
*                                                  *
*                                                  *
*                                                  *
*                                                  *
*                                                  *
*                                                  *
*                                                  *
*                                                  *
*                                                  *
*                                                  *
*                                                  *
*                                                  *
*                                                  *
*                                                  *
*                                                  *
*                                                  *
*                                                  *
*                                                  *
*                                                  *
*                                                  *
*                                                  *
*                                                  *
*                                                  *
*                                                  *
*  If you get down-right dumb at times, it's usually  *
*  one of two things:  what you are eating or what    *
*  you are breathing.  If you're always dumb, you'd   *
*  better check your detox chemistry.                 *
*                                                  *
****************************************************
```

ately, to make matters worse, sometimes the aldehyde pathway does not function well because of undiagnosed deficiencies. Aldehyde oxidase is a molybdenum dependent enzyme and most Americans consume an insufficient amount daily (especially since beans are one of the richest sources); likewise alcohol dehydrogenase is a zinc dependent enzyme and most people only receive about 75% of the RDA daily (since eating liver, for example, is equally unpopular).

```
***********************************************************
*                                                         *
*                                                         *
*                                                         *
*                                                         *
*                                                         *
*                                                         *
*                                                         *
*                                                         *
*                                                         *
*                                                         *
*                                                         *
*                                                         *
*                                                         *
*                                                         *
*                                                         *
*                                                         *
*                                                         *
*                                                         *
*                                                         *
*                                                         *
*                                                         *
*   Taking medications without finding the cause of       *
*   symptoms hastens the demise of the body.              *
*                                                         *
***********************************************************
```

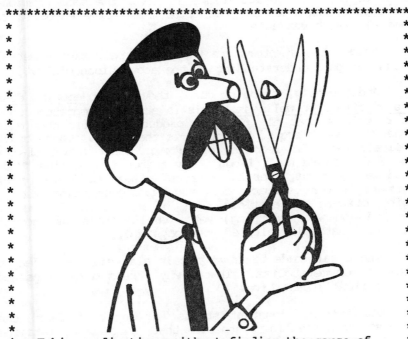

Taking medications without finding the cause of symptoms hastens the demise of the body.

So when these degradation pathways are ailing or blocked because they lack key minerals in the enzymes that make the pathway function (in order to clear these chemicals from the blood), an overload and backlog occurs. This is especially serious if not only are some key minerals deficient, but the path is further stressed by exposures to room chemicals that get changed into these very metabolites. The body looks for an alternative detox route and forms chloral hydrate. You'll recall this is the old "Mickey Finn" or "knockout" drops, and explains the precise symptoms that these people exhibit; dopey, dizzy, depressed, tired, unable to concentrate and focus, mood swings, etc. But the amount of chloral hydrate formed is never the same from one moment to another because the total cumulative exposure to chemicals is so variable.

Hence, the symptoms are thought to be strictly mental because of poor understanding of the above biochemistry.

B.   Additionally, frame of mind, thought, or emotion does have an effect on wellness. This is easy to comprehend when one remembers that all thoughts produce specific chemicals or neurotransmitters to be formed in the brain. These brain chemicals have far reaching effects in other areas of the body. You know this. I could say things to you like "Your child was just run over by a truck", that would make your heart race, your stomach sick and fill your being with a raging mixture of emotions. I haven't touched you or injected you with anything, yet with the power of thought you have drastically altered your physiology.

These self-made brain chemicals also vie for aldehyde pathways for metabolism. That's why stress makes a person more chemically sensitive.

Furthermore, constant stress (or anger or fear) can increase noradrenalin synthesis that increases histamine release from mast cells. Translation: stress also adds to the total load of the detox system, accentuating chemical intolerances, as well as regular dust or mold allergies.

An undiagnosed magnesium deficiency can make someone extremely irritable and edgey for no reason. When needless tranquilizers are prescribed, they further overload the detoxication pathways and further deplete precious magnesium. So there's a circle of worsening psychiatric symptoms just because of an unrecognized mineral deficiency. And with this worsening magnesium deficiency, as an example, there is less and less magnesium available to help metabolize and get rid of the stress hormones. So the neurotic simply get more neurotic. Or the criminal gets desperate.

Clearly, neurotransmitters must be metabolized, and because they actually contribute additional aldehydes that further overload an already compromised detoxification pathway, a bad thought can be as devastating as inhaling a bad chemical.

Now you understand how in the current drug-oriented, detoxication-ignored medical system, <u>the sick get sicker</u>. There is no way out until intelligent intervention breaks this vicious cycle.

Researchers all over the world have discovered that there are receptors for V.I.P. (vasopressor intestinal peptide, a special messenger protein in the gut) in the brain as well. In other words, the gut can talk to the brain and vice versa via these messenger proteins that get sent through the blood and other routes. This is exciting because it proves that the whole body communicates with itself. No organ is an island onto itself. <u>You can't have bad thoughts without harming your health.</u>

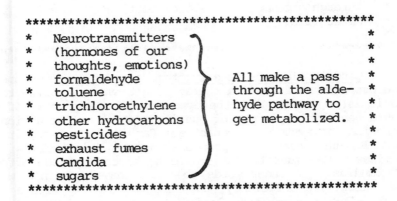

```
*************************************************
*    Neurotransmitters                          *
*    (hormones of our                           *
*    thoughts, emotions)                        *
*    formaldehyde          All make a pass      *
*    toluene               through the alde-    *
*    trichloroethylene     hyde pathway to      *
*    other hydrocarbons    get metabolized.     *
*    pesticides                                 *
*    exhaust fumes                              *
*    Candida                                    *
*    sugars                                     *
*************************************************
```

So remember <u>a bad thought can be as destructive as inhaling a bad chemical.</u> For they both have far reaching effects on the rest of the body and they both have to be metabolized eventually by the same aldehyde pathway in the detox system. That's precisely why I call this a biochemical bottleneck, because so much must get funneled through here. When it gets stopped up, overloaded, or backlogged, we are in serious trouble and having mental and physical symptoms that no doctor can accurately diagnose without this knowledge.

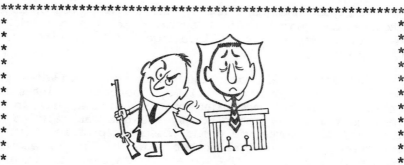

A bad thought can be as damaging to your body chemistry as a bad chemical, since they all pass through a common biochemical bottleneck to get metabolized.

C. <u>Candida albicans is a symptom, not a disease</u>. Some of the proponents of Candida therapy don't even recognize this, so it is no wonder that the opponents of it do not. If one has a healthy complement of nutrients and a well-functioning detoxication system, he cannot get Candida. In fact, it's a normal inhabitant of people's mouths, intestines and vaginas. One must be vulnerable to succumb to the effects of Candida. In other words they must have something wrong .... usually a deficiency; they are not playing with a full deck. Furthermore, once Candida has gained a foothold, the effects come about by any of over six different mechanisms: metabolic, immunologic, infectious, toxic, hormonal, or allergic. (Chapter 7 will discuss this.)

```
************************************************************
*    21st CENTURY MEDICINE NEEDS TO RECOGNIZE:           *
*                                                         *
*    Biochemical individuality                           *
*    Damaged detoxication system                         *
*    Total load varies daily                             *
*    Nutritional depletion from processed foods          *
*    Nutritional biochemical corrections are needed      *
*    Brain symptoms fluctuate                            *
*    Spreading phenomenon occurs anytime                 *
*    Heightened sensitivity occurs anytime               *
*    Genetic change has occurred                         *
*    Symptoms fluctuate to multiple organs               *
*    Adaptation (masking, bipolarity) occurs             *
*    Osmols penetrate blood/brain barrier                *
*    Backlogged chemicals can damage hormones, etc.      *
*    Many chemicals silently bioaccumulate               *
*    A bad thought can be as harmful as a bad chemical   *
*    Candida is a symptom, not a disease                 *
*    Lab animals do not react like humans                *
*    The environmental cause must be sought              *
*    The downward spiral results if the above is ignored *
*                                                       8
************************************************************
```

One example of the metabolic problem is that Candida elaborates acetaldehyde which further overloads the aldehyde path bottleneck. That is why, for example, a person can be dramatically less chemically or food sensitive once he has treated his Candida. He merely unloaded a common biochemical bottleneck through which metabolites of all those triggers had to pass. Isn't it exciting that an explanation for a long-standing observation is finally understood?

****

<u>Rogers' Rules Of E.I.</u>

1) Osmols of the environment are in the body.
2) The brain is the primary target organ.
3) An overload of the xeno-detox system damages detox and all other systems.
4) Windows of vulnerability/target organ varies.
5) Adaptation has two primary phases, <u>induction and depletion</u>.
6) Bioaccumulation proceeds unnoticed until poisoning.
7) The environment and total load are not constant.
8) Total load must be addressed for wellness.
9) All symptoms provide good clues.
10) As one is unloaded or detoxed, reactions are more clear-cut.
11) No two people will have the exact same causes.
12) Detox nutrients are usually deficient.

****

D.   <u>Provocation-neutralization principles are in evidence all throughout biology</u>. For every substance there is a bell-shaped curve of biological response. There is a dose that is too high and a dose that is too low, and both of these extreme doses can eventually be so deleterious as to be lethal (water, air, food, thyroid, vitamins, minerals, immune system complement, IgE, medicines, etc.). And there is an optimal dose that can turn off symptoms, (Diagnosing the Tight Building Syndrome, Rogers, SA, <u>Environmental Health Perspectives</u>, 76, 195-198,1987). For example too little vitamin A causes the exact same symptoms as too much vitamin A. But there is an optimal dose in the middle which promotes health.

Phenol (carbolic acid) is a common household chemical (in Lysol and other phenol containing sprays, cleaners, and room deodorizers, for example). The problem is it is in all conventional allergy injections to maintain sterility. Many people are sensitive to it. On single blind testing they duplicate many of their symptoms that persisted while they were on these injections. When it's neutralized the symptom disappears, and when they get non-phenolated injections for their other sensitivities, they clear all their symptoms and are able to tolerate injections for the first time.

Phenol has some other bad properties. It has a strong attraction or affinity for the blood vessel wall, and affects blood coagulation, and depresses the immune system (Nour-Eldin, F, Preliminary report: Uptake of phenol by vascular and brain tissue, Microvascular Research, 2, 224-225, 1970; LaVia, MF, LaVia, DS, Phenol derivatives are immunodepressive in mice, Drug and Chemical Toxicology: 2 (1+2) 167-177, 1979).

E.   Serial dilution titration is merely more scientific and logical than the canned "one dose for all" approach used by general allergists.   There is nothing wrong with their techniques; they have helped millions of people; I did them for 9 years myself. But for highly sensitive patients, like myself, they eventually only give us red sore arms, new symptoms, and dwindling help.

However, testing to several small dilutions to find the optimal individual dose for a person saves the day. It allows each individual's body to tell the physician the precise optimal dose of each and every antigen for that individual. When this "best" dose is found, it stays there, or in that vicinity. And it is safer since there is no arbitrary raising of the dose. If the dose that the general allergist uses for most people is not your best dose, it will make you worse. It's far safer to find your best dose in the safety of the office than crossing our fingers each time you get a higher dose in your regular injection and hoping this is not one of your "bad" doses. Ask any man on the street; would he rather be tested to one or two standard doses that everybody is receiving, or be titrated to a specific cut-off point, so specific that every further five-fold increment produces a two millimeter increment in skin wheal growth?   I have never met a man so illogical that he preferred the conventional doses.

F.   Cost effectiveness is evident when we have a once bed-ridden patient with say, rheumatoid arthritis, back to work because the sensitivities to foods, molds and chemicals and the nutrient deficiencies were addressed. And he is no longer on arthritis drugs that eat holes in his stomach.

G.   Life quality effectiveness goes hand in hand. Bed-ridden, pill popping people drain their families and society.

H.   It is quite clear there will be many opponents to this type of medicine who put their politics, finances and egos before the good health of their fellow man.
1.   The drug industry wants to sell drugs.
2.   The food industry wants to use additives, process foods, irradiate them, and use pesticides.
3.   The manufacturing industry wants to continue to pollute the air, water, and soil.
4.   Businesses want to continue to tighten buildings, eliminate windows, and conserve heat.
5.   Builders want to continue to use cheaper, outgas-sing synthetic materials.
6.   General allergists try to insist on the standard non-titrated allergy doses for all patients because it's quicker and does not require as specialized training. And they choose to ignore treating food, chemical, and Candida sensitivi-ties, since they require learning these same techniques.

But on the up side, government is starting to join this medical evolution. The National Research Council's 19-member panel recently concluded "that the American public could substantially reduce its risk of heart disease, can-cer, and many other chronic diseases through adoption of specific changes in eating habits. And it said, "this could be done by such simple measures as roughly doubling the per capita consumption of fruits and vegetables and starches." (Internal Medicine World Report, April 15-30, 1989). Of course they are far from recognizing the total picture, as you will learn, but it's a step in the right direction.

IV.   As we dawdle incorporating intelligent wellness medicine into the practicing twenty first century physician's
armamentarium, medical practice continues in the old way
(find a label, then a drug) and borders on serious negli-
gence, but survives under the outdated cry that there is not
enough evidence to warrant a change.   Meanwhile people are
given methotrexate for resistant asthma and systemic
steroids (prednisone) for eczema.   Children are given
Ritalin for hyperactivity and chemotherapy for rheumatoid
arthritis and colitis, when thousands of people have been,
and millions can be, cleared by environmental medicine techniques.   Dangerous drugs should be reserved for last ditch
efforts, after all possibilities have been ruled out.

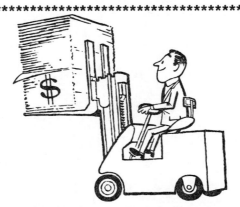

```
****************************************************************
*                                                          *
*                                                          *
*                                                          *
*                                                          *
*                                                          *
*                                                          *
*                                                          *
*                                                          *
*                                                          *
*                                                          *
*                                                          *
*                                                          *
*                                                          *
*                                                          *
*          It costs considerably less to find the cause   *
*      of arthritis, for example, than mask it with drugs  *
*      which can never give complete relief of pain and go *
*      on to damage the stomach, kidneys, eyes, and more.  *
*      Since there are over 30 million arthritis sufferers *
*      in the United States, can you imagine just the cost *
*      savings in drugs and the increased productivity     *
*      that that disease improvement alone would cause?    *
*                                                          *
****************************************************************
```

The bottom line is that the techniques of environmental medicine are logical, cost effective, and they work where all else fails. The time is ripe to put hi-tech medicine on the shelf when it comes to chronic problems and start incorporating intelligent (wellness-oriented) medicine into our armamentarium.

Chapter 5: IT $\underline{IS}$ ALL IN YOUR HEAD

Many of you undoubtedly are painfully aware that when medicine is stumped, in order to save face (and reinforce the unspoken message, "If I don't know what you have, then you probably don't have anything too important"), it frequently refers to psychiatry. Thousands of people yearly are told, "It's your nerves", "There's nothing wrong with you, so relax", or "It's all in your head".

Well, in this case, they are correct, but for the wrong reasons. For as you have already learned, many chemicals make a beeline to the brain. So that's one source of mental symptoms. Secondly, when the detoxication pathways become overloaded, aldehydes, chloral hydrate, and other metabolites produce direct brain symptoms to further baffle the physician who is untrained in environmental medicine.

Furthermore, as you now know, the body regularly makes many brain chemicals or neurotransmitters that mediate mood and memory (like serotonin, gamma aminobutyic acid, noradrenalin, acetylcholine, dopamine, histamine, adrenalin), and these must pass through the same biochemical bottlenecks as do many of the 20th century chemicals to get metabolized. Consequently, they may be dealt with too slowly or shuttle metabolites to new pathways that result in unexpected mood swings. You know, the metabolism of every chemical, once it is inside the body, influences the metabolism of all other chemicals, whether they are self-synthesized neurotransmitters, inhaled room chemicals, or ingested pesticides. And the major symptoms are exhaustion, depression, and inability to concentrate or think straight. Dizziness, spaciness, headache, body aches, and much more are just icing on the cake.

Lethal Legacy

As she reached out and touched the clear plastic covering on a magazine article I had written, her voice suddenly became hoarse, and it steadily worsened until she could barely speak. She then let go of the plastic, and her voice gradually returned to normal. This happened in just a few minutes' time.

Mary was demonstrating how sensitive she had become to ordinary chemicals. "I was normal until six years ago. I was at a new job at the bank and went on my coffee break. When I returned I began getting sick. I noticed my chair was wet, and I learned that the exterminator had just been through for his routine spraying of insecticide. Over the next hour I started feeling really sick. They told me to go home, that my symptoms would wear off. But each time I tried to return in the next few weeks, I felt so sick I couldn't stay."

"Gradually I started developing some of the same symptoms elsewhere, and becoming sensitive to some of the things that never before had bothered me. I had symptoms that baffled all my doctors until one finally diagnosed a possible pesticide poisoning. Meanwhile, my life is ruined. I can't touch any plastics, go in any stores, tolerate any medicines, and have to lead a very restricted life, in terms of my diet and environment. In order to control my symptoms, I have become a recluse."

And so the story goes for many victims of the unseen terror that can change your life as dramatically as any cancer: pesticide poisoning. You can see how the old way of viewing medicine would baffle any physician hearing Mary's symptoms. But with what you have already learned, you can see right through the problem and understand how it all came about.

Although pesticides are invisible, it would be extremely difficult for you to go through a day with no exposures to them. First of all, you awaken on them, for they are in all mattresses unless your doctor has written a prescription for a pesticide- and fire retardant-free cotton mattress. They outgas from other furnishings, carpets, paints, wall paper glues, adhesives, papers and boxes, cosmetics, toiletries, leathers and more. They can also be

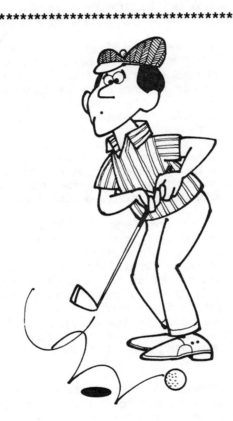

Pesticides in mattresses, offices, homes, and even on golf courses can effect brain function and coordination.

carried from thousands of miles away by way of airborne droplets from aerial spraying, as evidenced by measured levels in remote areas where the only access is by air (Insta-tape, appendix, lecture by Seba, D., at international symposium, Man and His World in Health and Disease, 1988).

They are deliberately added to the environment to kill some form of life, whether it be an insect, fungus, weed, algae, worm, barnacle, or rodent. There are over 1,500 pesticides and their nomenclature is conveniently an alphabet soup, so that even the smartest chemist would have to refer to several reference manuals to know what he is dealing with. And then no one is absolutely sure since many companies hide their contents under the cloak of "proprietary secret". As off-shoots from chemical warfare research, these derivatives of nerve gas and other enzyme inhibitors represent some of the most potent and simultaneously poorly reported chemicals on the face of the earth.

Even worse is the fact that the "inert ingredients" are often surreptitiously more potent than the ingredients listed, as they can often hide carcinogenic PCB's, EDB, dioxins, etc. in these "vehicles". For these are legitimate contaminants, and to refine the product to remove them would be foolhardy: (1) It would be too costly, (2) you'd have to figure out a way to dispose of the toxic leftovers, (3) it would reduce the power of the original product, giving its competitors the edge, and (4) the more contaminated the vehicle (the less refined), the cheaper it is as well as more toxic.

Although there have been many horror stories about isolated incidents of pesticide poisoning, the average physician does not have the training, nor the tests available, to diagnose this as the basis for the many chronic symptoms that it produces. Also many times, even when the inciting pesticide is known, it could not be retrospectively proven since often they are "hit and run" toxins. In other words, they can damage detoxication enzymes, or T suppresser cells, or hormone receptors, for example, and then be metabolized or biotransformed, so that no trace of their existence can be found. This doesn't bother the pesticide manufacturers, as many are also big name pharmaceutical companies that manufacture the leading prescription medications as well. So they are bound to get more of your business eventually. To further insure their share of the market place, they also have begun to corner the market on hybrid seeds, thus controlling the genetics of agriculture (and pesticide dependence) world-wide (Kulkarmi, AP, Hodgson, E, Metabolism of insecticides by mixed function oxidase systems, Pharmac. Ther., 8, 379-475, 1978; also Cassarett and Doull's Toxicology, chap. 18, Toxic effects of Pesticides, 519-581).

Thiram is a common carbamate fungicide. It has 26 trade names, very few of which would ever give you a clue as to what they represent. Take a look: Arasan, Thiramad, Thirasan, Thylate, Tirampa, Pomarsol forte, TMTDS, Thiotex, Fernasan, Nomersan, Tersan, Thiuramin, Tuads, AAtack, Aurels, CHIPCO Thiram 75, Fermide 850, Trametan, Hexathir, Mercuram, Polyram Ultra, Spotrete, Tripomol, Tersan 75, Tetrapom, Thioknock (ref. 3). You'd swear I had made some typing errors! Now multiply this by the 1,500 pesticides (Occupational Medicine, Zenz, C, chap. 46, Occupational health aspects of pesticides).

And let's look at how thiram works. It is the methyl analogue of disulfuram (Antabuse). This prescription drug is given to people who want to give up alcohol. Because its main action is to inhibit aldehyde dehydrogenase, it makes the person violently ill with horrendous vomiting if he slips off the wagon and takes a drink. Remember, the aldehyde path was one of the biochemical bottlenecks of the detox system. So aside from the regular pesticide symptoms of dermatitis, vomiting, diarrhea, psychotic reactions, exhaustion, trouble concentrating, peripheral neuropathy, dizziness, headache, and flu like achiness, this pesticide has an extra booster. Because the aldehyde detoxication pathway is one of the bottlenecks which is involved in manifesting sensitivity symptoms to multiple foods, molds, neurotransmitters and chemicals, this pesticide can mimic, potentiate, and/or create a chemically sensitive individual, or one with environmental illness, commonly known as E.I.

This explains why after an exposure some people will develop an avalanche of chemical sensitivities.

Thiram is a common fungicide which means it has no limits for its uses, since fungi are ubiquitous.

Another common type of fungicide is called phenyl-mercuric salts. These are extremely toxic compounds and have even produced symptoms resembling amyotrophic lateral sclerosis (Lou Gehrig's disease). Mercury (one of its components) is a known binder of sulfhydryl (sulfur, necessary for detoxication), groups and inhibits the enzyme aldehyde reductase, as well as glutathione, PAPS, and cysteine (all sulfur containing Phase II conjugators and the third bio-chemical bottleneck for detoxication). (Cassarett and Doull's Toxicology, chap. 19, Toxic effects of metals). This explains why so many people never had E.I. until after a specific root canal or dental amalgam filling. The mer-cury can bind these detox enzymes and conjugates, thus com-promising the person's future ability to handle chemicals. Then as further "normal" chemical exposures occur, the path-ways become backlogged. These backlogged chemicals begin to damage remaining parts of the detox system. And you guessed it: the sick get sicker. And any symptom is possible at this point. It just depends on where the weakest areas of the body are. So again, mercury exposure too can mimic and/or cause E.I.

Often people date the onset of their chemical sensi-tivity to after dental work where mercury fillings were used. Mercury is particularly toxic to the detox system (Are Your Mercury Fillings Poisoning You?, Stortebecker, M.D., Ph.D., see appendix).

Environmental illness, or E.I., can be manifested as just about any chronic symptom you can think of. The poorer the outlook and the less effective any attempts at diagnosis and treatment have been, the more likely it is that the symptoms are actually environmentally induced, meaning a cause and treatment are available.

Now let's say you decide to have a nice healthful lunch; you choose a salad of lettuce, tomatoes, carrots and onions, some french fries, and apple juice. Following are just the commonest pesticide residues found routinely in these foods (reference 3):

Foods	Pesticides*
lettuce	mevinphos endosulfan permethrin dimethoate methomyl
tomatoes	methamidophos chlorpyrifos chlorothalonil permethrin dimethoate
carrots	DDT trifluralin parathion diazinon dieldrin
onions	DCPA DDT ethion diazinon malathion
potatoes	DDT chloropropham dieldrin aldicarb chlordan

apples

diphenylamine
captan
endosulfan
phosmet
azinphos-methyl

*Again, remember each one of these has many other names that look and sound completely different but represent the same chemical.

Now this represents one supposedly "healthful" meal, and does not include pesticides which accumulate in even higher amounts in fats (salad oil and meat). Nor does it include any of the fungicides used on grains (bread).

Several points come to light readily as the uninitiated scans this list. First, several items are listed in more than one food (endosulfan, dimethoate, DDT, diazinon, dieldrin). So how does anyone compute whether you have exceeded your daily limit, when the limits are only imposed for singular items? To compound the problem, in setting up arbitrary limits for how much of a particular pesticide you can have on a certain food, someone who doesn't even know you guesses how much of a particular quantity you consume over a year. The average American eats eight pounds of carrots a year, but I eat 10-20 pounds a month, depending on whether I juice any as well. So you can see how fallacious this determination is.

Second, you will notice items like DDT that have been theoretically banned. We see measurable levels for three reasons: (1) Much produce originates in countries where we unload our banned pesticides, (2) pesticides like DDT and chlordane persist for decades in the soils where plants are grown, as they are not easily biodegraded (Cassarett and Doull's Toxicology), (3) there is always a market for illegal chemicals.

D.C. is a 38 year old man, who in his twenties, was a member of an eight man team of young men, all under 25, who were hired as pilots for aerial spraying of vegetables for a major food producer. He is the only one who hasn't yet died of cancer. He has suffered a barrage of symptoms that nearly disabled him in the last few years. He is improving for the first time on a program to reconstitute his health (You Are What You Ate, Prestige Publishing, PO Box 3161, Syracuse, NY 13220).

R.B. was a 42 year old surgeon, who monthly had his house pesticided. He began having what he thought was the flu, however it never left. A year, and many consultations later, he realized he had chronic indolent pesticide poisoning which now had damaged his immune and detoxication systems to the point where he reacted with symptoms when exposed to a variety of common indoor chemicals and commonly ingested foods that never before bothered him. His life was dramatically changed as he was no longer able to tolerate his home, the operating room suites, restaurants, nor many offices, hotels, and stores without suffering muscle aches, weakness, headache, dizziness, nausea, chest pain, fatigue and inability to concentrate (the diagnosis and treatment for this is covered in the 650 page book on environmental illness, The E.I. Syndrome, Prestige Publishing, PO Box 3161, Syracuse, NY 13220).

Certainly we have altered our ecology so severely that we could probably not stop all pesticide use tomorrow. But we can learn to use then more judiciously. For example, in many areas state office buildings, schools, groceries, restaurants, motels and even apartment buildings are pesticided on a contract basis. In other words, no one comes in to check to see if spraying is really needed, it is just done. For one, this is begging for the emergence of resistant strains, so that more potent pesticides will be required in the future.

To lower your family's exposure as much as possible check on the policies for your local school, church and office. Do not spray in your home or yard. Grow as much organic food of your own as you can, and scrub and peel those that you buy that are not organic. Try to avoid foods from countries that accept our cast off illegal pesticides, and eat more in season with your own local and gardening

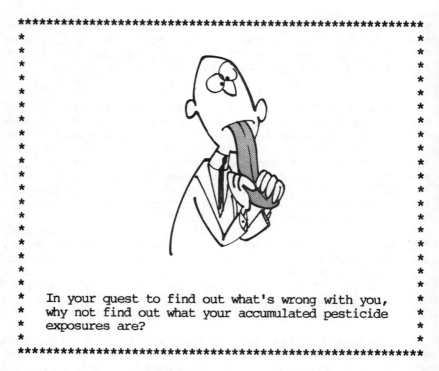

```
****************************************************************
*                                                              *
*                                                              *
*                                                              *
*                                                              *
*                                                              *
*                                                              *
*                                                              *
*                                                              *
*                                                              *
*                                                              *
*                                                              *
*                                                              *
*                                                              *
*                                                              *
*                                                              *
*                                                              *
*    In your quest to find out what's wrong with you,          *
*    why not find out what your accumulated pesticide          *
*    exposures are?                                            *
*                                                              *
****************************************************************
```

produce. For example, carrots, onions and squashes from
your garden will store well in a root cellar or cool area
and are more appropriate to the New England resident in mid-
winter than pesticided bananas, tomatoes and watermelon from
Central America.

In the meantime, our injudicious use of pesticides is
creating a lethal legacy in many respects. From dependence
on pesticides and creation of resistant strains, to persistence in the environment and damage to the 20th century
immune and detoxication systems. For as these systems are
already saddled with an unprecedented level of chemicals in
the air, food, and water, ubiquitous pesticides have particularly unique abilities to poison the vital enzymes and
pathways which determine how soon our biological time bombs
will go off. And when they do, they are capable of unleash-

ing the multitude of diagnosis defying symptoms collectively referred to as E.I. Or worse yet, pesticides are capable of uncorking the genetically linked time bomb to initiate cancer.

Most people have several pesticide residues in their bodies, including DDT. And studies abound showing the various nervous system damages, cancer initiation, infertility, and immune system defects that can arise from them.

So we have been left a lethal legacy from the purveyors of pesticides. We have picked up the ball and have carried it to lengths that could never have been dreamed of. Twenty years after Rachel Carson's warnings (<u>Silent Spring</u>), we continue to poison the earth and it's people. Combined with our current day 60,000 environmental chemicals, we are now creating new diseases with undiagnosable symptoms, many of which many result in cancer. The invisible and poisonous pillager is within the control of each person and the amount of pesticide he decides to use today is also passed on biologically, as well as environmentally, to his progeny. The type of legacy we decide to leave is up to us.

References

1. Wier, D, Shapiro, M, <u>Circle of Poison</u>, Institute for Food and Development Policy, 1885 Mission St., San Francisco, CA 94103, (1981).

2. Morgan, DP, <u>Recognition and Management of Pesticide Poisonings</u>, 3rd ed., EPA, Superintendent of Documents, United States Government Printing Office, Washington, DC, 20402 (1982).

3. Mott, L, Snyder, K, <u>Pesticide Alert: A Guide To Pesticides In Fruits and Vegetables</u>, Sierra Club Books, San Francisco (1987).

4. Klaasen, CD, Amdur, MO, Doull, J, <u>Casarett and Doull's Toxicology, The Basic Science of</u>

122

Poisons, 3rd ed., Macmillan, New York (1986).

5. Rogers, SA, The E.I. Syndrome, Prestige Publishers, Box 3161, 3502 Brewerton Rd., Syracuse, NY 13220 (1986).

6. Rogers, SA, You Are What You Ate, ibid (1987).

7. Ecobichon, DJ, Pesticides and Neurological Diseases, CRC Press, Boca Raton, FL (1982).

Do You Have The Pesticide Plague?

Agriculture boasts that bold new herbicides are on the way. In many studies of the commonest side effects of pesticides, forgetfulness and fatigue, have been way ahead of all the other symptoms (Metcalf and Holmes, Annals of New York Academy of Science, volume 160).

Pesticide poisoning can be one of the most insidious diseases. Chlorpyrifos (Dursban) is commonly sprayed in offices, schools, homes, apartment houses, churches, businesses and restaurants in the U.S. Studies show that in office occupants there was a wide range of individual susceptibility. In some the symptoms were abrupt, while in others they were gradual, slowly built up so that rarely did the victim relate cause and event. Exhaustion, poor memory, inability to concentrate predominated in some, while poor balance and loss of coordination occurred in others. These are two symptoms that are expected with age and not easily measured, proven or tested. Therefore they tend to be discounted.

Other studies confirm (Organophosphate poisoning in office workers, J. Occup. Med., 28, 1986, Hodgson et al) that once inside the body, these chemicals get stored in tissues that slowly release small amounts of the pesticide back into the blood stream over months! So a one-time exposure can give a dose that persists and causes continual baffling symptoms while the level in the blood is too small to be measured by regular medical tests. Meanwhile the level in the office air has dissipated, so there is no proof!

In addition, you can easily appreciate how this constant infusion of a potently toxic chemical can increase your vulnerability to all other chemicals. It's like standing on one leg; you are much easier to push over.

Some people have delayed symptoms (Neuro-toxic effects of organophosphorus insecticides, N. Engl. J. Med., 316, Senanayake, N., 1987) that don't appear for weeks after the exposure like vague numbness and tingling. With each subsequent exposure or dose, the person gradually deteriorates while medicine remains baffled. All the while, any new chemical or drug, even a simple aspirin or pain pill can become the final straw that pushes the detox system over, and suddenly we have a full-bloom case of E.I., reacting to everything (Interaction between acetaminophen and organophosphates in mice, Res. Comm. in Chem. Pathol. and Pharm., 44, 1984, Costa, L.).

In 1985 when Drs. Randolph, Rea, and I were lecturing through China, I took a photograph of a government worker pesticiding the trees along the side of the road. He was standing on the top of his truck with his hose aimed at the top of the trees. Unfortunately, just a few feet on the other side the tree tops were open apartment windows. The apartments hug the tree lined streets very closely in China. So some of this pesticide was being sprayed directly into the open unscreened apartment windows. But this invasion of one's health is minuscule when we compare it to what we have done in the United States to our citizens.

As scary as this scene appeared, what we do is even more ludicrous, in terms of pesticides and needless exposures to them. Businessmen who fly frequently on international flights are exposed to pesticides, as well as the air line staff themselves, as they run up and down the isles squirting a pesticide that is hardly going to make one bit of difference to an insect hiding inside a passenger's clothing or bags. The whole plane would have to be fumigated to the point that everyone would have tearing eyes and paroxysmal coughing to make this effective. But this amount of pesticide, especially repeatedly, adds to the total load or total body burden of other pesticides that people are exposed to nearly constantly in many different environments (homes, offices, stores, institutions, food, water, construction materials, clothing, books, plastics, and more), which have caused serious disease. Don't forget these bioaccumulate. That means the body just stores and stores these. And some it never gets completely rid of. So when you hear someone say, "Oh don't worry it's such a tiny amount it couldn't hurt you", you know they are utterly obtuse to the chemistry of pesticides. For example, one spraying of chlordane for control of termites lasts for 20 years in the soil. Its metabolism in the body is highly individual and some just can't get rid of it. And it's the lifelong accumulation of these "tiny" amounts that has caused undiagnosable depression, exhaustion, anxiety, poor balance, loss of nerve function, and death. Or have gone on to initiate E.I. with all of these symptoms and more as the person began reacting to molds, foods, and other chemicals.

Since the commonest pesticide poisoning symptoms are subtle, most people do not even know that they have been exposed. They consist of confusion, fatigue, poor concentration, poor memory, irritability, poor libido (sex drive), and slow thought process (Feldman, American Journal of Industrial Medicine, 1980). If you complained of these to a doctor untrained in environmental medicine, you're more likely to be handed a tranquilizer, after an exam.

A commonly sprayed pesticide like diazinon is used routinely in apartment buildings, schools and offices. Its residues and inhibition in lab animals were highest in the kidney and brain (Tomokuni, K, et al, The tissue distribution of diazinon and the inhibition of blood cholinesterase activities in rats and mice receiving a single intraperitoneal dose of diazinon, Toxicity, 37, 1-2, 91-98, Oct., 1985). Again it depends on the individual whether he will have long range, short range, or no effect. Bear in mind it is usually accompanied by another pesticide as well as the "inert" solvent vehicle. The cumulative and synergistic effects are unknown, and pose a dual problem: (1) many pesticides cannot be completely metabolized and excreted by the body, so they accumulate in the body with each exposure, and (2) the action of two different pesticides when combined together can be more damaging to the body than the sum of the two given individually. This is possible, for example, when one inhibits the metabolism of the other and causes a build-up (or biochemical bottleneck for other chemicals).

The "inert" ingredients, which are the vehicle or carrier, contain even worse chemicals than the pesticide itself. This is the liquid in the bottle which the potent poison is riding in. The poison is so potent, that only a small volume can be used. In order to disseminate it widely throughout a room, for example, it is put in a larger volume of "inert" diluent so it can be sprayed about. For many of these, less than a teaspoon of the undiluted pesticide can be lethal to a 200 lb. man. The label makes this diluent appear harmless when it reads "99% inert ingredients". But diluents or "inert ingredients" are far from being truly inert, as they frequently contain acetone to methyl cyanide, benzene, toluene, phenol, kerosene, xylene, dioxin, formaldehyde, ethylene dibromide, trichloroethylene, chloroform, carbon tetrachloride, methyl methacrylate, and much more. Yes, you have learned that these are some of the very same chemicals that outgas from our modern homes and offices that cause E.I. Only now they are linked with even more toxic chemicals (the pesticides), often causing cumulative and irreversible nervous system damage (Cassarett and Doull's Toxicology). Frequently even outlawed pesticides are hiding in these inert ingredients, and add power to the punch. Plus if they are classified as inert, they become part of the proprietary trade secret. So it is to the manufacture's benefit to have as contaminated a product as possible when it comes to "inert" carriers or solvents.

****
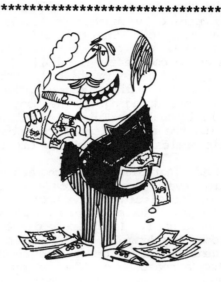

Anyone who tries to convince you that pesticides
are harmless is either uninformed or has an
ulterior motive from which he will reap the
rewards.
****

You'll recall that common solvent symptoms (not only
from regular hydrocarbon inerts, but from the home and
office) are also poor memory and inability to concentrate,
confusion, paresthesias (numbness and tingling), dizziness,
hyperacusis (average noises seem uncomfortably loud),
nervousness, depression, compulsion, irritability, apathy,
weakness, tremor, ataxia (poor equilibrium or balance), and
exhaustion. Panic disorders are also caused by these
solvents (Dager, SR, et al, Panic disorder precipitated by
exposure to organic solvents in the work place, Am. J.
Psychiatry, 144:8, 1056-1058, Aug., 1987). So not only can
everyday chemicals make you an exhausted space cadet, but so
can the pesticides, and so can their "inert carriers"! It's
a wonder that anyone can think and emote with all their

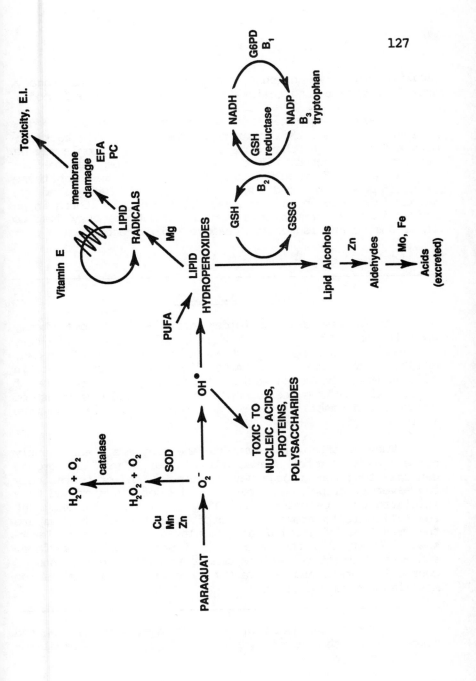

faculties (and we haven't even talked about the sugary breakfast cereals and their effect on brain power and mood).

Finally, if the person has a dysfunctional detoxication system, this results in these chemicals backlogging and causing further damage, whereas other people may be seemingly unaffected. This resultant and often severe illness is nearly impossible to diagnose, since many of these pesticides are "hit and run". They do their damage and are metabolized into an unrecognizable form, or are stored in an unidentifiable form in some tissue. Sometimes they just do their damage and leave (get changed and excreted).

QUICK STOP SUMMARY

So in essence, pesticides are like a triple whammy when it comes to the damage they can do. Ironically they frequently cannot be smelled as other chemicals often can, and they are usually commercially sprayed at night in offices with the housekeeping chores so you are unaware of their existence. Most people have multiple sources of exposure and generally the more public a place is, the more it is sprayed.

They do often bioaccumulate and many are predominantly nerve toxins, but of course all of your glands and organs can only function through nervous input. And of course they can severely cripple many parts of the detox system and have initiated many persons' E.I. They are often "hit and run" and difficult to prove, and worst of all some of them are the most poorly studied and regulated toxic chemicals we know. After all, they are derived from chemical warfare, and most at least potentiate cancer if not cause it. And of course the brain and the rest of the nervous system is the most favored target organ.

Everyone has heard of Agent Orange, Love Canal, and Times Beach: the culprit was dioxin {2,3,7,8 - tetrachlorodibenzo-p-dioxin, or TCDD}. It is reported to be one of the deadliest substances produced by man. Even the lowest measurable levels produced cancers in laboratory test animals. Yet municipal incinerators produce it when they burn plastics of polyvinyl chloride (just the garbage and leaf bags themselves are enough of a world burden, not to mention their contents and other plastics like saran and styrofoams that we discard daily.

Dioxin is also a contaminant in the wood preservative pentachlorophenol (PCP) and is spewed into the air by the U.S.'s 104 paper mills as a result of the bleaching process. Nearly all white papers contain some dioxin; these include baby diapers, coffee filters and cups, paper plates, food packages like milk cartons, toilet paper, and paper towels. There are many scientific papers showing that benzene is a potent cause of some leukemias. Well TCDD is a double benzene ring structure. This makes it more than doubly difficult for the body to get rid of and so it is stored in fat of the membranes of cells which function like the computer keyboard of the body (Greenpeace, vol. 14, #2, Mar/Apr 1989, 1436 U St. NW, Washington, DC 20009).

But as long as the average consumer stays unaware and unconcerned, these and hundreds of other practices will continue. Isn't it silly that we need bleached white paper products when the natural tan and off-white shades would suffice just as well? We seem to consistently put cosmetic appeal ahead of health.

For example, pesticides silently damaged a young nurse's kidney tubules. She slowly lost magnesium (the kidneys could not absorb 95% of it as they should), and she developed multiple severe chemical sensitivities with depression, pains, seizures and other debilitating symptoms. All were uncontrolled by hospitalization and drugs as she got progressively worse. Her improvement came when it was discovered that she needed daily intravenous magnesium to keep up with the renal loss (Rea, pers. comm.).

Another factor that should be appreciated is that, suppose a person has a certain level of chemical in his

blood stream after a day at work. He goes home and clears
out if the house is clean enough. When he returns to work
the next day, he gets another dose, and then goes home

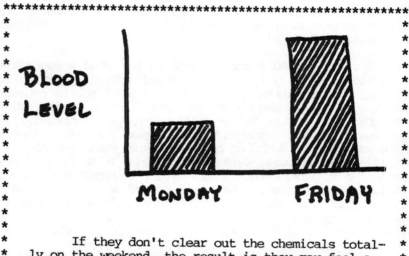

If they don't clear out the chemicals totally on the weekend, the result is they may feel a
little better on weekends but get progressively
sicker with time. Some don't feel sick until the
over all accumulation reaches a critical level
months or even years down the road.

and clears out. But what if he doesn't clear out totally at
home? What if at home he has new carpeting, fresh paint,
gas heat, a new mattress and furnishings that outgas the
myriad of xenobiotics that you are now aware of? By Friday
his level may be much higher than it was on Monday. Hopefully he can clear out by getting some exercise outdoors
over the weekend. But if he doesn't, his levels are going
to go higher and higher every week, until he finally has
some terrific end organ failure. It may take months or
years. Meanwhile all the physicals, blood tests and x-rays

are negative if he consults a physician untrained in environmental medicine.

Or imagine this scenario. Someone goes to work and has a specific blood level of xenobiotic; by noon the liver starts attempting to detoxify it and gets overwhelmed, and some of the chemical gets stored in the fat. He goes home at night and soon the blood stream is fairly empty of the chemical, so it starts coming out of the fat and back into the blood stream so that it can be further metabolized and excreted in the urine or the bile. The problem is that every time it is in the blood stream, that's when the worst symptoms occur. So these people are having symptoms when they load up in the office, and then when they get home again they are having them when they unload. This makes the determination of where they are getting sensitized very difficult to ascertain if symptoms are experienced in both places.

You can see that pesticides can produce symptoms that can run the gamut of barely noticeable and chalked up to aging, to devastating flu-like achiness accompanied by scores of other symptoms. But because medicine cannot keep up with the pace of technology, these indolent poisonings get ascribed to such things as "a virus", or "Yuppie fatigue", when in essence it's THE PESTICIDE PLAGUE.

The metabolism of pesticides, although not fully worked out, is very complex, and calls into play many of our precious nutrients. A 1981 Science (vol 212) publication showed that there was sequential decrease in mortality as vitamins essential to the detox pathways were plugged in. First they reduced the percent mortality with vitamin B3 {niacin, which goes on to form NADP}, then even more with B1 {thiamine, which helps G6PD form NADP and recycle glutathione for reuse}.

Since we are all exposed to unseen pesticides from multiple sources on a daily basis, it is really ludicrous for anyone to suggest that Americans do not need vitamins.

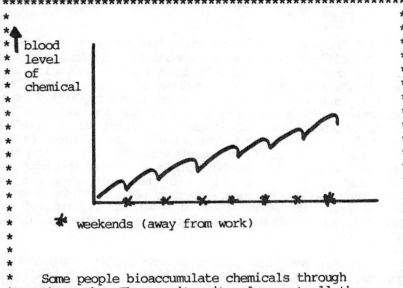

blood
level
of
chemical

✳ weekends (away from work)

Some people bioaccumulate chemicals through
the week. They can't quite clear out all the
chemicals in one day that they have accumulated

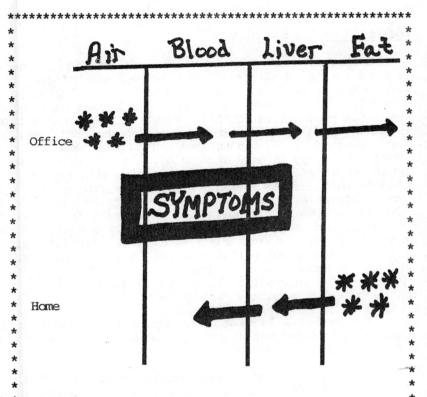

Symptoms are at their peak when the chemical is in the blood.

Understanding The Big Picture

Collating and interpreting scientific research involves reading hundreds of publications and bringing them down to a practical level of "so what?" Once I give you a minuscule idea of how it works, you'll see how easily scientific progress is stifled. First it is extremely time-consuming to gather the papers, even more to read them, and then they need to be interpreted. But interpretation of a paper's relevance is only as meaningful as the experience of the interpreter. If he is not a clinician with thousands of patients with bizarre symptoms, then much goes by the way-side, unappreciated for its relevance. The problem is, the clinician's time is already spoken for, being busy treating patients. But she in reality is the only one who has the knowledge of all aspects that enable the scientific jargon to be interpreted and pulled together in a meaningful way so that it can explain what is observed on a daily basis in the clinic. This leaves her doing double duty: clinician by day, scientific researcher/writer by night.

For example, look at four papers on organophosphate pesticides I pulled out at random from a recent pile of over 100 on my desk:

(1)   Interaction between acetaminophen and organo-phosphates in mice (Costa, LG, et al, Research Communications in Clinical Pathology and Pharmacology, 44 (3) p 389-400, June 1984).

(2)   Neurotoxic effects of organophosphorous insecti-cides (Senanayake, et al, New England Journal of Medicine, p 761-763, 316, March 26, 1987).

(3)   Toxicity of organophosphorous esters to laying hens after oral and dermal administration (Francis, et al, Journal of Environmental Science and Health, 20 (1), p 73-95, February 1985).

(4)   Organophosphate poisoning in office workers
       (Hodgson, et al, _Journal of Occupational_
       Medicine, 28 (6), p 434-437, June 1986).

(1)   Shows that, as we suspected, extra drugs in one's body
       compete in the detox path and interfere with the
       detoxication of pesticides. The drug was
       acetominophen (Tylenol).

(2)+(3) Show that symptoms from pesticide poisoning can be
       delayed for 2-3 weeks, and can be as severe as
       neuromuscular weakness, ataxia (poor coordination and
       balance), paralysis or death. When symptoms take
       weeks to occur and most people are not aware anyway of
       when their office or apartment is sprayed, pesticide
       poisoning would not be considered.

(4)   Shows us that the recovery curve is not a constant
       rate, but an exponential curve. That means there is a
       leveling off so that the rate of getting better
       diminishes with time; there is some permanent residual
       defect. And if re-exposure keeps occurring there is a
       slow and dangerous accumulation.

This exponential curve suggests redistribution of the
pesticide to a body compartment (fat storage) where it is
slowly released over time back into the system to get
detoxed and eliminated.

So how do we apply this information to a practical
scenario that we see daily?

Take a secretary at the bank who takes Tylenol for
headaches. Now suppose her apartment house manager, unknown
to her, sprays the organophosphate Dursban (chlorpyrifos) in
her apartment hallway during the day once a month to control
roaches. The same is done at the bank once a month in the
evening. She is unaware of either event. She doesn't detox
as well as everyone else because she has a double dose and

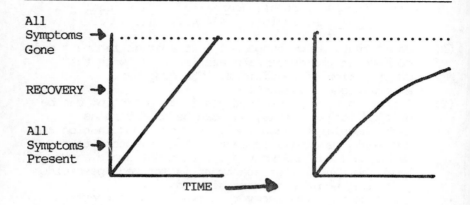

This is not how recovery from pesticide poisoning occurs.

This exponential curve is how recovery really proceeds, never to reach 100%.

takes drugs (birth control pills, which lower B2 necessary to regenerate glutathione, and maybe has some sinus and headache pills) that compete with detox enzymes. The result is she is slowly accumulating progressively higher doses of pesticide all the time, because her detox system total load is too high.

Since all of this happens in small doses that accumulate over months and years, she is not aware that anything is wrong: until she tries to learn to water ski one summer. She learns that she is very uncoordinated and can't balance well. She doesn't think much of it and eventually gives up trying to get any exercise and besides she is always tired. (A good test of whether your balance is going is to stand on one leg and then close your eyes. You should be able to keep standing for at least ten seconds. Try it and see. you might be in for a surprise. Please have protection around you in case you fall.)

With accumulating levels of pesticide, she slowly becomes more weak, more clumsy, tired, depressed, develops poorer memory: all the symptoms of insidious pesticide poisoning. These pesticides require extra metabolic energy as well, so she develops a few nutrient deficiencies. Since she feels so lousy, she eats more goodies to try to make herself happier and gets further depleted. It becomes a vicious circle of eating foods that deplete nutrients and as nutrients are depleted less of the accumulating pesticide can be detoxed. As more accumulates, she feels worse, is able to do less and eats more junk food in attempt to find happiness.

As physical exams are normal, the doctor just thinks she is an overweight, under exercised boring person with some deep seated hang-ups. Tranquilizers might be prescribed.

What she really needs is a thorough environmental history. She has to find out what sprays are used in her environment. And every symptom she has, regardless of how seemingly inconsequential, should be elicited, for they are all clues. They suggest to us whether other competing influences are at work, such as hidden mold allergies causing the headaches she's taking the Tylenol for. She needs vitamin and mineral blood levels and an assessment of her detox capabilities. For she can't detox if her machinery isn't in good working order. Last, she needs a detox program.

Now you can begin to appreciate how long it will be before this type of medicine becomes the standard of care. Few physicians have the personal interest, time, energy and health themselves to carry it off.

This chemical sensitivity affects every aspect of our lives. For example, an air plane cockpit has trichloroethylene from the dry cleaned clothes (capable of being metabolized to chloral hydrate which causes brain fog), styrene from the plastics (produces impaired concentration and diminution of manual dexterity) and jet fuel (poor nerve conduction velocity, anxiety, mental depression, and reduction in reaction time). (Grasso, P, Neurotoxic and neuro-behavioral effects of organic solvents in the nervous system, Occupat. Med. 3:3, 525-539, Sept. 1988). Now this doesn't include the dozens of other chemicals and pesticides in there, nor take into account the pilot's home environment, nutritional status, nor diet.

Dizziness is a complaint that frustrates many physicians. The victims describe it in a variety of ways from the feeling that they have to hang on to the walls and furniture to walk, a feeling they are going to fall over, a feeling of unreality or spaciness, to overt severe vertigo with nausea and spinning rooms. Often when these people elude diagnosis, a tranquilizer is prescribed.

One indicator of dysfunction of the vestibulo-oculomotor (balance system, which is intimately connected with vision) system is nystagmus. To test someone, have them follow your finger about 10 inches from their face, move it from one side of the face to the other, 10 inches past the ear and hold it. If the eye jerks or bounces back and forth this is nystagmus. It can be a sign of magnesium deficiency, or other problems. But it can also be a sign of chemical toxicity (often from plastics and glues) in the vestibular system. When it is, it clears once you have helped that person heal (Tham, R, et al, Electronystagmographic findings in rats exposed to styrene and toluene, Act. Otolaryngol., 93, 107-112, 1982; Odkuist, LM, On the mechanism of vestibular disturbances caused by industrial solvents, Adv. Oto-Rhino-Laryng., 25, 167-172, 1979; Odkuist, LM, et al, Vestibulo-Oculomotor disturbances in humans exposed to styrene, Acta. Otolaryngol., 94, 987- 993, 1982).

Since 1945, some 15,000 individual compounds and more than 35,000 different formulations have come into use as pesticides (Davis, JE, Changing profile of pesticide poisoning, N. End. J. Med., 316:13, 807-808, Mar. 26, 1987). How many of those do you think have been adequately tested, much less tested for synergistic (additive) effect with one another and the other chemicals and prescription medications we are exposed to?

Common, everyday pesticides have caused schizophrenic and depressive reactions, severe memory impairment and difficulty in concentration (Gershow, S, Psychiatric sequelae of chronic exposure to organophosphorous insecticides, Lancet, 1371-1374, June 24, 1961). Next time you blame this on life's stresses, bad genetics, or age, you'd better think twice (provided you're still able to). These pesticides that you breath and eat every day of your life have far-reaching and often unsuspected effects.

Multiple other studies confirm that the central nervous system takes the brunt of this insidious poisoning, documenting again poor concentration, slowed though process and computation, failing memory, difficulty speaking, depression, anxiety, and irritability (Levin, HS, et al, Behavioral effects of organophosphate pesticides in man, Clin. Toxicol., 9:3, 391-405, 1976). But if the physician is unaware of this or lazy, it's quicker to write you an Rx for a tranquilizer and pat you on the shoulder, reminding you that you're not getting any younger. He probably has the same problem. I know I did!

Sometimes these effects of nerve damage are irreversible or permanent (Petty, CS, Organic phosphate insecticide poisoning, Am. J. Med., 24, 467-470, 1958). And don't forget the class of organophosphates is the safest and least dangerous of the pesticide classes. I'm telling you what the weak ones do.

So how are you going to detoxify yourself and restore your personality, mood and memory to normal? First you have to be sure your detox chemistry is in healthy shape.

In the meantime, don't let anyone tell you it's all in your head!

Depollution Enzymes: How To Test Your Detox System

How can your doctor determine if you have an overloaded or dysfunctional detoxication system? He can check the enzymes that are working to clean up chemical pollution in the body and stave off resultant disease.

Signs of xenobiotic detoxication exhaustion, or exhaustion of the detox pathway, are decreased levels of glutathione peroxidase, elevated blood level of lipid peroxides, depressed super oxide dismutase, increased mercapturic acid and/or D-glucaric acid, and an elevated formic acid.

Unfortunately, these tests are not found in all labs, but can be found by the persistent physician at these labs:
1. Monroe Labs, Southfields, NY.
2. Doctor's Data, Chicago, IL.
3. National Medical Services, Willow Grove, PA.

You already know why the glutathione peroxidase would be low. It is necessary to quench dangerous (free radical) peroxides (generated from chemicals) before they eat holes in precious membranes. Glutathione peroxidase is a selenium-requiring enzyme. If this is low, it is a good sign that the detox pathways are over stressed, as it is being depleted. Knowledge of this is just starting to creep into the allergy literature, but the majority have not put it to practical use (Bibi, H, et al, Erythocyte glutathione peroxidase activity in asthmatic children, Ann. Allerg., 61, 331-340, Nov. 1988).

A urinary metabolite of glutathione conjugation is mercapturic acid (Tate, SS, Enzymes of mercapturic acid formation, Enzymatic Basis of Detoxication, Vol. II, Jakoby, WB, ed., chap. 5, 95-120, Academic Press, NY, 1980). The majority of organophosphate pesticides and many other chemicals pass through this route. After preliminary Phase I steps, a molecule of glutathione (GSH) attaches to the pesticide or chemical. Then acetyl CoA attaches. (This is composed of cysteine and pantothenic acid and GSH contains a molecule of cysteine so you can see why it's such an important antioxidant detox amino acid). The GSH is lost with the xenobiotic as it gets carried into the urine where it can be measured.

Mercapturic acid is a better overall measure than D-glucaric acid, since the majority of pollutants tend to go this route, and D-glucaric acid is unaffected by benzene and toluene, commonly encountered xenobiotics.

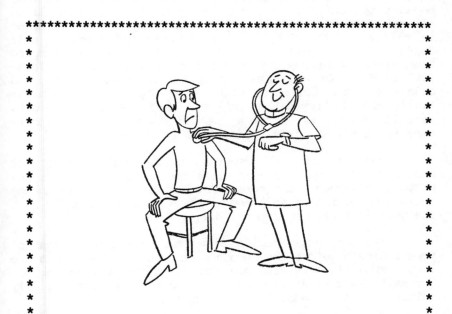

If a doctor insists there's nothing wrong with you because your blood tests and x-rays are negative, he is most likely untrained in environmental medicine. When in doubt, ask him to name one of five tests that could show whether your detoxica- tion system is functioning (depollution panel).

Excess lipid peroxides are a sign that the lipid mem- branes of cells are being destroyed by backlogged chemicals. Chemicals and free radicals (crazy naked destructive elec- trons resulting from the body's attempt to get rid of foreign chemicals) are actually eating destructive holes in them like battery acid on a silk dress. As membranes are destroyed, levels of peroxidized (burned up, destroyed) lipids (important structural fats in cell membranes) become raised. So elevated lipid peroxides are another good indication of a detox system approaching serious exhaustion, because not only is it not able to handle, or metabolize, all the chemicals presented to it, but they are eating holes in the cells, thereby creating sickness and eventual cell death. The sickness can manifest as literally any symptom from vague exhaustion to over twenty symptoms as is classical in E.I. Or with more unifocal destruction, we see end organ failure. In other words, one organ gets preferentially more destroyed than others. If the organ is the gut, we call it colitis; if it's the kidney, we call it nephritis; if it's the joints, we call it arthritis.

Damage to the cell membrane is extremely serious for herein resides the receptor sites for hormones, neurotransmitters, allergens, and more. Also if it's defective, chemicals can penetrate and damage areas inside the cell like the genetics (causing cancer, E.I.).

Likewise, super oxide dismutase attempts to control free radicals before they produce damage. If the levels are low, you're in deep trouble for they are inadequate for "normal" day to day exposures, making the body particularly vulnerable to any additional exposures.

D-glucaric acid, if it is elevated, also means that the hepatic (liver) pathway for detox is accelerated due to overload of chemicals (Hunter J, et al, Urinary D-glucaric acid excretion as a test for hepatic enzyme induction in man, Lancet, 1 (699) 572-575, Mar. 20, 1971). If it is lower than normal, however, it indicates that (depending on the levels) the cytochrome P450 detox system is overworked or ready to shutdown because it has become seriously exhausted. (It does not get stimulated by benzene or toluene exposures, however).

Suffice it to say, the excess lipids resulting from unbridled destruction of membranes, must also be metabolized. If they get hung up in the aldehyde path, more chloral hydrate and aldehyde backlog symptoms can result, not to mention a myriad of other cerebral symptoms.

Finally, no average physician could ever diagnose whether a person's symptoms are all in their head. If he has ruled out that free radical pathology, abnormal biochemistry, nutrient deficiencies, and environmental sensitivities are not operant, then he can justifiably begin to consider it. But to diagnose it just because one has failed to take an adequate dietary and environmental history and is ignorant of environmental triggers and detoxication biochemistry is indicative of a lack of education in this field.

```
**************************************
*                                    *
*     Depollution Panel              *
*     Glutathione peroxidase         *
*     Lipid peroxides                *
*     Superoxide dismutase           *
*     D-glucaric acid                *
*     Formic acid                    *
*     Mercapturic acid               *
*                                    *
**************************************
```

However, none of these tests are absolute proof of detox overload, but rather indicators, just as current liver enzymes do not tell us that you definitely have hepatitis or gall bladder obstruction. They are indicators that must be taken into account with the entire clinical picture. These enzymes likewise tell us the detox paths are being stressed. But they don't differentiate if it's from a poor diet, too much smoking, cumulative pesticide damage or other xenobiotic overload. They are more sensitive than current liver tests, however, and they help us see that we're headed for trouble early on in the course, not when it's too late.

Until the time that your doctor can gear up to get these tests, there is a simple (but simple is never fool proof) test of your detox function that can be done in any medical office. Have him draw a formic acid level. If it is normal or below, it just suggests you are handling your aldehydes fairly well. It does not say anything about your other detox pathways.

If on the other hand it is elevated, you're like an accident waiting to happen. It says you have a back log of formic acid (a metabolite of formaldehyde) and therefore are not handling your everyday exposures as well as possible. So it is backing up and bathing the rest of your system, including the detox enzymes in a toxic material. It puts excess burden on the body and gradually weakens the detox system. Then when some seemingly innocuous event occurs (they paint at the office, you buy a new carpet at home, you visit a pesticided hotel), you're the only one who falls apart and has symptoms, because you were ripe all along for a catastrophe. (By the way, if you smoke this raises levels greatly, as does having abnormal amounts of intestinal flora or microbes).

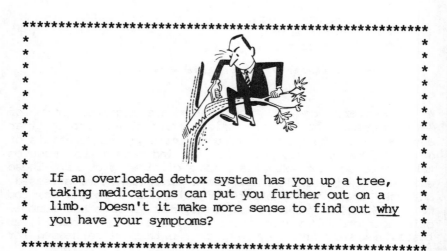

```
**********************************************************
*                                                        *
*                                                        *
*                                                        *
*                                                        *
*                                                        *
*                                                        *
*                                                        *
*                                                        *
*                                                        *
*                                                        *
*    If an overloaded detox system has you up a tree,    *
*    taking medications can put you further out on a     *
*    limb.  Doesn't it make more sense to find out why   *
*    you have your symptoms?                             *
*                                                        *
**********************************************************
```

These five tests make a "depollution panel" that enables a physician to begin to check how a person is handling his ambient environment. As more physicians become aware of the need for this, they will put pressure on commercial laboratories to make these more readily available. Right now your biggest problem will be to locate a physician who knows what they are for and how to use them.

Many people have a home environment that is even worse than work. On the flip side of that, many people have a home environment, that once they learn how to make it relatively pollution free, unloads their detox pathways so well, that they are now able to tolerate the environment at work. We have witnessed this over and over again. Likewise, there are some people who are so overloaded by the ambient air of their community, that they will never clear until they move 30-50 miles out of the vicinity. Then they are suddenly able to tolerate many more chemicals, and eventually heal and become symptom free. The pollution panel won't tell you which environment the chemicals emanate from. It only tells you whether the detoxication system is in trouble. If being out of the suspected environment for a few weeks corrects these values, that gives you a good clue. But before and after work and home blood levels will tell you what chemicals you pick up from each environment, while the provocation-neutralization test will help tell you what symptom a particular xenobiotic or foreign chemical may be causing.

Having figured all this out with your specialist in environmental medicine, you are on your way to reducing those blood levels of chemicals. Further on, you'll learn how to minimize the total load through diet and environmental controls. Once you don't present your overtaxed detox system with so much burden, it can start to use those corrective nutrients to heal itself as opposed to seeing them as an additional part of the total burden and reacting adversely to them, as well.

Because chemicals can derange brain function and cause psychiatric symptoms, once again they become a double edged sword. For bad emotions do bad things to the body and even create disease. People with high anger can cause the output

146

```
*************************************************************
*                                                           *
*    The Air In Your City                                   *
*           May Prevent You From Testing Accurately         *
*                                                           *
*    Case Example:  One engineer came from his home town    *
*    (out of state) for single blind testing to chem-       *
*    icals to prove sensitivity for disability.  When       *
*    we tested normal saline in the first four tests        *
*    over the first hour, he reacted to every one of        *
*    them.  There is no way we could prove anything         *
*    for him because he was in such an overloaded           *
*    state (a constant state of reaction).  We              *
*    suggested he get more unloaded, so he stayed           *
*    with friends in the country over night.  The next      *
*    day he beamed that he had just had the most rest-      *
*    ful sleep that he had had in three years since his     *
*    symptoms began.  We proceeded to test him and the      *
*    placebos were negative.  But chemicals could turn      *
*    him on and duplicate his symptoms.  Then the neu-      *
*    tralizing dose (still single blind) turned him off     *
*    just as quickly.                                       *
*                                                           *
*         The moral of the story is that before we          *
*    label anyone as a malingerer, or tell them it's        *
*    all in their heads, the total load should be           *
*    reduced sufficiently to make testing possible.         *
*                                                           *
*************************************************************
```

of more norepinephrine which in turn can cause high blood
pressure (Dinsdale, JE, Anger and blood pressure, Drug
Therapy, 105-109, June, 1989). In fact, I have never seen a
chemically sensitive person heal who has not first gotten
rid of hidden anger.

In the same vein, painful emotional stress can induce
lipid peroxidation resulting in inactivation of Na, K-ATPase
in the heart (Meerson, FZ, et al, The role of lipid peroxidation in inhibiting cardiac Na, K-ATPase during stress,
Biull. Eksp. Biol. Med., 96:12, 42-44, Dec. 1983). This
translates into the fact that emotions can impair the

heart's (or brain"s) sodium pump and create damage and disease. Look at the healthy people who suddenly died shortly after their spouse of decades died. In another study they actually found that strong emotional pain led to the accumulation of lipid peroxides in the brain and even the formation of anti-brain antibodies (Prilipko, LL, et al, Activation of lipid peroxidation: a mechanism triggering autoimmune response, <u>Acta. Physiol. Pharmacol. Bulg.</u>, 9:4, 14-50, 1983).

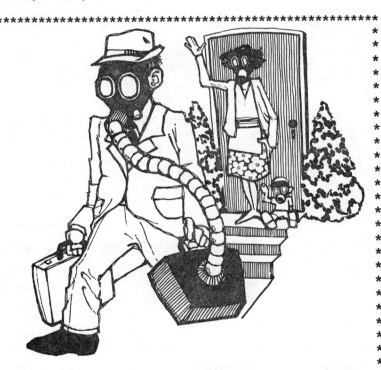

If you can't feel well at home, you'll never give your body enough rest to detox what you've inhaled at work. Top priority: make your home as safe as possible.

And on the flip side, nutrients like vitamins can change our intelligence (Denton, D, Roberts, G, Effect of vitamin and mineral supplementation on intelligence of a sample of school children, The Lancet, 140-143, Jan 23, 1988). Likewise, amino acids which are the precursors to brain hormones or neurotransmitters can influence our moods.

Sleep, mood and appetite have been known for years to be under the control of brain neurons and their neurotransmitters that are influenced by precursor amino acids. In other words, the availability of specific types of building blocks of proteins determines in part how much of a brain hormone is available (Wurtman, RJ, Nutrients that modify brain function, Scientific American, 246:4 50-60, Apr. 1982).

For example, tyrosine is necessary to form dopamine, norepinephrine, and epinephrine (adrenalin, the "fight or flight" hormone). Serotonin, a mood hormone, (and vitamin B3 for detox) depends on tryptophan, while choline availability influences the amount of acetyl choline, which in turn affects the firing rate of neurons (memory).

Amino Acid	Forms Neurotransmitter	Sample Association
tyrosine	dopamine norepinephrine epinephrine	Parkinsonism hypertension depression anxiety energy
tryptophan	serotonin B3, NADPH	depression, mood pivotal in detox
choline	acetylcholine	memory Alzheimer's

It becomes clear that the brain should never be considered a separate entity as it has been in medicine. It has powerful effects on the rest of the body, and likewise the body, the nutritional status and the environment have powerful effects on the brain. So if you're tired, dopey, dizzy, confused, or depressed, plagued by inability to concentrate, poor memory and embarrassing mood swings, read on, MacDuff. There is hope.

Chapter 6:   ARE YOU PLAYING WITH A FULL DECK?

If this chapter is too technical for some readers, breeze through it anyway. You will be amazed at how much you assimilate and every little bit of knowledge further strengthens your understanding of how to get and remain healthy. Anyway, be sure to read about vitamin L at the end.

Having been around for decades, E.I., or environmental illness, is nothing new. It is just that we needed to have a new term so that you can remember that we are no longer stuck in the era of highly specific names or diagnoses for constellations of symptoms. For it doesn't matter if a person who hurts is labeled rheumatoid, lupus, degenerative, osteo, or traumatic arthritis. We have found the causes in many people who bore any of these labels. And they all had different triggers, dependent upon the individuality of the person, not the disease name. The mere fact that there is a label that can be applied means symptoms have been ignored and/or suppressed so long that there is identifiable end organ damage. The body has struggled to rid itself of toxic matter and failed miserably.

Environmental illness is clearly now the product of three factors. First, we are the first generation of man exposed to such an unprecedented number of chemicals. Second, we are the first generation of man to tighten build-ings and thereby amplify the effect of these many chemicals. Third, we're the first generation to consume such a nutri-tionally inferior diet, and to do so progressively. This produces an overload in a system that may not already be functioning optimally. For reasons of overload or nutri-tional deficit or both, we have in many people a maladapta-tion of the detoxication system; a system that we really never looked at before because we had no need to. We didn't even know it existed. But, to practice medicine today (including allergy), without a knowledge of the biochemistry of the detoxication system, is to practice medicine without all of the necessary tools.

```
****************************************************
*                                                  *
*    ENVIRONMENTAL ILLNESS (E.I.)=                  *
*                                                  *
*    (1) The first generation of man exposed to     *
*        such an unprecedented number of chemicals. *
*                                                  *
*    (2) The first generation of man to extensively *
*        tighten his buildings to accentuate the    *
*        effect of these chemicals.                 *
*                                                  *
*    (3) The first generation of man to eat such a  *
*        nutritionally inferior diet.               *
*   +   _____ *
*    The result is a dysfunctional or maladapted    *
*    detoxication system, (overloaded and ailing)   *
*    capable of producing any symptom and breaking  *
*    all the current rules of medicine.             *
*                                                  *
****************************************************
```

Biochemical Bottlenecks That Lead To The Downward Spiral

R.A. is a 52 year old female who had worked 15 years in the same factory. For 11 years she had excruciating headaches that were getting worse, and she was chronically fatigued. For the last four years she had had many workups and had seen neurologists and had had two CAT scans. An ENT allergist gave her injections for four years; they were of no help. Then a conventional allergist tested her and told her that she was not allergic. Her family doctor told her she needed a psychiatrist.

We tested her, single blind, in the office to some chemicals. She knew that the headaches were excruciatingly worse at work, although she was never clear of them even out of work. We could turn her on and off with xylene and tri-chloroethylene, by the provocation technique, (we published this in the NIH Journal, Environmental Health Perspectives, volume 76, also appears in The E.I. Syndrome, and has been done in horses to provoke and relieve heaves (asthma), Clinical Ecology, Rogers, SA, 5:4, 185-187, 1988/1989).

We then looked at the chemical levels in her blood after a day at work. Her level of tetrachloroethylene (TCE) was 26.9 ppm (parts per million); normal is 1.1 ppm in the current day population; of course, normal should really be zero, but in this era normal is called 1.1 ppm, because there are very few "normal" or unpoisoned people left. After two weeks at home, her level was 18 ppm. So we had her go home and stay there for 8 months to see if her detoxication system could heal. It couldn't. She couldn't tolerate any stores, and she was miserable at home and could not do her house work, because she felt so ill.

We looked at several nutrients and found that the only one that was significantly low was the rbc zinc at 870 (normal is 880-1600 ng/dl). So we corrected it and in one month she was totally clear; all the headaches were gone, and the TCE level had dropped to 1.3 ppm. Her detoxication enzymes were finally able to kick in and work. She could tolerate stores, she could do her house work, she was happy, she was healthy and full of energy.

But here is a lady who could have been committed to a life at home with miserable daily symptoms just because nobody understood the needs of the detoxication pathway. Her doctor and friends would continue saying, "Poor gal, she hasn't been well for years and there's nothing that can be done for here. No medicines help her, and if we send her back to work she gets even worse. She'll just have to learn to live with this for the rest of her life". When medications make one worse, it seems logical that someone would have thought of an overlooked and nutritionally deficient detox system; but don't forget it's not taught in medical schools.

So it is clear that our patients are not playing with a full deck; a full nutritional deck, that is. They don't have a full complement of nutrients; most likely overwork of the detox system has helped to deplete these, as well as the nutrient depleted standard American diet (appropriately abbreviated SAD).

There are many biochemical bottlenecks in the detox pathway. You learned a very stylized, very over simplified view of how many xenobiotics, or foreign chemicals, are detoxified. They can be metabolized into an alcohol stage, and then alcohol dehydrogenase becomes one of the key enzymes. Then the metabolism proceeds into an aldehyde (so that aldehyde oxidase or aldehyde dehydrogenase becomes a key enzyme), and then into an acid and excreted.

In Phase II, foreign chemicals or xenobiotics are usually conjugated with something like cysteine, PAPS, glucuronic acid, or glutathione. Lack of minerals like magnesium and the amino acid cysteine in these pathways will also severely compromise the system and cause a biochemical bottleneck.

Magnesium Deficiency Can Cause Sudden Unexplainable Death

Magnesium is one mineral that is in just about every single phase of the detox pathway. In fact, magnesium is in over 300 enzymes and metabolic pathways. It is the most under-recognized electrolyte disorder in the U.S. One magnesium authority suspects 80% of the population is deficient (Science News, vol. 133, June 1988). It is responsible for the resistance of many therapies, like hypokalemia, (uncorrectable low potassium, as from using diuretics, "fluid pills", heart and blood pressure pills), uncorrectable vitamin D3 deficiencies (as with osteoporosis and osteomalacia), or resistant iron deficiencies. I suspect it accounts for much of the sudden death in athletes. Several joggers and other athletes who were very healthy and had no coronary arteriosclerosis, suddenly dropped dead. When one sweats, much magnesium is lost. But if the cardiologist or family doctor doesn't check it and replace it (protocol for physicians in Appendix), a mystifying death results from cardiac arrhythmia (irregular heart beat that becomes so chaotic that it becomes fatal as insufficient blood is pumped to the rest of the body).

The average American consumes less only 40% of the RDA (recommended daily allowance) of magnesium, a recent United States government survey has shown (<u>Science News</u>, volume 133, June 4, 1988). This causes no overt symptoms, but can not be considered benign when over 300 enzymes depend on it. In laboratory animals, for example, merely supplementing magnesium has cleared salt induced hypertension, chemically induced pulmonary hypertension, and high cholesterol induced hyperlipidemia. Dr. Mildred Seelig, one of the country's leading authorities on magnesium (along with Dr. William J. Rea), suggests that 80%-90% of the population is notably magnesium deficient. This is truly an epidemic in disguise in its own right, since this deficiency can cause nearly any symptom one can think of (see Chapter 7).

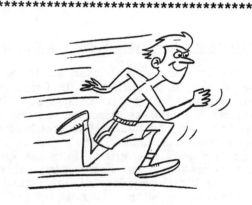

****
Jogging is one way to commit the perfect crime if you don't know your magnesium status. For sweating causes excessive loss of magnesium and sets the runner up for developing a fatal cardiac arrhythmia. Please do the magnesium loading test, for your sake.
****

How We Become Deficient In Magnesium

There are many factors that contribute to the lowering of magnesium and other minerals in the diet:

1. Poor soils, which become depleted as we feed much of the world. You know that a tomato from your garden doesn't taste the same as one from the grocery store because they don't have the same minerals in them. Commercial growers fertilize with the minerals that make the tomato look plump and red, but not necessarily the minerals for good taste or good nutrition. Studies now demonstrate what we know through taste: Commercially grown produce often has less than 75% of the nutrients that organically grown produce has. With organic produce, man-made chemical formulations are not relied upon to restore what was taken from the soil. Instead mother nature makes the formula, since real manures and compost materials are used. There are many trace minerals, some of whose roles in plant physiology are not yet understood. Mother nature always has the wisdom to include them, but man hasn't yet reached her level of biochemical sophistication.

2. Acid rain will leach out minerals from the soil just as water softeners remove them from our drinking water.

3. Cooking, destroys some vitamins and removes minerals that are lost to the water.

4. High fat diets.

5. Aging depletes nutrients.

6. Chronic exposure to chemicals (which we are all getting more of).

7. Chronic diseases deplete nutrients.

8. High phosphates in soda or soft drinks; as well as in other processed foods, compete for absorption of minerals.

9. Medications (diuretics, digitalis, etc.) use up or deplete nutrients.

10. Competitive inhibition from many other minerals by not balancing them. For example, you may read about zinc and decide to take some, but in an unbalanced form, you will eventually create an iron or molybdenum or copper deficiency. Too high a dose of vitamin C will inhibit the uptake of many minerals, and high levels of calcium (commonly prescribed in an unbalanced form by gynecologists and family doctors) can actually cause a magnesium deficiency.

```
***************************************************************
*                                                             *
*                                                             *
*                                                             *
*                                                             *
*                                                             *
*                                                             *
*                                                             *
*                                                             *
*                                                             *
*                                                             *
*                                                             *
*                                                             *
*                                                             *
*                                                             *
*                                                             *
*                                                             *
*                                                             *
*                                                             *
*   Every time you have a food that has low nutrient          *
*   density (very low vitamin/mineral to caloric              *
*   ratio), you fall further behind in nutrient debt.         *
*                                                             *
***************************************************************
```

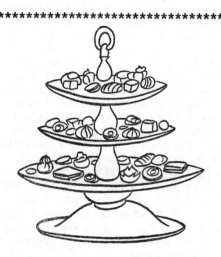

How To Diagnose Magnesium Deficiency

So how do we diagnose magnesium deficiency? It is difficult. Blood tests like the rbc or red blood cell magnesium and the plasma magnesium are practically useless because if they are positive that is wonderful; but they miss about 80% of the people who are magnesium deficient. Dr. Jon Pangborn, Ph.D. suggests that if specific amino acids are low in a 24 hour urine amino acid analysis, that you can be pretty sure that you have a magnesium deficiency. This is probably a better criteria, but the best one is published in volume IV, issue 4 of Clinical Ecology, 1986 (Rea, W.J., Magnesium Deficiency and Chemical Sensitivity). Dr. Rea presented cases that had symptoms suggestive of magnesium deficiency, but whose rbc (red blood cell) magnesiums were normal. He then gave them an intravenous (injected into the blood stream) challenge of magnesium and their symptoms cleared. This showed that they were indeed magnesium deficient, and that the blood test was useless. Before and after urine tests for magnesium also further proved that they were deficient.

One of the commonest symptoms of magnesium deficient patients are back and neck pain. In fact, at one time I had chronic back pain with insufferable spasm for months. I foolishly blamed it on old horseback and lifting injuries of 20 years earlier because I had x-ray evidence of a destroyed disc, collapsed vertebral bodies (back bones) and arthritic spurs. But when Dr. Rea suggested I give myself an I.V. trial of magnesium, the constant pain of months miraculously melted away. Once more this shows us that regardless of what blood tests and x-rays demonstrate, there is usually a correctable abnormality in the here and now. We just need to be smart enough to find it.

The other common symptoms, besides chronic pain, relieved by the magnesium challenge test in this study were fine tremors, muscle spasms, anxiety, panic disorder, and nervousness, Raynaud's spastic vessels (cold white fingers), arrhythmia (irregular heart beat), and of course, you guessed it: fatigue.

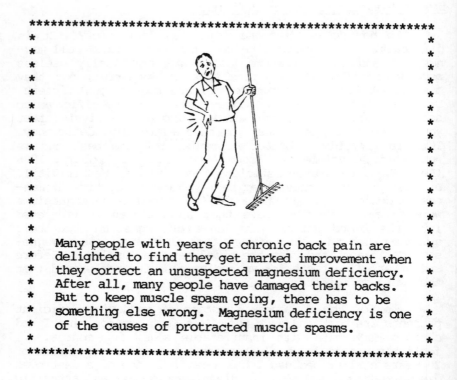

```
*************************************************************
*                                                           *
*                                                           *
*                                                           *
*                                                           *
*                                                           *
*                                                           *
*                                                           *
*                                                           *
*                                                           *
*                                                           *
*                                                           *
*                                                           *
*                                                           *
*                                                           *
*                                                           *
*      Many people with years of chronic back pain are     *
*      delighted to find they get marked improvement when   *
*      they correct an unsuspected magnesium deficiency.    *
*      After all, many people have damaged their backs.     *
*      But to keep muscle spasm going, there has to be      *
*      something else wrong.  Magnesium deficiency is one   *
*      of the causes of protracted muscle spasms.           *
*                                                           *
*************************************************************
```

Any neurotic symptoms can result from a magnesium deficiency since not only the synthesis but the breakdown of brain chemicals or hormones is critically dependent upon it. The toxic brain syndrome symptoms (spacey, dizzy, dopey, confused, depressed for no reason, can't think straight, irritable, depressed, abnormally aggressive, and more) can be duplicated by a magnesium deficiency just as easily as by a chemical exposure.

```
**********************************************************
*                                                        *
*                                                        *
*                                                        *
*                                                        *
*                                                        *
*                                                        *
*                                                        *
*                                                        *
*                                                        *
*                                                        *
*                                                        *
*                                                        *
*                                                        *
*                                                        *
*   Top Drawer treatment of any cardiac arrhythmia or    *
*   chronic muscle spasm should include assessment of    *
*   magnesium status.  Since several scientific papers   *
*   demonstrate that blood tests are worthless in        *
*   ruling out a deficiency, a magnesium loading test    *
*   followed by a therapeutic trial is recommended.      *
*                                                        *
**********************************************************
```

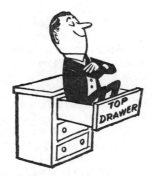

Magnesium deficiency also causes mast cells to release much more histamine. This is the stuff responsible for much hayfever misery. So the more deficient one is, the worse the allergies. Obviously correcting a solitary magnesium defect can often greatly improve one's allergies.

So a trial of magnesium is indicated for any spastic condition. Remember, in order for a muscle to contract, it needs calcium. In order to relax it needs magnesium. Many people have spastic conditions which smack of magnesium deficiency, like asthma, migraine, colitis, angina, chronic back pain, muscle spasm, arrhythmia, vasculitis, hypertension, cystitis, eye twitches, tremors, seizures, Raynaud's, infertility and nystagmus. But vertigo, psychosis, confusion, depression, eclampsia, diabetes, phlebitis, exhaustion, TIA's (small strokes), refractoriness to potassium therapy and insulin can also be due to magnesium deficiency.

The bottom line on magnesium is, the physician should think about it in everybody. Because chances are he is going to be right. Then an oral or injectable magnesium loading test will provide the proof (see Appendix for magnesium loading test). Studies now show that the blood tests are not sensitive enough to diagnose magnesium deficiency with certainty. Only a therapeutic trial can do that. For if the blood test is abnormal that's wonderful information. But if it's "normal", it does not mean the other unmeasured storage sites of magnesium are, for the magnesium in the blood serum accounts for only 1% of the body total. We must remember the blood test is only measuring one area where magnesium "hangs out" {homeostasis}. And only before and after urine tests (see Appendix) will show you when you have finally saturated all the pools or storage sites.

But each nutrient has an optimal dose for each person, and on either side of this optimal dose is a dose that becomes progressively more harmful. Furthermore, each nutrient must be in balance with all the others.

Manganese Deficiency Can Cause The Senile Brain

Manganese is important because sometimes you will do an I.V. magnesium challenge and the patient won't improve because he is deficient in manganese. You'll know this when giving manganese suddenly makes the magnesium click in and work. Of course, manganese is also important in SOD (super oxide dismutase) which is a protein in the mitochondria (where energy to run the detox pathway is synthesized). The function of SOD here is to keep the energy-producing machinery free of free radicals (those dangerous naked electrons that run rampant through the body trying to accelerate degeneration or aging and create destruction and disease).

Manganese is necessary for the function of glutathione synthetase, an enzyme needed for the body to make the predominant Phase II detox conjugator, glutathione.

Also it's in the brain enzyme glutamine synthetase (which accounts for 80% of the manganese in the brain). This enzyme is needed to make glutamine which is needed for conversion to the neurotransmitters glutamate and gamma amino butyric acid (GABA). It's the GABA receptor in the brain where many tranquilizers like Valium fit in; hence the calming effect sometimes observed when people correct a manganese deficiency (Prohaska, JR, Functions of trace elements in brain metabolism, Physiolog. Rev., 67:3, 858-901, July 1987). Likewise, chronic manganese toxicity can lead to neurological signs similar to Parkinson's disease. So as always, measurement of levels, balancing nutrients, and monitoring of effectiveness of a program are tantamount.

Manganese is also important in adrenal function (and we're certainly a stressed society, stress being one of our major environmental pollutants). The adrenal gland produces our stress response hormones like adrenalin (epinephrine). And one of the more important enzymes requiring manganese for its action is choline acetyl transferase. It forms acetylcholine which triggers the firing rate of nerves: it's like the spark plug of the nervous system. With a deficiency of manganese, researchers find the same pathology they find in Alzheimer's disease {senile plaques, neurofibrillary tangles (the nerve cells actually become tangled up with one another), and progressive deterioration of dendritic processes (the long exteriors of nerve cells)}. Clearly a manganese deficiency is one of the potential causes of pre-senile brain function loss in some individuals. And because a deficiency and resultant senility occur so slowly over years, it's important to know your manganese status now.

Formaldehyde Is Just Like The Tip Of The Aldehyde Iceberg

Aldehydes, as you have seen, represent a second block or a biochemical bottleneck in the detox pathway. Many xenobiotics, or foreign chemicals, break down into an aldehyde stage. Alcohols are degraded into aldehydes (acetaldehyde); the yeast, Candida, that grows in vaginas and intestines makes acetaldehyde; vinyl chloride (saran wrap type plastics), formaldehyde, industrial and auto exhausts, and much more, all go through an aldehyde breakdown stage. Aldehydes are extremely toxic to the body; they are free-radical initiators that cause cross linking (accelerate aging), they are mutagens (they cause permanent changes in the genetics; this creates new diseases), carcinogens (start the process of cancer), and they are highly toxic to the systems of the body, including detoxication.

```
*********************************************************
*                                                       *
*                                                       *
*                                                       *
*                                                       *
*                                                       *
*                                                       *
*                                                       *
*                                                       *
*                                                       *
*                                                       *
*                                                       *
*       Are you tearing your hair our because you're neu-  *
*       rotic, magnesium deficient, or toxic?  Let's find  *
*       out.  Remember everything has a cause.  One of the *
*       commonest findings when someone corrects a magne-  *
*       sium deficiency is they can't get over how relaxed *
*       they feel; for after all, magnesium is nature's    *
*       tranquilizer.                                      *
*                                                       *
*********************************************************
```

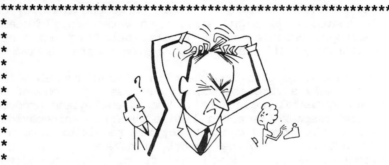

To give you an idea, acetaldehyde itself can explain the whole spreading phenomenon of chemical sensitivity. You know those people who just seem to get worse and worse constantly? They become more and more sensitive to more chemicals, but in smaller doses. If their aldehyde pathway is bottlenecked, they get a build-up of aldehydes; let's just look at some of the things this does:

1.   Aldehydes cause the release of vasoactive substances (make blood vessels contract or dilate), like catecholamines. Examples of catecholamines

are epinephrine and norepinephrine which can
cause nervousness, panic, fear, and edginess
(many of the same symptoms a magnesium
deficiency can mimic). How many chemically
sensitive people are on tranquilizers because
they are so nervous? Is it from aldehydes?
2. Aldehydes cause flushing (red hot face or body).
3. Tachycardia (fast heart beat).
4. Chilling (inappropriate coldness of hands and
feet when everyone else is warm).
5. Paresthesias (numbness and tingling).

These aldehyde symptoms are the exact symptoms that
many highly chemically sensitive patients get when exposed
to certain chemicals. And chemical overload (like formaldehyde from traffic exhaust or a new carpet or couch) can add
to the overload or build up of aldehydes. When odorless
everyday chemicals overload the aldehyde pathway, it can no
longer function; suddenly you have a patient who complains
of flushing, numbness and tingling, and spaciness. But
people unknowledgeable about the biochemistry of detoxication will perceive them as neurotic.

6. Aldehydes also condense with catechols (brain
hormones or neurotransmitters like adrenalin and
serotonin) and form tetrahydro-isoquinolines;
these are false neurotransmitters that are
thought by some researchers to be the cause of
addiction. And we certainly know about
addiction in our patients. Many are unknowingly
addicted to the very foods and chemicals that
make them so sick.
7. Aldehydes also form adducts (stable chemical
bonds that can produce damage) with liver
membranes and proteins thereby causing abnormal
function of cells and enzymes.
8. They activate the complement sequence (stir-up
the immune system and start it acting on itself)
explaining the inflammatory symptoms like
arthritis and colitis, etc. that we see in our
patients.
9. Aldehydes also injure mitochondria (this is

where energy is produced inside the cell and
nearly all of our patients have low energy).
10. Decrease the redox ability (and nearly all of
our chemically sensitive patients are aging
faster and/or exhibiting progressively more
trouble dealing with chemicals). Redox is short
for reduction and oxidation, which are
simultaneous chemical reactions that aim to
balance our chemistry so we don't get cancer, or
age overnight, for example.

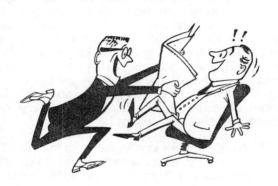

I don't expect you to be overjoyed with this
chapter. I know it may be over your head now,
but you'll see the relevance for at least a
familiarity with these terms which will enable you
to understand the big picture later on. In the
future you are going to be hearing many of these
terms as medicine evolves, so I want you to be
familiar enough with them so that you'll have an
idea that they are involved in detoxication. Then
when you encounter these terms again, you'll know
you have a place that you can refer back to in
order to learn more about them.

11. Aldehydes also bind with glutathione (GSH)
     (remember that was the third biochemical
     bottleneck), one of the Phase II conjugators
     that helps to pull chemicals out into the bile
     so the body can get rid of them.
12. Aldehydes can also bind with cysteine (another
     very important conjugator by itself), so that it
     is not available for synthesis of glutathione,
     PAPS, or for N-acetyl cysteine conjugates. For
     when the body lacks sufficient GSH and cysteine,
     the result is more peroxidation (destruction of
     membranes through oxidation or actually burning
     electrons off the delicate cell membranes,
     leaving dysfunctional holes). The consequence
     is that this initiates a domino effect of
     orphaned electrons that buzz around aimlessly
     destroying more membranes, with consequent
     further production of aldehydes. Hence, another
     route for the sick to get sicker: the never
     ending, every worsening downward spiral. You
     will find that that is a recurring theme in the
     mechanism of how chemical hypersensitivity and
     all disease works, and that it explains what we
     see in our patients. They keep getting more
     symptoms until the process is arrested.
13. Aldehydes have other effects, like decreasing
     the storage of B6 which is necessary for zinc
     absorption, as well as neurotransmitter (brain
     function hormones) synthesis.

So here is just one tiny pathway, an overloaded aldehyde pathway, that can explain the full toxic brain syndrome. Suddenly all the symptoms that we see in our
patients, such as being spacey, dopey, dizzy, unable to concentrate, can't think straight, depressed for no reason,
exhausted, and the numbness and tingling that no one can
explain are not only understandable, but treatable.

Aldehydes accumulated from the bottleneck create free
radicals that punch holes in cell membrane, creating disease

in whichever organ is most vulnerable. This sets off a cascade of destruction.

Now you can see why the sick get sicker. As parts of the detox system are overwhelmed and damaged by 20th century chemicals, the xenobiotics float around unmetabolized and cause further damage. If this were not enough, undiscovered nutrient deficiencies cause a further downward spiral as they further compromise the detox system. As it gets sicker, more and more parts of it are damaged. The only way out of this downward spiral is to find a doctor who is very knowledgeable in environmental medicine.

In addition, just that one little bottleneck in the aldehyde pathway can explain the heightened sensitivity and the spreading phenomenon that we see in people who just get progressively worse and worse. Nothing you do seems to make them better. Because they have a constant supply of aldehydes from Candida in their intestines (from years of antibiotics and sweets), they have a constant supply of aldehydes from the xenobiotics in their food, water, and from the plastics that abound in their homes, from their metabolism of excess stress (like epinephrine) and depression (like serotonin) hormones, and from the polyaromatic hydrocarbons in the office, and even their prescription drugs. All of these things must be degraded or metabolized through the same aldehyde pathway.

But once this is understood, it is clear why when one goes on the diet in chapter 8, often they become less chemically sensitive. Or when one detoxes his physical environment as we will describe, he becomes more tolerant to foods. They are related because they funnel through the same bottleneck.

Now we can explain in biochemical terms why they also get increasing symptoms from smaller and smaller amounts of the same chemicals that prior had no effect. Everything in their 20th century lifestyle adds to the total load. Aldehydes can bind with cysteine and glutathione and tie them up so that other xenobiotics cannot use those proteins for Phase II conjugation. When chemicals cannot be degraded, they can be metabolized into chloral hydrate in the brain. Chloral hydrate you remember is the old "Mickey Finn" or ""knockout drops". And that is exactly how these people act; spacey, dopey, dizzy, and can't concentrate. When the pathway gets overloaded, one option for the body is to make this chemical in the brain. And so you get the bizarre fluctuating cerebral symptoms as they pass in and out of this phase.

You now know three powerful mechanisms that can make a person appear neurotic when they are actually dangerously ill:
1. Overloaded aldehyde pathways, from chemical exposures and Candida.
2. Secondary synthesis of chloral hydrate (from overloaded detox pathways).
3. Magnesium deficiency.

The Mineral Maze

Molybdenum (pronounced: mol lib' den um) is a key mineral in the enzyme aldehyde oxidase. Where do people get molybdenum? They don't! Peasant foods like beans, are generally not in vogue, and those are the types of foods that are high in molybdenum. Rbc or wbc (red blood cell or white blood cell) molybdenum is the best measure of its adequacy. The 3 laboratories below offer this test:
1. Doctors' Data, Chicago, IL
2. Monroe Laboratories, Southfields, NY
3. National Medical Services, Willow Grove, PA

Remember the common chemical, trichloroethylene? It is usually in everybody's blood stream on a daily basis because of dry cleaned suits and upholstery, and dry cleaned carpets. This chemical takes the first pass through the alcohol dehydrogenase enzyme (a zinc dependent one), and then becomes an aldehyde, which is highly toxic, as you saw. Now if there isn't enough molybdenum for the aldehyde enzyme {aldehyde oxidase}, then it cannot be degraded. What happens is, as the pathway becomes blocked, it switches now to making the old foe, chloral hydrate. Chloral hydrate has the added ability to actually inhibit aldehyde dehydrogenase (another aldehyde enzyme), and so, yet another example of how the sick get sicker.

You might say, "Well that's easy. I'll just take magnesium and molybdenum and I'll be in great shape." But there are a host of problems with this. For example, take zinc. It is on a delicate teeter totter or balance with many other minerals such as copper, molybdenum and iron. So, if for example, you take too much zinc, you may knock the bottom out from under the copper in a couple of months. Then you'll have copper deficiency symptoms.

What enzymes are dependent on copper? The polyphenol oxidases are, in fact most oxidases in the body are copper enzymes. Without this enzyme, you have a malfunctioning of the detoxication system again, as the body is unable to metabolize phenols (common in household cleaning products, for example, and in conventional allergy injections; see The E.I. Syndrome).

Monoamine oxidase in the old biochemical literature was shown to be a copper-dependent enzyme in some animals. It found its way into some current biochemistry books as such, but in men it is not copper dependent, but instead vitamin B2 {FAD} dependent. Vitamin B2 is shown throughout the literature to be often low, for example, with use of birth control pills. Monoamine oxidase is why when a thought makes you laugh, you don't continue laughing for the rest of your life. The neurotransmitter gets metabolized. Likewise you don't stay nervous or depressed unless the enzymes are not around to metabolize your neurotransmitters. But with a B2 deficiency, it's apparent how you could have crazy, psychiatric symptoms, that persist.

The tyrosinases and dopa oxidase are copper-dependent enzymes responsible for neurotransmitter (brain hormone) synthesis. Another copper dependent enzyme cytochrome C oxidase, is in the energy synthesis pathway. So with an unrecognized copper deficiency, you have a patient who is tired and has bizarre mental symptoms, and yet he is taking vitamins (albeit too much zinc in proportion to copper in many multiple vitamin preparations), so he can't understand why he is tired. And this doesn't begin to show you any of the silent long-range effects of copper deficiency like high cholesterol or aortic aneurysms (a ballooning of the main heart artery; when the balloon bursts, you bleed to death internally within minutes).

```
***********************************************************
*                                                         *
*    Copper-Dependent        Affect Metabolism of         *
*         Enzymes                                         *
*                                                         *
*    polyphenol oxidase      chemicals                    *
*    SOD                     free radicals                *
*    tyrosinase              neurotransmitters            *
*    dopa oxidase            neurotransmitters            *
*    cytochrome C oxidase    energy                       *
*                                                         *
***********************************************************
```

Now you can begin to appreciate why so often our patients are told by doctors that their symptoms are all in their heads. Usually this can be interpreted to mean that this necessary chemistry is not in the doctor's head. I personally prefer to tell someone I'm not yet smart enough to figure out the cause of their symptoms. Fortunately in this field, we keep discovering new information every few months. That makes it very exciting, for as people check back every 6 months or so, we often find we have new answers that didn't exist even 3 months prior. I'm sure this scenario will be repeated a thousand fold as conscientious physicians world wide struggle to learn the whole new world of molecular biology. It is a constant learning process, involving constant study and growth. But the result can be the progressive ability to understand and correct a multitude of problems that have eluded us for so long.

Iron

If you have a resistant iron deficiency, always check magnesium, nickel, copper, zinc and manganese, because these are sometimes the reasons why a deficiency cannot be corrected. Just as with a magnesium deficiency, when it could not be incorporated and work until the manganese deficiency was corrected, the same thing occurs with iron deficiency. If there isn't enough of the accessory or other minerals, you are not able to incorporate it into the enzymes to correct the deficiency. Another fact about iron that really surprised me was the very high frequency of an undiagnosed deficiency. This is partly due to the fact that we were taught over 20 years ago in medical school to suspect it if the cbc (complete blood count) was abnormal {low hemoglobin, hematocrit or microcytic hypochromic indices}. But over 90% of the people with low iron that we see have totally normal cbc's. So no wonder it is overlooked.

Zinc

You'll recall zinc was pivotal in the first biochemical bottleneck, the Phase I conversion of alcohols via zinc dependent alcohol dehydrogenase to aldehyde. If this is low, the same backlog scenario can occur with a shift to chloral hydrate and toxic brain symptoms. But more importantly it's another case of how the sick get sicker as backlogged xenobiotics aimlessly float around and further damage other parts of the detox system in the process. The same endless downward spiral of more new symptoms and gradual worsening of the old ones results. And all the while the tiredness never improves.

Molybdenum

Molybedenum is essential in only four known enzymes: the very important aldehyde oxidase which metabolizes aldehydes, xanthine oxidase which, if the system is stressed, can pinch hit for aldehyde oxidase in Phase I detox reactions, sulfite oxidase and some of the many sulfo transferases.

The latter two are important for several reasons:
1.   They help metabolize the sulfur containing amino

acids (methionine, cysteine, taurine), which are very important in detoxication.

2. They contribute to the metabolism of some steroids, hormones and neurotransmitters.

3. They metabolize sulfurous acid gas which has been regarded as one of the primary causes of air pollution and photochemical smog. Sulfurous gases are known contributors to lung disease like chronic bronchitis, emphysema and asthma, being strong enough to dissolve the faces of some of the world's most cherished historic buildings, monuments and statues.

4. Sulfite oxidase also handles the sulfites in foods (beer, wine, French fries, salad bars, shrimp, etc.) that were meant to keep foods fresh. Unfortunately some asthmatics who lacked sufficient sulfite oxidase (molybdenum deficiency?) died from sulfite ingestion.

This has triggered interest in sulfite metabolism and indeed Scadding (B.M.J., 297, 105-107, July 9, 1988) found that patients with food allergies were poor sulfoxidisers. When deficiency of sulfite oxidase is severe, it is associated with brain damage, which is not surprising with the compromise of essential compounds like cysteine to protect against xenobiotic damage. And nerve sheaths depend upon this chemistry, for inorganic sulfate is the precursor of the organic sulfate ester in myelin (Shih, VE, et al, Sulfite oxidase deficiency, N. Engl. J. Med., 297:19, 1022-1028, Nov. 10, 1977).

The enzyme sulfite oxidase can be inhibited by such compounds as phenols (found in home cleaning solutions) or in pentachlorophenol, a common wood preservative (Mulder, GJ, Scholtens, E, Phenol sulfotransferase and uridine di-phosphate glucuronyltransferase from rat liver in vivo and in vitro, Biochem. J., 165, 553-559, 1977). And, of course, without sufficient molybdenum the enzyme is dysfunctional. Diets high in copper (self-selected vitamins, copper leaching into drinking water from copper pipes) and calcium (the current calcium craze) can competitively inhibit molybdenum.

The defect in one studied case with severe brain damage was traced to a defect in synthesis of the enzyme. (Johnson, JC, Rajagopalan, KV, Human sulfite oxidase deficiency, J. Clin. Investig., 58, 551-556, Sept. 1976).

What concerns us is the numbers of asthmatics unable to handle sulfites in foods and sulfur in air pollution. It stands to reason that the metabolism of sulfur-dependent detox amino acids (cysteine) and neurotransmitters are most likely vulnerable. Also, a partial defect could be present that would not be as devastatingly fatal, but lead to a slow unrecognized brain damage. Even more disconcerting is the fact that the efficiency of the enzyme decreases as the sulfite load increases, (Gunorison, AF, Palmes, ED, A model for the metabolism of sulfite in mammals, Toxicol. and Appl. Pharmacol., 38, 111-126, 1976): so the sick got sicker.

Dr. Jonathan Wright, through urinary tests for sulfates via Meridian Labs (appendix), has also found that a substantial number of asthmatics are indeed poor sulfite metabolizers. This provides us with one more clue to help "impossible" cases respond to environmental insults.

It is apparent that minerals are all interacting with one another, as though in a maze. You can't take one without affecting others. On the same note, when one is deficient, most likely there's another one somewhere that is deficient also. Or on the other hand, it may be one we do not yet have an adequate test for or are yet unaware of.

When you are trying to decide what nutrient deficiencies to consider, I suggest you start by looking at minerals. Look at an rbc zinc, a selenium, serum iron, copper, and do a magnesium loading test. The minerals take far longer to correct than vitamin deficiencies in general, because they often have to be incorporated into an enzyme over a period of months.

Let's take a very sketchy look at several key minerals and just one example of each one in terms of where it is useful in the detox scheme:

1. Molybdenum is in the aldehyde oxidase enzyme.
2. Manganese in SOD and glutathione synthetase.
3. Magnesium is necessary for glutathione synthesis.
4. Zinc in gene repair (DNA polymerase and thymidine kinase) and Phase I alcohol dehydrogenase.
5. Selenium in glutathione peroxidase to recycle GSH.
6. Sulfur in the PAPS for Phase II conjugation.
7. Copper in the cytosolic SOD.
8. Iron in the cytochrome P450 (where Phase I detox occurs).

```
*****************************************************************
*                                                               *
*    Examples of Minerals        In Detox Pathways              *
*                                                               *
*    molybdenum . . . . . . . . . aldehyde oxidase              *
*    manganese  . . . . . . . . . SOD, glutathione              *
*                                     synthetase                *
*    zinc . . . . . . . . . . . . .DNA polymerase, alcohol      *
*                                     dehydrogenase             *
*    selenium . . . . . . . . . . glutathione peroxidase        *
*    sulfur . . . . . . . . . . . PAPS                          *
*    copper .. . . . . . . . . . . SOD                          *
*    iron . . . . . . . . . . ... cytochrome P-450              *
*                                                               *
*****************************************************************
```

Remember that when you start correcting minerals, always get follow-up blood work in about three months, because you are vulnerable for knocking the bottom out of other minerals that are reciprocally related. It's as though, for example, zinc were on a teeter tauter with iron, molybdenum, and copper. It will lower these as its level gets raised. We like to stop the correction right at the horizontal balance point but sometimes we accidentally over-shoot the mark. Then, whether or not you stay on minerals once your deficiency is corrected, you must check the level again in about a year, because the deficiency may have recurred. Remember, we don't have all the answers yet, and in particular we don't know precisely what made you low in the first place, nor how long you had been low before it was discovered. Your new healthier diet changes should assist in maintaining an appropriate balance.

So, in essence, to heal E.I., or environmental illness, you need to diagnose and then correct resistant nutritional deficiencies, unload the system with environmental controls and diets (as we describe in The E.I. Syndrome), and then the body will detox and start to heal itself.

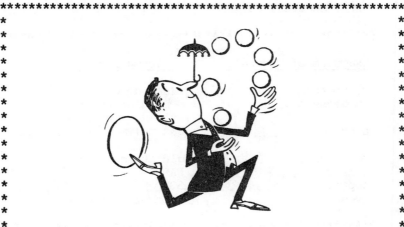

Orchestrating your nutritional biochemistry is quite a balancing act. It requires a specialized knowledge and periodic monitoring, for nothing is static.

The Other Neglected Nutrients

Besides the minerals, many other nutrients are crucial for the detoxication system: vitamins, amino acids, essential fatty acids and accessory nutrients. For physicians who may want examples of where the vitamins fit into the detox scheme:

```
****************************************************************
*       EXAMPLES OF VITAMINS IN DETOX PATHWAY                  *
*                                                              *
* Vitamin A ..... Antioxidant to protect membranes of endo-    *
*                 plasmic reticulum, promotes healthy intes-   *
*                 tinal mucosa for absorption of other         *
*                 nutrients                                    *
*            B1 ..... Needed for G6PD for GSH regeneration,    *
*                 energy for synthesis of conjugates,          *
*                 aldehyde carrier                             *
*            B2 ..... Glutathione reductase (to recycle        *
*                 glutathione), FAD                            *
*            B3 ..... NADPH (electron transfer)                *
*            B5 ..... Aldehyde control via acetyl CoA          *
*            B6 ..... Metabolism of methionine for GSH         *
*            B12 .... Synthesis of cysteine from methionine    *
* folic acid                                                   *
*       choline ... Helps to synthesize methionine,           *
*                 phosphatidyl choline for membranes, and      *
*                 acetyl choline for memory, and maintaining   *
*                 peristalsis in intestines                    *
*            C ..... Scavenger for free radicals, electron     *
*                 transport                                     *
*            E ..... As a 2-electron donor, intercepts and     *
*                 scavenges free radicals from membranes       *
****************************************************************
```

Paraquat is a pesticide so potent that half a teaspoon is lethal in a few hours. Yet the mortality rate was markedly reduced, as a sample example by the addition of vitamin B1 (thiamine necessary for energy synthesis of detox paths) and further reduced by the addition of vitamin B3 (niacin used many times over as NADP/NADPH, an electron donor-acceptor, in the detox path). Obviously with our daily exposures to sublethal but often bioaccumulative doses, a healthy nutrient system is vital to longevity.

Sometimes a vitamin level may be too high, but the person is not taking supplements. Many of us initially fell into the trap of thinking that this indicated abundance of a nutrient. But more often, an abnormally high level (without supplements) means there is a block in the metabolism and the vitamin has difficulty getting to the next usable stage and backs up.

Such is the case often with B6. The person may lack sufficient ability to convert it to pyridoxal-5-phosphate (P-5-P), and so we must give that form (P-5-P) and not B6.

This reminds me to warn you about what you learn on T.V. or the newspaper. There are some circles that would prefer that nutritional medicine go away. So they are forever highlighting the negative aspects of it. Example; a New England Journal of Medicine article a few years ago received great press as a warning against taking B6. It made the 7 a.m. news programs and major newspapers.

But when one read the article, it was a case study of a few people who must have been deranged, for they took exorbitantly high levels of B6 for many years. Some of the doses were so high I wondered how they fit all the capsules in their mouths. Remember the bell-shaped curve? Everything has a good and bad dose. And remember the concept of biochemical balance? These people obviously didn't for they developed the expected problems of massive B6 overdose of brain and nervous system diseases. The sad part of this was that it was perceived by many lay people as meaning they should never take any B6. And as you now know, if through the standard processed diet and the use of medications one is deficient, the lack of B6 potentiates arteriosclerosis and mental disease.

Soft signs of B6 deficiency may include wakening with "pins and needles" or the sensation that your arm is asleep when you know you didn't sleep on it. Carpel tunnel syn-

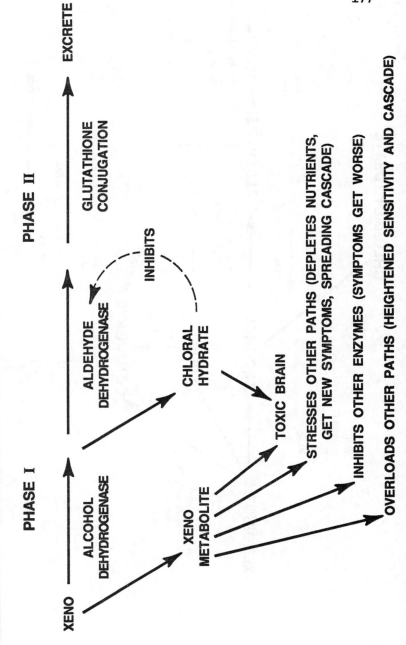

BIOCHEMICAL BOTTLENECKS OF DETOXICATION

PHASE I   PHASE II

EXCRETE

GLUTATHIONE CONJUGATION

ALCOHOL DEHYDROGENASE

ALDEHYDE DEHYDROGENASE

XENO

XENO METABOLITE

CHLORAL HYDRATE

INHIBITS

TOXIC BRAIN

STRESSES OTHER PATHS (DEPLETES NUTRIENTS, GET NEW SYMPTOMS, SPREADING CASCADE)

INHIBITS OTHER ENZYMES (SYMPTOMS GET WORSE)

OVERLOADS OTHER PATHS (HEIGHTENED SENSITIVITY AND CASCADE)

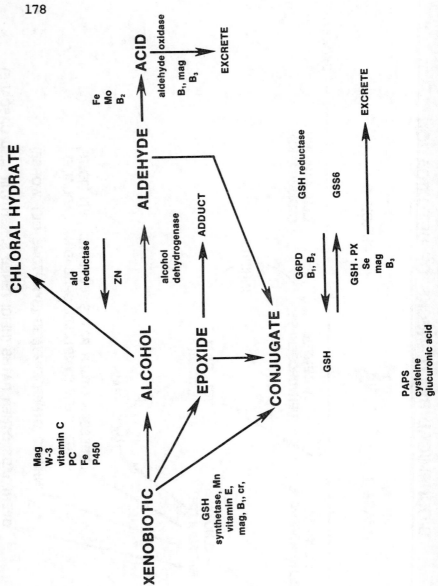

drome, PMS, depression and much more respond to B6 treatment if it is the deficiency involved.

And of course, sometimes the vitamin level is normal, but its functional assay (the enzyme that depends upon adequate levels of that vitamin for its function) is abnormal. An abnormal functional enzyme assay provides several clues:
(1) A therapeutic trial is in order.
(2) Another important nutrient (like magnesium, for example) is low and impeding conversion.
(3) The vitamin itself cannot be metabolized because of toxic, genetic, or nutrient deficiency reasons. For example, some people cannot convert vitamin B6 to pyridoxal-5-phosphate. Instead the vitamin B6 metabolite, pyridoxal-5-phosphate must be given (Klaire Laboratories, Vital Life products, see Appendix).

Some of the more common functional assays follow and are all available through Monroe Laboratories, Southfields, N.Y.

```
***************************************************************
*      Examples of Functional Assays For Vitamins            *
*                                                            *
*      VITAMIN            TEST                                *
*      B1                 rbc transketolase                  *
*      B2                 rbc glutathione reductase          *
*      B3                 1-N-methyl nicotinamide            *
*      B6                 rbc glutamate pyruvate             *
*                         transaminase                       *
*      B6, tryptophan     xanthurenic acid, kynurenic acid   *
*      B6, Zn, Mn         kryptopyrole                       *
*      B12                methylmalonic acid                 *
*      folic acid         formiminoglutamic acid             *
*      selenium           rbc glutathione peroxidase         *
***************************************************************
```

Amino Acids

Besides minerals and vitamins, amino acids may be deficient and mimic any symptom. Amino acids are the building blocks of all proteins.

Amino acidodopathies, or abnormalities of amino acid metabolism can be secondary to nutrient deficiencies (without enough magnesium you can't convert methionine to cysteine, for example), food allergies, faulty intestinal absorption, and/or genetic abnormalities. Most commonly the symptoms of amino acidopathies are vague tiredness, weakness, body aches, digestive problems, inability to concentrate and many of the same symptoms of food, chemical, and mold sensitivities.

```
**********************************************************
*                                                        *
*                                                        *
*                                                        *
*                                                        *
*                                                        *
*                                                        *
*                                                        *
*                                                        *
*                                                        *
*                                                        *
*                                                        *
*                                                        *
*                                                        *
```

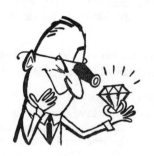

```
*                                                        *
*   The more valuable something is, the more it be-      *
*   hooves you to understand it.  What is more valuable  *
*   than your body?  If you don't understand that the    *
*   symptoms of nutrient deficiencies can mimic those    *
*   of any disease including chemical, food and mold     *
*   sensitivities, how will you ever begin to learn to   *
*   sort them out in your journey toward wellness?       *
*                                                        *
**********************************************************
```

As your doctor is getting started, he may need help in interpretation of the amino acid reports. They require extensive biochemical knowledge and often we will enlist the help of a "consulting biochemist" in difficult cases (see Appendix).

There are many clues to abnormal function that can be obtained through a 24 hour urine quantitative amino acid analysis coupled with a plasma quantitative amino acid analysis.

Example: Veronica was an attractive 42 year old who after having had some dental work, experienced 2 years of burning in her mouth that had left her threatening suicide. Obviously she had made the rounds of many dental and medical specialists.

Her nutrient levels were surprisingly normal, but a 24 hour urine amino acid analysis suggested that she had a deficiency in her vitamin B12 metabolism. But her blood levels had been 350 (normal 200-900). The anti-parietal antibody was negative as well. We gave her a trial of B12 injections and it immediately gave her what she described as 70% relief for the first time in years.

Moreover, she requires 1000 mcg every week to maintain this improvement; this, of course, told us there were further deficiencies. The point is, we never would have considered the B12 trial without the abnormal amino acid analysis. Meanwhile, for the person who is chronically tired, or chronically symptomatic, when many of the more common preceding abnormalities have been ruled out, don't overlook abnormal amino acid metabolism. It provides great clues to general body biochemical dysfunctions and whether someone is playing with a full deck.

Recall how different magnesium deficiency is to diagnose without a cumbersome retention test? Often a 24 hour urine amino acid analysis will offer clues to support a magnesium trial.

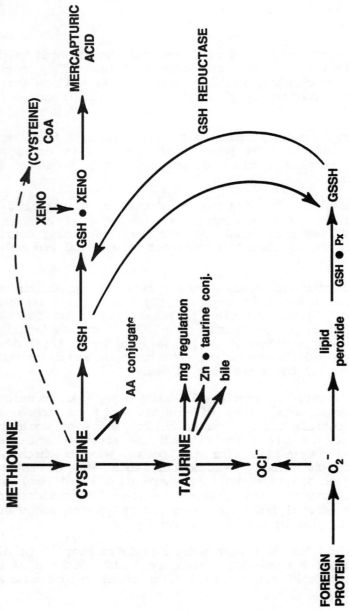

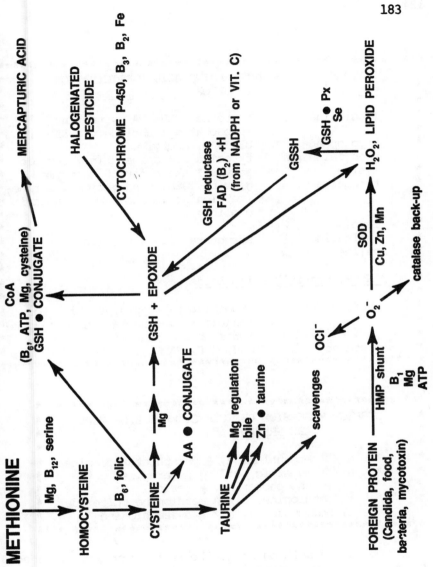

```
*****************************************************************
*                                                               *
*       EXAMPLES OF ESSENTIAL AMINO ACID PARTICIPATION          *
*       ---            IN DETOX                                 *
*                      ----------                               *
*       methionine          cysteine, GSH, PAPS, taurine,       *
*                           {phosphatidyl choline via SAM}      *
*       tryptophan          B3, NAD, acetyl CoA                 *
*       phenylalanine       tyrosine for epinephrine, thyroid   *
*       lysine              enzyme linkage for B6 coenzyme       *
*       threonine           glycine (GSH, conjugation), serine  *
*                           (methionine metabolism and acetyl   *
*                           choline)                            *
*       leucine                                                 *
*       isoleucine     }    structural liver proteins           *
*       valine                                                  *
*                                                               *
*       "Non-Essential" Amino Acids                             *
*                                                               *
*       taurine             hypochlorite scavenger, bile for    *
*                           conjugation, zinc-taurine conjugate *
*                           for membrane stability              *
*       cysteine            GSH, GTF, PAPS, taurine             *
*****************************************************************
```

```
***********************************************************
*                                                         *
*       SUSPECT MAGNESIUM DEFICIENCY WHEN 2 OR MORE        *
*                  ARE PRESENT                            *
*                  -----------                            *
*                                                         *
*    *   nl/↑ ethanolamine, ↓ phosphoethanolamine         *
*    *   nl/↑ aspartic acid, ↓ asparagine                 *
*    *   nl/↑ phosphoserine, ↓ serine                     *
*    *    ↑ methionine, nl/↑ methionine sulfoxide         *
*        nl homocysteine, nl/ ↓ cystathionine            *
***********************************************************
```

Obviously methionine is the most important amino acid since it gets metabolized to cysteine, the major source of sulfhydryl groups for detoxication, and because it is a major source of methyl groups for synthesis of neurotransmitters and for detoxication, for example. From methionine, cysteine is formed which not only conjugates directly by itself {or as N-acetyl cysteine}, but is the pivotal amino acid for synthesis of other conjugators like glutathione, PAPS, taurine, as well as pantothenic acid and glucose tolerance factor {GTF is actually GSH}.

```
***************************************************************
*                                                             *
*     THE DOWNWARD SPIRAL:  HOW THE SICK GET SICKER           *
*                                                             *
*     Many nutrient deficiencies cause tiredness and vague    *
*        symptoms, especially of the nervous system.          *
*     Many chemical sensitivities cause the exact same        *
*        symptoms.                                            *
*     Put them together and the already malfunctioning        *
*        (deficient) detoxication system becomes further      *
*        overloaded (by chemical exposures).                  *
*     Backlogged chemicals and their metabolites cannot be    *
*        disposed of, so they linger and cause further        *
*        loss of precious nutrients and destruction to        *
*        the detox mechanisms.                                *
*     The result:  the sick get sicker.                       *
***************************************************************
```

Think Zinc

So let's just take a peek at merely one trace mineral. And mind you, "trace" means the body only requires very small levels of it to function. Zinc is commonly low due to mainly commercial farming and food processing practices as well as people being hooked on sweets, salts, and fats. We found 54% of 350 patients were deficient in rbc zinc. But look at what an unsuspected zinc deficiency can cause: (zinc dependent enzymes are underlined)

(1)   Genetic change:
       Zinc deficiency can account for the seemingly overnight change to E.I. since it's necessary in DNA polymerase and thymidine kinase, the gene repair enzymes. Genetic material is continually breaking down as old worn out parts {purine bases} are replaced. When the DNA strand with it's new parts is ready to be reassembled, if the

reassembly enzyme is defective, chances are the reassembly will be also. Hence you have altered genetics.

(2) Poor healing:

RNA polymerase is active in making new proteins for healing, and alkaline phosphatase is the enzyme in white blood cells that helps them destroy foreign organisms (bacteria).

(3) Defective detoxication:

Alcohol dehydrogenase, a major Phase I enzyme changes alcohols to aldehydes. It is the first biochemical bottleneck. If this is deficient in zinc, chemicals can backlog and further damage the detox areas. Meanwhile the spreading phenomenon or cascade begins. The victim reacts more quickly and to more things and with less of a dose. Formate dehydrogenase and carbonic anhydrase are necessary for aldehyde (formate dehydrogenase can metabolize formaldehyde) metabolism, glucuronic acid is a Phase II conjugator, catalase and SOD control free radicals, RNA polymerase helps synthesize detox enzymes, glutamate dehydrogenase is needed for glutathione peroxidase synthesis and transmethylation of methionine is necessary for cysteine synthesis.

(4) Brain fog:

There is a zinc-taurine conjugate that stabilizes membranes, carbonic anhydrase buffers pH, and GABA synthesis is also zinc dependent.

(5) Defective nutrient metabolism:

Retinol binding protein is zinc dependent and necessary to get vitamin A out of liver storage, alcohol dehydrogenase to metabolize vitamin A from retinol to retinaldehyde so you can begin to use it, pyridoxine kinase to metabolize vitamin B6 to pyridoxal-5-phosphate (it's first usable stage), lipase to absorb essential fatty acids and vitamin E for membranes, and carboxypeptidase, thermolysin, and amino peptidase for amino acid metabolism (they help proteins get broken down so they can be absorbed from the intestine).

(6)   Poor metabolism:
      Zinc is necessary for <u>insulin storage</u>, and
      <u>carbonic anhydrase</u> for pH buffering and aldehyde
      metabolism.

Although we didn't get anywhere <u>near</u> listing all 90
metalloenzymes that require zinc, this represents how perva-
sive and all encompassing one out of over 40 essential
nutrients is.

Truly, "nutrition is the single most important component of preventive health care". Diet has been associated
with cancer, heart disease, diabetes, stroke and hypertension, arteriosclerosis and cirrhoses of the liver. (Implications of nutritional status on human biochemistry, physiology, and health, Sauberlick, HE, <u>Clinical Biochemistry</u>,
vol. 17, Apr. 1984, 132-142). And the ability of the human
to respond to life stresses from trauma, surgery, and infection can be influenced by nutritional status.

For example, a recent study shows that 39% of hypertensives were able to use nutrition in place of blood pressure medications to keep their pressure normal for over four
years (Cardiac status after four years in a trial on nutritional therapy for high blood pressure, Stamler, R, et al,
<u>Arch. Intern. Med.</u>, 149, 661-665, March 1989).

But identifying and correcting nutrient deficiencies
is only the start. You can't hope to balance your chemistry
on vitamins, minerals, and amino acids. You need to address
your diet so you can stay corrected without supplements.

NOTE:

Whenever you have nutritionally oriented medical care,
you must become much more involved and organized. To each
visit you should bring a notebook and chart. The chart
should be on-going. Along the left hand margin you should
put all your products. You can cut and paste, subtract and
add all you want, or use your computer. The important point
is that both you and the doctor should always be able to

tell at a glance what your total intake is. This is a sample of what I suggest: Suppose you are taking only two products: multiple minerals and extra magnesium. Your chart would look like this:

Date Started:_____

PRODUCTS:	Multiple Mineral (mg)	Magnesium (300 mg)	Total Daily Dose
DAILY DOSE:	2	1	
CONTENTS of EACH:			
Magnesium	83x2-166	300	466
Calcium	83x2=166		166
Chromium	83x2=166		166
Selenium	33x2=66		66
Molybdenum	83x2=166		166
Zinc	9x2=18		18

This is the only way that both you and your physician will have a clear picture of what you are taking on a daily basis and to avoid mistakes. You must have every single supplement you take on your list in order for you or your physician to quickly spot incompatibilities, overdoses or imbalances.

Is Part Of Your Problem A Sluggish Adrenal Gland?

I really don't want to turn this into a textbook of general medicine, but sometimes people with E.I. are so overwhelmingly loaded with undiagnosable symptoms, that regular medical problems get overlooked. One of these is an adrenal gland that is suboptimally functioning. In other words it works normally day to day, but give it a smidge of stress and it cannot rally.

I don't know if these glands were target organs to toxins, fail because of just being worn out, or are depleted in some nutrient especially important to their function like manganese or vitamin C.

Some individuals, due to severe or chronic environmental stresses and/or nutrient deficiencies, have prematurely worn out their adrenals. Symptoms usually include fatigue and can often include low blood pressure, and inability to gain weight. The adrenals make a background amount of hormones daily but during any period of stress must rise to the challenge and suddenly make more, or the individual suffers.

Furthermore, the adrenal has really no storage mechanism. There's no big fat analogue of a gall bladder storing all this precious corticosteroid, ready to squirt it into our systems when we have an emotional, physical, or toxic stress. In fact "the amount of corticosteriods found in the adrenal tissue is insufficient to maintain normal rates of secretion for more than a few minutes in the absence of continuing biosynthesis. For this reason, the rate of biosynthesis is tantamount to the rate of secretion" (Goodman, LS, Gilman, A, The Pharmacological Basis of Therapeutics, 5th ed., 1477, MacMillan Publ. Co., NY, 1975).

The adrenal glands, which sit on top of the kidneys, are the body's primary glands that enable us to respond to stress.

Dr. William Jeffries, former professor of medicine in the endocrinology department at Case Western Reserve Medical School, has written a book about sub-clinical hypoadrenalism (Safe Uses of Cortisone, Charles C. Thomas Co., Springfield, Il, 1981). As we are all trained, prednisone, cortisone and other adrenal hormone derivatives can be dangerous, causing ulcers, depression, osteoporosis, hypertension, cataracts, and much more.

But Dr. Jeffries has discovered that some people have depleted their adrenal reserves over the years. Besides environmental chemicals, toxins, pesticides, heavy metals like mercury, and nutritional deficiencies, excessive stresses like anxiety, worry, grief, and depression can precipitate wearing out or degeneration of the gland. Furthermore, he has shown how depleted adrenal reserves can be diagnosed and treated. Dramatic improvement has resulted in a variety of conditions for which there was no help. Furthermore, his studies in over one thousand patient years show the doses of hormones used are very safe. Borderline adrenal reserves can masquerade as any symptom from chronic fatigue, arthritis, infection and hypoglycemia, to chronic mono, colitis, thyroiditis, diabetes, allergies and menstrual abnormalities.

The cortrosyn stimulation test tells us whether the gland functions optimally. Cortrosyn is a synthetic peptide corresponding to {amino acid residues 1 to 24 of human} ACTH, the hormone made by the pituitary (master) gland to turn on the adrenal.

An intramuscular dose of 0.25 mg of cortrosyn should double the cortisol blood test value in half an hour. And that's how simple the test is to diagnose whether one has sluggish adrenal metabolism. A cortisol (hormone from the adrenal gland) blood test is drawn. Cortrosyn is given, and in 30-45 minutes a second level is drawn. If it does not double, a trial of 5 mg cortisol every six hours is in order. For some of the most severely toxic people this has been another step up the ladder of wellness.

What Tests Should I Have Done?

We're asked this so often, and now you most likely understand that it's highly individual. Also many tests are not yet available in some areas. So you do the best you can. For the average person, these tests would make a good start:

Test	Rationale
rbc zinc (NOT PLASMA OR SERUM, NOT PROTOPORPHYRIN)	low in 54% of our patients, needed for gene repair, detox (alcohol dehydrogenase), antibody synthesis, vitamin metabolism.
formic acid	a guide to whether you can metabolize your average exposures to formaldehyde, or if it gets backlogged.
thiamine (B1)	necessary for energy metabolism and detox.
GGT (gamma glutamyl transaminase)	an indicator of liver detox overload.
copper	in detox, energy and neurotransmitter synthesis.
rbc chromium	insulin metabolism, vascular structure.
pyridoxine (B6)	amino acid metabolism.
folic acid	amino acid metabolism.
cobalamin (B12)	amino acid metabolism.
serum iron	in detox cytochromes.
MLT (magnesium loading test)	low in 50% of our pts., in over 300 enzymes.

glutathione reductase   detox (vitamin B2, FAD).

selenium   detox (glutathione peroxidase). Due to homeostasis, when this is low in serum the patient is often seriously stressed by a toxin.

Then if needed, you could progress to more sophisticated tests:

Quantitative amino acids	Specific pesticide levels (e.g. malathione)
Specific chemical levels (e.g. toluene)	Gastric analysis for HCl
Special stool exams for foreign flora	Depollution panel
Vitamins A, C, D, E, K, B3	rbc Molybdenum
rbc Manganese,	EFA (essential fatty acid levels)

24 hr. urine for hydroxyproline

There are many more useful tests, but space limits their inclusion.

What Should I Take?

We're asked this question frequently, and by now you appreciate that it is highly individual. There is no Rx for everyone. Bearing that in mind, here's a general hypothetical outline:

Nutrient	Rationale
Multiple mineral (with iron, chromium, molybdenum, vanadium, selenium, copper, zinc, manganese, magnesium, potassium, calcium, iodide, cobalt, silicon, for example.	people get progressively fewer minerals from food.

You won't find one with all of
these).

Antioxidant (with A, C, E, L-cysteine or N-acetyl cysteine, glutathione, selenium, B, P-5-P, B3, B5, or PABA, beta carotene, lipoic acid, for example. You won't find one with all of these).	most people have free radical overload.
Multiple B (B1, B2, B3, B5, B6, B12, folic acid, P-5-P, PABA, inositol choline, biotin).	this is the most commonly low vitamin group.
Multiple vitamin/mineral (some have strange imbalances. Avoid ones with over 2 mg copper per day, less than 5 mg manganese, less than 15 mg zinc, or magnesium to calcium ratio of less than 3:4, etc. Be sure to tally with multiple minerals).	to balance out the others.
Organic flax oil in opaque, dated bottle.	many are in need of an oil change.

At the next stage when you sit down to correct deficiencies discovered through the blood work, you may need a variety of additions:

Betaine HCl.	to correct hypochlorhydria
Pancreatic enzymes.	also to enhance digestion of supplements.

Amino acids (total or individual).

Omega 6 oil.

Individual vitamins or their metabolites.

Individual minerals.

Phosphatidyl choline.

There are scores of exceptionally useful nutrients. But there is also a limit as to what the stomach can hold, and a limit to the amount of capsular material and filler (like magnesium stearate that keeps capsular material from sticking in the machine) that we want to tolerate. After all, that has to be detoxified too. Therefore this must be individualized.

Some of these nutrients are difficult to find. All can be obtained by mail from N.E.E.D.S. (see appendix, 1-800-634-1380). Following is a very brief example of specialty nutrients that have been available for some people, and the houses we have found to supply the most hypo-allergenic products we can get:

Allergy Research Group: (Nutricology)	liquid selenium germanium egg lecithin

Cardiovascular Research Lab:
  (Arteria, Ecological
  Formulae)
	lipoic acid
	Psorex-fumaric acid
	L-carnitine
	lipothamine
	magnesium chloride solution

Probiologic (Neesby):	aqueous chromium
Vital Life (Klaire Labs):	alpha keto glutaric acid Micel E Micel A Vital plex

There are many others, such as: N-acetyl cysteine, DMG, P-5-P, Co Q10, taurine, digestive enzymes, etc., etc., not to mention Chinese herbals and homeopathic remedies.

Remember, supplements are potent medicines. A deficiency should be diagnosed, corrected, and rechecked for correction and balance. Meanwhile your lifestyle and diet should be modified so the deficiency does not recur and you don't need supplements the rest of your life.

But when you get hormonal and nutritional deficiencies corrected, and your life detoxed, there is one last vitamin you will need daily, forever........vitamin L.

THE LAST VITAMIN ---- VITAMIN L

There is one more vitamin you haven't heard of yet, and it is the most pivotal one for health and the detoxication of stress. For along with an increasing chemical overload, this era has stressed man to untold limits psychologically.

Vitamin L is the most important nutrient of all. You can have all the others at excellent levels, and without this one you can die. You have read about it or observed it. A couple is married for 50 years; the husband eventually dies of a long standing illness, six months later his wife is dead; only there was nothing wrong with her ------ except that she had a lethal deficiency of vitamin L.

LOVE AND LAUGHTER are very real nutrient needs, in spite of the fact that we can't yet measure them directly with a commercial laboratory test. But if you don't think that thoughts and emotions have a powerful physical effect on the body, then how does a man have an erection? How does a person blush or faint, or have a heart attack or a stroke from merely being told a story? What is behind the chemical reaction when you laugh so hard you think you will burst? Or when you love so intensely you are overwhelmed?

There is a certain set of people who will never get well until they get rid of anger that they perennially carry. Most of them don't even consciously know that they emit it, but it is unmistakably there at every encounter. For special occasions it can get relegated to the basement, but sooner or later it comes back upstairs to make its presence known. It usually requires professional help, but can be dealt with quickly depending upon how honest you can be with yourself. Remember, bad thoughts produce bad neurotransmitters that sooner or later must be metabolized just like any other chemical. And just like any other chemical, they can over-burden the aldehyde detoxication pathway.

Love and laughter are necessary for a healthy detoxication and immune system, as they can speed healing even against all odds, as Norman Cousins so beautifully demonstrated (<u>Anatomy of an Illness</u>). So you need to take an honest, hard look. Do you have someone <u>and</u> something in your life that you can love immensely? Do you get as much love as you want? Without giving love, you will rarely receive enough. And without a burning interest in something, you will rarely be interesting enough to be around. For people derive a certain amount of spark and enthusiasm from what they do. If you can't get any spark from what you do, how do you bring zest, newness and energy into a relationship? Like a garden, it must be tended and fertilized. It needs sunlight or an energy source. When you get a "lift", or enjoy what you are doing to the point of raising your energy level, you are not only re-energizing yourself and bringing more "elan vital" to your loved one, but you are fostering beneficial chemistry in your body.

If you don't believe it, I will bore you with more biochemistry. But I think you have learned enough, so just take it as fact. Just think of Maurice Chavalier singing, dancing, funning at womanizing, loving life to the point that it filled him with energy into his eighties.
Try awakening with a song ----

"Oh what a beautiful morning
Oh what a beautiful day!"
or

"Zippity do da, zippity day
My, oh, my, what a wonderful day!
Plenty of sunshine heading my way!
Zippity do da, zippity day!"

or

"When Irish Eyes Are Smiling!
All the world is bright and gay!"

Feel the lift you get already? This is real neuro-chemistry in action. You can learn to turn this energy on anytime you need it. You have a little control knob in your brain and you can jack the energy thermostat up whenever you desire.

Some people do better with dance. Turn on the music you like to dance to best and energize yourself every morning. Then if you need a boost during the day, just close your eyes and relive this experience.

As your body gets progressively detoxed and cleared out, you will be more attuned to these abilities. You have within you the power to buoy yourself and others up to untold heights of mental and physical wellness, at almost anytime you wish to exercise your talents. But it takes practice to learn how to turn it on. If you are loaded with coffee, sodas, medicines, cigarettes, sweets and meats, you won't be able to do this yet. But sooner or later you will be ready to detox yourself (Chapter 8).

Now back to love. Do you get enough? Are you demanding of one person that they supply your total quotient of love? Isn't that pretty heavy duty? Shouldn't you try to get it from other sources as well? What can your fertile brain come up with?

Last but not least, LAUGHTER. If you cannot see the humor in yourself, and much of life, most likely you are not having much fun, and are not too much fun to be with. How can you lighten up? Can you give yourself permission to be happy? Are you waiting until life is perfect before you can be happy? You know where that will lead you. Even though it is less than perfect, can you give yourself a trial day

of not taking things so seriously? See what it feels like.
What treat can you do for yourself that would relax you so
that you can back off and get another perspective? How can
you begin to see the comedy about you?

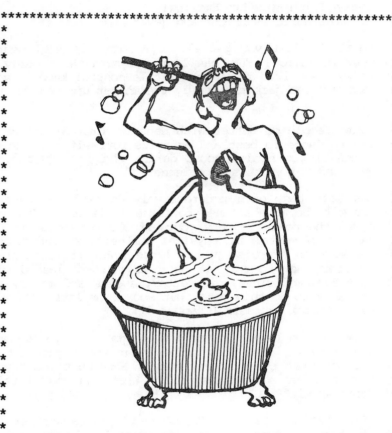

Why not start every day with a song to rev up your
happy hormones (endophins) in the brain?

If you have difficulty getting in the laughter mode, read comic books, watch Saturday morning cartoons, start surrounding yourself with humor, bring a cartoon or joke to friends, and soon it will become a part of your life. Read books on how to become a comedian --- not because you are going to make a living at it, but because you want to train your psychic eye to appreciate the many chances to laugh that we overlook daily.

Laughter is somewhat like an orgasm. It has beneficial effects on the organism, but the chemistry has yet to be fully worked out. Don't be afraid of it, but use it as one of many God given tools with which to heal. After all, with the "Future Shock" type stress and unprecedented chemical load, plus increasingly inferior nutrition of this century, we need all the help we can get. One thing is for sure, at this rate we will never run out of material for comic relief.

Last, before you turn in at night, as you are laying there about to drift off, fill your head and soul with good appreciative thoughts. It's difficult to be angry or worried when you are full of appreciation. Did you tell someone you appreciate them today? Before you go to sleep, actually count your blessings, yes, one by one. And when you awaken, count them again. Make your mental plans for the day and then begin your song or dance to rev up your enthusiasm and energy level. Remember, it is infectious and you will be revving up your partner (or later on in the day, your other friends) as well. At least it will provide some comedy and laughter with which to begin your day. Remember to bring some glimmer of happiness into the lives of as many as you can each day. It takes surprisingly little effort - a smile, a gesture, a hug, a thoughtful gift or remark of appreciation. See how it makes you feel.

If at this point you are just too miserable to think about making yourself happy, or you are too blocked to be able to do it, try a different tack that often works. Concentrate on making someone else, or several people, happy. Think of as many ways as possible, of making a certain person happy. Sometimes this has a magical effect on turning things around. And don't put all your eggs in one basket.

```
***********************************************************
*                                                         *
*                                                         *
*                                                         *
*                                                         *
*                                                         *
*                                                         *
*                                                         *
*                                                         *
*                                                         *
*                                                         *
*                                                         *
*                                                         *
*                                                         *
*                                                         *
*                                                         *
*                                                         *
*                                                         *
*                                                         *
*                                                         *
*   If you're so miserable that you can't get yourself    *
*   happy, forget it. Make someone else happy.            *
*                                                         *
***********************************************************
```

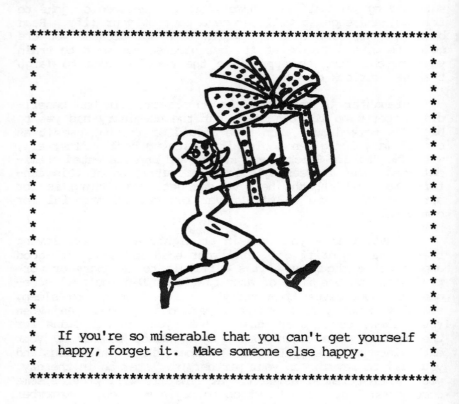

Exercise after skin brushing is another beneficial adjunct. Skin brushing is merely taking a luffa sponge, or wash cloth, and rubbing the body all over briskly to stimulate, open and facilitate drainage of stagnated lymphatics. Exercise then carries this one step further. It not only helps discharge bad emotions and accumulated mental stress, but it is part of the actual detoxication system. You see, chemicals stored in the fat can be discharged through sweat. Exhaled air, and excreted urine and stool are not the only outlets for chemicals. Sweat, seminal, vaginal discharges, and saliva are other avenues for getting rid of accumulated toxins. There is now a program you can attend for several weeks of special exercises and sauna and sweat out many toxins (p. 395). Of course very strict attention is paid to your nutritional balance during such a forced cleanse. (Root, DE, et al, Diagnosis and treatment of patients presenting subclinical signs and symptoms of exposure to chemicals which bioaccumulate in human tissues, Health Effects of Hazardous Materials, 150-153, Proceedings of Hazardous Wastes and Environmental Emergencies, Hazardous Materials Control Research Inst., 9300 Columbia Blvd., Silver Springs, MD 20910, 1985).

Being physically limber is tantamount to being mentally open and agile. Has rigor mortis begun to set in prematurely? Can you stand on one foot and hold the heel of the other foot to your pelvis for ten seconds with your eyes closed? Do this in an area where you'll be protected for you may fall the first time. Can you touch your toes without bending your knees or throwing your back out? Can you even see your toes? A stiff body can lead to a stiff, stagnated mind; and that can make a rigid, boring person; one not easily brought to laughter.

Because of the emphasis on having a healthy attitude, you might think that a lot of this is merely mind over matter. But remember that when the amassed effect of these modern day chemicals takes our detox system down, they take along with it many other systems. No system is an island onto itself. We are damaging as well, the immune system, the endocrine system, the reproductive system and more. But the primary system to be secondarily effected by all of this chemical overload is the nervous system. So anything we can do to unload it and give it a boost back into function is fair game.

```
***********************************************************
*                                                         *
*                                                         *
*                                                         *
*                                                         *
*                                                         *
*                                                         *
*                                                         *
*                                                         *
*                                                         *
*                                                         *
*                                                         *
*                                                         *
*                                                         *
*                                                         *
*                                                         *
*   Exercise not only discharges harmful chemicals        *
*   in the sweat, but discharges malignant emotions       *
*   which can otherwise overburden the detox pathways.    *
*   Also a stiff body may reflect a stiff mind, unable    *
*   to grow.                                              *
*                                                         *
***********************************************************
```

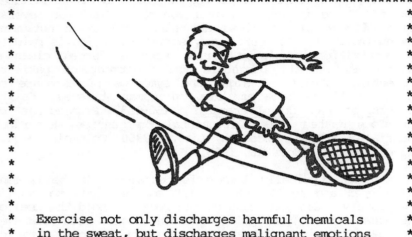

Only mono-organ directed doctors will think that because you got something better after your attitude improved, that it must have been all in your head to begin with. Some people will never be able to appreciate the intricacies of the total body all at once. It is too overwhelming. And you just saw a glimmer of how overwhelming it is in this chapter. That is precisely why the environmental medicine specialty has not taken off with a bang; it is too overwhelming. The last time I was giving board exams for doctors taking their oral exams for specialty certification by the American Board of Environmental Medicine, I was shocked as were many fellow examiners. Here were men who had been to many of the courses and meetings for years, but could not pass the exam. Why? It is an overwhelming specialty. Much is not even synthesized and written down yet, and in addition, it places a tremendous burden on the

physician to know a great deal about many aspects of the
body. We are all pioneers on the cutting edge as a new leaf
of medical history begins to unfold. It is not easy. My
hat goes off to these men ..... at least they tried. And I
have no doubt most will eventually succeed. No wonder medicine compartmentalized itself into specialties a long time
ago. It sure makes the practice of medicine a whole lot
easier having to know only certain areas well.

In this era of easy, one organ focus, who needs all
the aggravation of learning environmental medicine? Life is
too short. So to ease the burden and to get yourself out of
the overwhelmed stage, merely remember to compartmentalize
your total load and whittle through it until you have no
symptoms left (Chapter 8).

The only road to real health is through education of
physicians and patients alike. When we join forces in the
battle for wellness, then health is no longer an overwhelming possibility. And as first priority, you must be playing
with a full biochemical deck of nutrients.

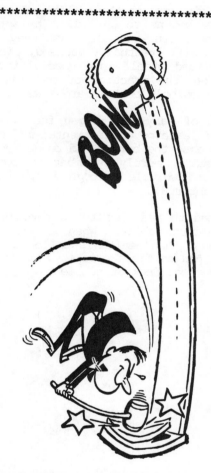

```
***********************************************************
*                                                         *
*                                                         *
*                                                         *
*                                                         *
*                                                         *
*                                                         *
*                                                         *
*                                                         *
*                                                         *
*                                                         *
*                                                         *
*                                                         *
*                                                         *
*                                                         *
*                                                         *
*                                                         *
*                                                         *
*                                                         *
*                                                         *
*                                                         *
*                                                         *
*                                                         *
*                                                         *
*                                                         *
*                                                         *
*                                                         *
*                                                         *
*                                                         *
*                                                         *
*   You have accomplished a miraculous feat!  You have    *
*   broken the 20th century health barrier and entered    *
*   into 21st century concepts.                           *
*                                                         *
***********************************************************
```

Chapter 7: COMMON CURRENT MEDICAL BLUNDERS

Like a butterfly in metamorphosis, when I stopped thinking drugs and started thinking biochemistry, the whole world of medicine changed. But what really startled me was that much of this had been known for many years, albeit by non-physician scientists. And what concerned me the most was the fact that if I hadn't been forced into learning (and collating this with what we had discovered in environmental medicine about detoxication) because I was sick, I'd still be on the other side of the fence denying this and pushing (prescription) drugs.

Are You Due For An Oil Change?

Most people never think of oil in terms of having a need for it in their bodies. But oils, or lipids (specialized body fats), are actually essential for life itself. Beyond lubricating the body and providing enough fat to hold up your pants, oil (lipid) is critical for the function of every cell membrane and for the nerve sheath that protects and nurtures the function of your delicate nerves. These cell membranes are like the computer keyboard and direct the actions of the cell. Furthermore, the brain is a highly lipid structure as well. So three vital areas of the body --- cell membranes, nerve sheaths and the brain are composed of a specialized fat, called lipids.

Aside from the cell membrane protecting the internal environment of a cell, you'll recall there is a series of membranes inside cells which have pivotal functions. The mitochondria are membranous cigar-shaped areas within the cell where energy is actually manufactured. Another membrane structure called the endoplasmic reticulum (ER) or the microsomes is the site where chemicals are detoxified: chemicals that occur in foods, water and air, and that if left undetoxified, damage body chemistry and create disease.

Most people's membranes contain a percentage of wrong oils, called trans fatty acids. These act to interfere with normal cell membrane function and structure. Trans fatty acids come from years of ingesting grocery store oils, such as polyunsaturated corn oils, and other grocery store "poly- unsaturated, hydrogenated" vegetable oils, such as safflower oils, and margarines. Margarines have the highest percent- age of trans fatty acids (often 15-35%) and actually, there- fore potentiate arteriosclerosis. For the body views this changed chemical (called a trans form), produced by high temperatures in processing, as foreign and harmful. Therefore, margarines and other products high in trans fatty acids are not recommended for anyone, much less the cardiol- ogy patient, for whom they are most often prescribed.

Another source of wrong oils are the fried foods, especially those commercially done, like french fries. Not only is the oil heated once to destroy the precious essen- tial fatty acids, but many times over as it is reused, thereby increasing the percentage of bad oils. As well, wrong oils are in most processed foods, but are especially high in baked goods and candies. Any foods containing "hydrogenated vegetable oil" or "shortening" have some trans form oils.

What is wrong with trans oils? They started out in nature in "cis" form. This is the form that is user- friendly to the body and necessary for life. But with the high heat necessary to hydrogenate margarines and oils, the fat molecule actually undergoes a permanent twisting in its shape that actually straightens it out. It now is viewed as unnatural by the body and interferes with function. For example it acts much like a broken key when inserted into living tissue like the cell membrane, nerve sheath or brain. It fits in, but does not function optimally. Furthermore it blocks the correct or good form from being taken in. And most importantly, trans fatty acids inhibit the enzyme delta-6-desaturase (D-6-D) which you'll learn makes good things happen in the body.

It is clear, now, that in the last century man has changed his eating dramatically. He has gone from wild game, seeds, roots and leaves, to refined foods. In doing so he has not only added these trans oils, but changed his ratio of oils. Fatty acids are of two types: (1) Saturated oils which are solid at room temperature and come from butter, lard and coconut, for example. (2) Unsaturated oils that are liquid at room temperature which can further be categorized as either non-essential oils, like olive oil, or essential fatty acids (EFA's).

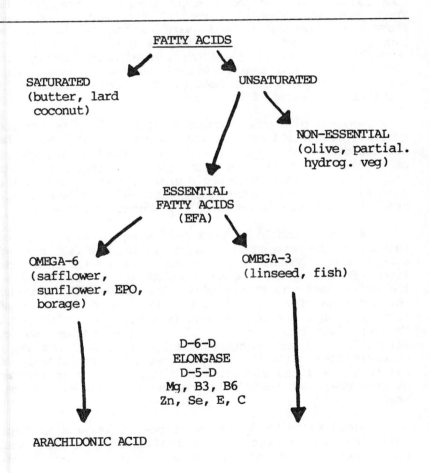

From the EFA's above, prostaglandins are formed which regulate inflam- mation, blood clotting, vessel and bronchial tone, and other disease processes.

Essential fatty acids (EFA's) mean just that. The body cannot make them and must get them from ingesting them. There are two types of essential fatty acids, or EFA's. These are called Omega 6 and Omega 3 (named because of their biochemical structure). The Omega 6 oils come from mainly vegetables and nuts, (safflower, sunflower, sesame, corn and almond oil are some). Oil of evening primrose, oil of borage and black currant seed oil are good sources of high percentages of Omega 6 fatty acids.

Omega 3 oils come from cold water fish, like sardines, halibut, trout, salmon, herring, mackerel, and tuna. These are foods Eskimos eat and they have a notoriously lower rate of heart attack than other Americans ..... until they change their diet to ours. Also whole grains, beans, chestnuts and pumpkin seeds are substantial sources. Flaxseed (food grade linseed oil) is an excellent source of Omega 3.

All oils should be packaged in an opaque, dated con- tainer, as the more nutritious an oil is, the faster it will deteriorate. Absence of light and heat retard this oxida- tion. So buying small quantities at a time and storing in the refrigerator is recommended. You can readily appreciate how stripped of nutrients your grocery store oils are when they come in clear bottles and last forever in the pantry. The mere fact that they are colorless and odorless to begin with tells you much nutrition, like vitamins E and B6, and minerals like magnesium and manganese, are practically non- existent. And the advertisements thrive on your ignorance as they brag that their oils are clear, odorless, and taste- less.

Blood tests to determine if one is Omega 6 or Omega 3 deficient are not yet readily available on a wide scale. But a good rule of thumb would be a trial of Omega 3 first, since these oils have been drastically cut from the diet in the last century. If there is worsening, a trial of Omega 6 would be in order, the second commonest essential fatty acid deficiency.

As with any nutritional correction, a wide spectrum of symptom relief is possible, since we are all biochemically unique and each nutrient generally has a wide range of biochemical effects. With the proper oil change, common improvements occur with skin problems like eczema and psoriasis, and can extend to the psychoneuro immune system since the prostaglandins, neurotransmitters, hormone receptors, and enzymes depend on the proper ratio of EFA's for maximal function. For example, the ratio of Omega 3 to Omega 6 plus nutrients that metabolize them, determine the amounts of various types of prostaglandins that are made. Some are good and some are bad. They direct the activity and severity of all inflammatory diseases like asthma, migraines, colitis, arthritis, arteriosclerosis, prostatitis, etc. (The Omega-3 Phenomenon, Rudin, DO, Felix, C, Avon Books, NY 1988; plus Fats and Oils, Omega-3, The Fish Oil Factor, and Essential Fatty Acids and Immunity in Mental Health, see appendix). So as with any essential nutrient, any symptom (improvement) is possible when the system malfunctions. Likewise we have the knowledge to begin to manipulate the chemistry in our favor and turn off diseases.

For metabolism of either EFA, adequate levels of magnesium, zinc, selenium, and vitamins B, C, and E must be present as well as other nutrients.

Years ago, oils were extracted from seeds with heavy pressure, such as with roller presses. With the discovery of chemical processing, extraction procedures called hydrogenation replaced the roller or cold pressed methods. Hydrogenation exposed the seeds to extremely high temperatures over a thousand degrees Farenheit, which can change the normal cis form to trans form. The abnormally high heat causes an untwisting of the molecule, which now the body views as undesirable since it no longer is compatible with its chemistry. These deformed molecules just do not fit

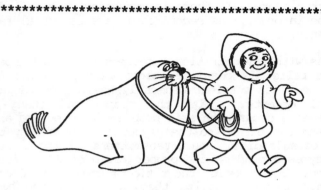

****

One of the reasons Eskimos can eat a higher fat
diet and not have the heart attack rate that we
do, is that cold water fish oils have a protective
factor, eicosapentaenoic acid (also known as EPA,
an Omega-3 oil) that fosters protective prostaglandins {PG-3 series}.

****

into the lipid or fatty matrix of cell membranes as a cis
configuration does.   In fact their fit into the cell membranes is analogous to trying to cram your right hand into a
left-handed bowling ball.   The overall effect is that the
body chemistry is stressed, so aging and degenerative
disease is accelerated.

It cannot be overstressed that this unnatural trans
form is highest in margarines (that are supposed to be
healthy substitutes for butter).   So margarines, plastic
creamers, "plastic" eggs (substitutes), and many other processed foods are helping you to dig your grave faster with
your teeth. And plastic foods lead to plastic hearts.

At this juncture your confusion is understandable.
After all, the cardiologists of the country recommend margarines and hydrogenated polyunsaturated oils for reducing

cholesterol. True they will reduce it, but at the time all this cholesterol information was coming out, very few biochemists knew of the deleterious effects of the hydrogenation procedure. They did not know that these trans processed oils actually accelerated arteriosclerosis and degenerative change and inhibited the D6D enzyme (which is necessary to convert them into body compounds that fight arthritis and arteriosclerosis). For example, in one study, eating margarines caused the trans fatty acids to be deposited in the heart itself. As more accumulated, there was, of course, a decrease in the good or protective fatty acids, and hence an essential fatty acid deficiency was induced in the heart muscle by dietary margarine intake (Hill, EG, et al, Intensification of essential fatty acid deficiency in the rat by dietary trans fatty acids, J. Nutr., 109, 1759-1765, 1979). Nor did the cardiologists know there were healthier ways to decrease cholesterol.

Meanwhile the food manufacturers learned there were great profits to be reaped. So they started educating physicians just like the drug industry does. So we have the science of health taught (and research funded) by industries that profit from the use of their products. Don't hold your breath for the margarine mistake to be corrected tomorrow (just don't eat any ever again, please).

If the "trans" formation were not bad enough, the processing procedures that accompany hydrogenation remove many precious nutrients like vitamin E, B6, chromium and magnesium that are also crucial to reducing arteriosclerosis and preventing early heart attacks (Fats and Oils, see appendix). And these are not replaced; only the cheaper B1, B2, B3 and iron are usually replaced. For example, frozen vegetables are often treated with EDTA to retain their color. This process strips much of the zinc from these foods (Mertz, W, The effects of zinc in man: nutritional considerations, in Clinical Applications of Zinc Metabolism, Pories, WJ, Strain, WH, Hsu, JM, Woolsey, RL, Eds., Charles C. Thomas Publ., Springfield IL, 1974).

You can read on any label the amount of nutrients that were added to "fortify" the product. Just remember: good whole food doesn't need to be fortified. If they hadn't stripped the nutrients so badly, there would be no laws about reconstituting. And you know when you have to legislate a supplement, that the minimum is what will be implemented. The source of these B vitamins is often merely yeast fermentation of left-over peels, juices and garbage. It is inexpensive to do, whereas adding correct amounts of non-rancid vitamin E, essential fatty acids, B6, molybdenum, boron, silica, zinc, etc. (which are not mandated, but are the cornerstones of preventing arteriosclerosis), would take some doing and be more expensive. Also I hope by now that you realize that when it says "provides 100% of the RDA (recommended daily allowance)" that what was 100% 30 years ago no longer holds. It only serves to confuse medicine all the more. For instead of people developing signs of easily diagnosable frank vitamin deficiencies, now people get subtle, vague, "subclinical" symptoms that defy diagnosis. In addition, the foods are even more processed, so people are getting less and our detox systems working harder, so we need even more!

Anyway, the removal of these nutrients from oils lengthens the shelf-life, but unfortunately the shelf-life of a product is inversely proportional to it's beneficial effects on your life. With the removal of nutrients, microorganisms find the food less nourishing and do not grow in it nor make it turn bad, or rancid as quickly. But if the bugs do not want it, why should you?

In essence, we have hydrogenated oils and margarines, and extended their shelf-lives by removing most of their nutrients, like vitamins E and B6 which actually protect against heart disease. These products are cloaked under the guise of lowering cholesterol, but so does wood fiber! Meanwhile they serve to further stress an already overstessed and nutritionally inadequate 20th century body.

In the wake of the cholesterol craze, bad press was given to the egg. This is an excellent and inexpensive source of lecithin, necessary, for example, to ward off changes like those seen in Alzheimer's presenile dementia. If you are on the correct vitamins, you can most likely tolerate eggs, and you can always have your cholesterol level checked to be sure. But there are very few places in the country where you can check the adequacy of your brain lecithin levels. By the time your short term memory is shot, it's too late.

You see, again, it's no longer a simple problem, but a complex series of blunders combined with megabucks Madison Avenue advertising hype that has gotten us into the wrong trend. The power of this is evident when intelligent people go out of their way to follow advice that they trust, only to be actually accelerating their journey down the path of degenerative disease. But again, a historical perspective will make it all blatantly clear:

(1) Man was originally a hunter/gatherer. He gathered herbs, fruits, vegetables, seeds, nuts and grains; and hunted (ran his butt off!) for wild game. For example, wild game is about 30-60% polyunsaturated fatty acids, while domestic (commercial) meat is 2-17% (New England Journal of Medicine, vol. 312, page 283-289, 1985). So his diet was high in Omega 3 oil and high in exercise. It was also

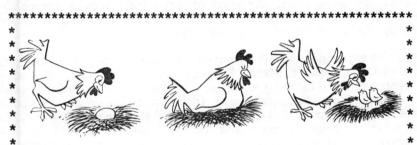

****
* *
* *
* *
* *
* *
* *
* *
* *
* *
* *
* The poor egg has been unfairly denigrated. When *
* you have healthy levels of chromium, magnesium, *
* and other nutrients, you can usually metabolize *
* your cholesterol. The egg (as are soybeans) is a *
* good source of lecithin, one of the nutrients *
* essential to prevent Alzheimer's disease. *
* *
****

devoid of processed foods and chemical overload.

(2) As this century evolved, man had the means to eat what
he liked, over what was available. So every night Mr.
Suburbia was seen out in the backyard grilling hamburgers,
steaks, and hotdogs. And these came from feed lot animals
with inferior levels of fatty acids (2-17%). Breakfasts
were a lumberjack's feast of sausages and eggs. But instead
of trudging off to the forest, he rode to work in a car and
sat at a desk all day. On weekends he watched football.

(3) Meanwhile eating all this meat turned on his sweet
tooth for balance and he began increasing his sugar and
white flour with resultant vitamin and mineral loss, thereby
making it more impossible for him to properly metabolize or
break down his excess cholesterol. Remember many people eat
very high cholesterol diets and have no arteriosclerosis.
Is it because they do not have the hidden mineral and essential fatty acid deficiencies that prevent their systems from
functioning optimally? They eat real whole foods with all
the nutrients intact, not processed foods loaded with fat,
salt, and sugar, and stripped of arteriosclerosis preventing
vitamins like E and B6, and minerals like magnesium, manganese, chromium, zinc, and vanadium.

(4) Margarines were invented to save money for us poor
folks who couldn't afford butter. Then along came the polyunsaturated oils with nearly all the vitamins and minerals
stripped from them, packaged in clear bottles so you could
see just how pure this devitalized, tasteless oil was. The
vitamin E they removed was often repackaged with a mold
retardant and sold back to people in the form of petrochemi-
cal glycerinated vitamin capsules.

(5) When the cholesterol craze hit, eggs, butter, and beef
were blamed. Little did anyone know that the unnatural
hydrogenation density of margarine was not good for the body
and accelerated degeneration, for it had not yet been tested. Nor did they realize that the full complement of vitamins and minerals was no longer present in many foods to
metabolize this cholesterol. Nor did they understand that

the #1 cause in the rise of cholesterol was due to lack of nutrients and exercise to properly metabolize it (as proven by many studies where, for example, the correction of a chromium, B6, fatty acid, or magnesium deficiency corrected the cholesterol level: Chromium deficiency as a factor in arteriosclerosis, Schroeder, HA, Mason, AP, Tipton, IH, <u>J. Chron. Dis.</u>, 23: 123-142, 1970; there are many more recent articles but this gives you a hint at the fact that this information is not brand new!).

An excessive diet of red meats was properly identified as one cause of high cholesterol, while nutrient depleted processed foods and sugar were virtually ignored for years

Instead of an occasional feast on a wild animal that he had chased and hunted, sedentary Mr. Suburbia is out in his backyard nightly grilling feedlot beef with inferior levels of protective essential fatty acids. No wonder he has high cholesterol.

in their ability to greatly potentiate arteriosclerosis. As the years rolled by the the lack of exercise was picked up on and you saw the jogging craze.

But for some who were marginal in some nutrient, for example magnesium, this just served to push them over the edge and they died (of cardiac arrhythmia, for example).

(6) Meanwhile more people ate packaged foods, ate in restaurants, and fast foods took over. Fried foods were at the top of the popularity list and the stage was set for the decline in ingestion of Omega 3 fatty acids. People rarely ate fish or fresh seeds, but had plenty of corn and safflower oils. The worst and most popular oil was "100% pure vegetable oil", for this added other problems in addition to hydrogenation. This broad term of vegetable provided a license to include less desirable oils such as:
1. Peanut (often contaminated with a tasteless, odorless toxin from molds, aflatoxin, that is a potent cause of cancer and is not destroyed by cooking).
2. Cottonseed (contaminated with special pesticides because cotton is not considered a food).
3. Coconut oil (which is saturated and as bad as lard for you).

In essence, man is no longer the hunter; he is rarely even a gatherer. Eat butter and eggs occasionally if you like, but have your fasting cholesterol checked periodically to assess the correctness of this for you. In the meantime reduce red meat to 1-2 times a week if you need it, increase naturally grown, deep water fish (not commercially raised on dog food - like pellets or caught near shore by river mouths that carry heavy industry toxic wastes to the ocean) to over twice a week and attempt to gradually make meals 50-50 whole grains (not flour products) and vegetables. Avoid all margarines and grocery store oils. Use only olive oil for occasional high heat cooking or unrefined sesame oil for low heat cooking. Give yourself a trial oil change of Omega 3's. If you worsen, switch to Omega 6's. After a 3-6 month trial of either, back off to a more balanced routine. Your nutritionally oriented physician should guide you in this endeavor, for there still remains much for you to know.

Being aware of advertising hype is the most important step, but difficult unless you plan on forfeiting your weekends to search the biochemistry journals in the local medical school library. For now you have learned much that will help you interpret the trick wording that capitalizes on people's ignorance:

(1) Any oil or shortening that says its "great for cooking, frying, baking" is always of low quality because no oil is good for this since heat destroys EFA's.

(2) "Contains no preservatives" is meaningless because cold pressed oil has its own natural preservative, vitamin E, and bad hydrogenated oil has been so destroyed that no self respecting bug would set foot in it. Hence, it lasts for years in the pantry without preservatives because it is dead.

(3) "No cholesterol" is redundant, since no plant oils contain cholesterol anyway. Also you cannot live without cholesterol; your body makes it to enable all membranes, nerve sheaths, sex and adrenal hormones, skin oils, bile acids, vitamin D and more to function.

(4) "High in polyunsaturates" is meaningless because it can contain as little as 2% to qualify for this misnomer. Likewise, even though the essential oils are polyunsaturated (contain double bonds that promote more fluidity in your membranes), so do many nonessential oils that your body manufactures.

(5) "100% pure corn oil" margarine does not tell the unsuspecting buyer that yes, it is made from corn oil, then hydrogenated to saturate bonds and hardened it into a margarine that is 25% unnatural trans oils (which inhibit the D-6-D enzyme that

would normally promote the synthesis of body hormones to protect you against arteriosclerosis and heart disease).

(6) "100% natural" has been over exploited, recognizing that people are getting a smidge more educated. Cyanide is 100% natural.

(7) Look for "organic, cold-pressed" oils. If the manufacturer is knowledgeable and proud of his product, it will be in an opaque package because he knows light accelerates rancidity. It will also have an expiration date, since all vital oils deteriorate with time. Lastly, it will be found in the refrigerator of the health food store, since heat accelerates deterioration, and that's where it will go when you get it home, too.

(8) And watch out for any products that boast "high in fiber". They know that you know a high fiber diet lowers your cholesterol by decreasing the gut transit time. What you don't know is that often the words "methyl cellulose" will appear in the fine print of the ingredients list. This is wood fiber or sawdust! So unless you're part beaver, you won't get much nutrition from it. A much better form of fiber, complete with real live vitamins and minerals, is the fiber of whole grains and fresh vegetables.

Medicine has gone full circle. In the turn of the century doctors used herbs and vitamins, and shunned patent medicines and snake oils. As antibiotics took over, pharmaceutical companies learned that megabucks and power over medical practice were theirs with marketing. Subsequently, the food industry hitched up with Madison Avenue advertising and jumped on the wagon. The overworked doctor had little time to keep up with advances, much less do independent biochemistry research to check the validity of all this. Now we know that how we eat and think is capable of producing far greater health than any processed food or pills. And with modern day assay techniques, we have even discovered that snake oil is a great source of essential fatty acids!

Scientists all over the world are now learning that they can manipulate many inflammatory and allergic conditions by directing the chemistry with better oils (lipids) and gradually changing over the oils in cell membranes to the preferred forms. They first became interested in this when they learned that Eskimos eat an extremely high fat diet, but do not have early coronary artery disease until they come to the United States and eat our diet. They learned that there was a protective factor in fish oil that lowered cholesterol. Scientists also now know that the trans oils that are in margarines and regular grocery store oils inhibit an enzyme called Delta 6 Desaturase (D-6-D), which is important in metabolizing good oils so that they can become incorporated into the membranes where they belong for optimal function.

Remember cholesterol (eggs are a good source) is not bad. In fact you must have it in membranes to be alive; it makes them rigid (to keep the cell contents from spilling all over). Likewise, you must have lecithin (phosphatidyl choline, from eggs and beans, for example) for that makes the membranes fluid (for messenger molecules to pass in and out easily). It's the cholesterol to phospholipid ratio that is crucial, as well as all the other nutrients like vitamin B1, etc. We must remember balance is the key. When the proper nutrients are on board, cholesterol can be metabolized the way it should, and incorporated into the membrane. Cholesterol does not just aimlessly shoot around until it lays down and dies whereever it finds a spot, like in arteries! Abnormal deposits of cholesterol, or calcium, or anything else happen because the necessary nutrients are not available for the body to do what it is supposed to do with it. It's really quite logical when you think of it. Now we need to break out of this Madison Avenue trap that keeps recommending more drugs and more plastic foods to correct the ills of 20th century man.

I am reminded of a tiny Caribbean island that is my favorite, for it has some of the loveliest people I've ever known. When I became familiar with their cooking techniques I couldn't understand how they had such good health using coconut oil for years for cooking. After all, it's a saturated oil and should potentiate degenerative disease. But their years of isolation from the rest of the world is what saved them. For they were essentially seamen and lived on fish and vegetables they were able to grow. The balance of good oils was sufficient.

Then when an airport was constructed, things changed. I saw that the children no longer came home from school and opened a fresh coconut, but instead went to the tiny store and bought a soda. American-type groceries appeared with processed foods and people fell in love with beef and sugar. Now children (in their 50's and 60's) of parents who died of natural causes in their 90's, have diabetes, cataracts, arthritis, hypertension, and cancer. And there is no longer a local market where you can daily buy fresh, unfrozen fish. Their dream has come true: they have become Americanized.

How To Do Your Own Oil Change

At this juncture you may want to take 4-6 months and see what effect changing your oils over to the good form will have. The Omega 3 oil change is the most likely to benefit. Cook only with olive oil, since it is less easily changed to a trans form when heated. (It is neither Omega 3 nor 6, but Omega 9 and is less easily damaged by high heat). Do not ever use margarine or regular grocery store oils again. Never eat fried foods nor buy prepared food containing oils (candy, baked goods like breads and cookies, ice cream, oil roasted nuts, packaged mixes, commercial salad dressings, packaged dinners, etc.). Use butter on the table if you want, and be sure to get one or two tablespoons of cold pressed food grade linseed or flaxseed oil daily (available from N.E.E.D.S. (Drumlins Pharmacy), 1-800-634-1380 or Allergy Resources, 1-800-USE-FLAX).

To use this oil you can simply pour it on granola, rice, potatoes or squash, or you can put it in a blender with garlic, parsley, and lemon to make a dressing (a few anchovies makes it a Caesar's dressing), or you can just drink it plain. Do not heat the oil, for heat destroys the Omega 3 functions. If you are sensitive to linseed (flax-seed), it requires a bit more planning to get a couple of grams of Omega 3 oils in per day, but it is possible. Consider using cold pressed walnut or soy oil. A teaspoon of old fashioned cod liver oil is also a good source, but be sure to reduce your vitamin A and D from other sources. Or snack frequently on chestnuts and pumpkin seeds and have a can of sardines in sild oil a few times a week.

Make sure all oils you ingest are cold pressed. Also to make this program successful, you must reduce sugars and red meat to once or twice a week, maximum. And eating oily, cold water ocean fish (like salmon and mackerel) a couple a times per week, minimum, helps make this change come about, as they are high in Omega-3. If you must eat red meat, try to find undomesticated wild animals. They have higher amounts of beneficial EFA's than commercially grown animals who are not naturally grazed but fed a synthetic commercial-ized diet. Additional Max-EPA, one or two capsules 2-3 times per day might also be used depending on your require-ments and tolerances. You should see your doctor for direc-tions in incorporating this into your diet and for a calcu-lation of the proper doses; assess your blood levels of vital companion nutrients, whose status will be greatly aided by trading in white flour and white sugar for whole grains (like brown rice) and vegetables (like kale and col-lards, squash, carrots and onions).

Studies show that many people with severe arthritis who are put on very high doses of Omega 3 precursor oils are having no pain, and require no medication after a 6 month oil change. This is because it promotes the synthesis of nature's own anti-inflammatory prostaglandins. Remember it takes 3-6 months to change your oils over from the bad kind to the good kind. For the moment you may want to see what effect just changing your oils over to the correct type has on your body chemistry.

With all the research that is coming out, it is pretty exciting that we are able to manipulate the body into becoming less reactive to environmental insults. So isn't it about time that you had your oil changed?

```
*************************************************************
*                                                           *
*                                                           *
*                                                           *
*                                                           *
*                                                           *
*                                                           *
*                                                           *
*                                                           *
*                                                           *
*                                                           *
*                                                           *
*                                                           *
*                                                           *
*                                                           *
*                                                           *
*                                                           *
*                                                           *
*                                                           *
*                                                           *
*                                                           *
*                                                           *
*                                                           *
*         Aren't you due for an oil change?  Let's get      *
*         rid of all those damaging trans fatty acids from  *
*         years of margarine and other processed foods and  *
*         change over to protective oils.                   *
*                                                           *
*************************************************************
```

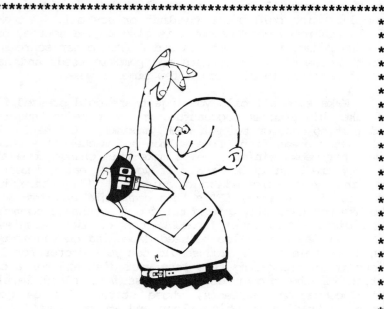

QUICK STOP SUMMARY

<u>Omega 3 Oil Change</u> (Many people have improved migraine, asthma, cardiac disease, hypertension, arthritis, psoriasis, etc.)
    1. For six months replace red meat and dairy with

cold water ocean fish, no white sugar or white flours are allowed either.

2. 50% of every meal, and/or every plate, should be vegetables, raw or cooked.
3. At least 1/3 of each plate, and/or meal, should be organic whole grains (brown rice, oats, millet, barley, quinoa, amaranth, or teff, etc.), and/or beans.
4. Cook with olive oil, or unrefined sesame oil.
5. Use 1-3 tbsp (depending upon your doctor's advice and your blood work results) of flaxseed oil per day (opaque, dated refrigerated bottle).
6. Be sure your vitamin/mineral levels are excellent and do the magnesium loading test, for you will never convert the flax oil to eicosapentaenoic acid without sufficient magnesium.
7. See the doctor if you need substitutes for any of the above.
8. Consider an Omega 6 trial if the above makes you worse.
9. Eat no processed foods, no grocery store oils or margarines.

A salmon a day may keep a coronary away!

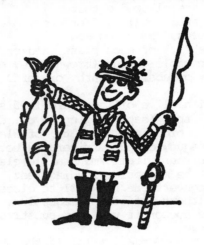

A salmon a day may keep a coronary away!

<u>Omega 6 Oil Change</u> (This has helped many people have improved PMS, eczema, hyperactivity, learning, disorders, psoriasis, etc.)

1. For six months you may have dairy and red meat once or twice a week if desired.
2. Eat 50% vegetables every meal, or plate, and at least 30% whole grains, and/or beans.
3. Cook with olive oil, use cold pressed safflower, corn, soy, sunflower, or almond for uncooked oil source, or take it plain, 2 tbsp per day.
4. Oil of evening primrose capsules (Efamol is best) 2 capsules, 2-4 times per day, depending upon the doctor's advise. Oil of borage or black currant seed oil may be substituted.
5. Avoid peanut oil, as it can be contaminated with unassayable carcinogenic mycotoxins. Likewise, avoid any "vegetable oil", since these blends may also contain cotton seeds (many potent pesticides allowed on cotton, as it is not considered a food), and/or coconut (a saturated oil like lard).

****

The Myth Of Degenerative Disease

A degenerative disease is supposedly part of natural aging, the result of the wear and tear of life on our bodies. It has a steady but slow downhill course. But did you know that you can actually <u>cure</u> some degenerative disease processes and not only stop them, but get rid of the symptoms entirely? And for those who want, you can go to the next step and actually cause regeneration or turn back the hands of time and make the tissue/organ as healthy as it was years ago. In short, you can make degeneration become regeneration. Of course, it takes knowledge.

The commonest degenerative disease is arteriosclerosis, or "hardening of the arteries". It is also the number one cause of death in the U.S. With time, arteries become dry and brittle, and get plugged up with deposits of cholesterol, calcium, and (as you have already learned) many of the junk chemicals that the detox pathway could not transform and eliminate. So these aging, damaged arteries appear to become the dumping ground or toxic waste site for excess substances the body has no use for.

As a consequence of arteries becoming rigid, blood pressure goes up. And as a consequence of their becoming plugged and narrowed with deposits, the end organs they supply become sick, as they no longer get as much blood supply for oxygen and nutrition as prior. So we commonly see heart failure which in turn leads to swollen ankles and shortness of breath as the major pump (heart) becomes flabby and swollen. We see angina (chest pain), strokes, claudication (severe pains in abdomen and legs because not enough oxygen can get through these clogged vessels to the muscles), senility, undesirable personality change, poor function of glands (like the pancreas leading to diabetes, or poorly functioning thyroid leading to the sluggish exhaustion of hypothyroidism), impotency (inability to have an erection because the vessels cannot supply enough oxygen and nutrients) and a host of other symptoms.

But when you understand the many biochemical glitches that lead to degenerative disease, various levels of correction are possible, all the way up to regeneration.

The Chromium Catastrophe

You probably associate chromium with your car bumper. You know it is added as a protective covering that will prevent rust or oxidation of the underlying steel. Remember you learned that "rusting" or oxidation (mediated by those nasty electrons called free radicals) is also the cause of aging and degenerative disease in the body.

Free radicals are produced as a byproduct of many chemical reactions in the body. Inhaled chemicals, rancid oils, and aldehydes which spill over from the aldehyde bottleneck are only a few of the many causes. These free radicals bounce around and chew holes wherever they can. The commonest place is in the blood vessel wall. Once an injury has occurred, the body tries to patch it up. It uses anything that is handy ..... left-over calcium (because someone forgot to balance the prescription with other nutrients so it could be laid down in the bone), left-over cholesterol (because the owner is stuffing himself with high cholesterol food and/or because he doesn't have all the proper nutrients that will enable him to metabolize the cholesterol properly), and chemicals (that have overwhelmed the detox pathways. The overflow ends up also floating freely in the blood, waiting for a nice (free radical) damaged spot to lay down to rest in). Chromium is a protector of rust, if you will, in the blood vessel lining just as much as it is on your car bumper. If you have enough of it

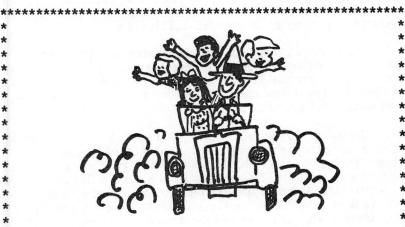

Just as chromium protects your bumper from pitting and rusting, it protects the lining of your arteries from the very same thing. For when pits form here, cholesterol is laid down in attempt to patch the holes.

and other nutrients, the vessel wall will not develop cholesterol deposits, because there is no scratch for the rust
(cholesterol) to begin in (no blood vessel lining tear,
known as an intimal defect). It is only damaged, unprotected vessels that use cholesterol to patch up (free radical or rust) holes. If there's no hole, there's no need for
the patch.

So it's a down-right catastrophe that this knowledge
has not been disseminated to the American public, where
arteriovascular disease is the #1 cause of death. But then
you'd have to have physicians checking rbc chromium levels,
magnesium loading tests, rbc zinc, etc.; this is just plain
not taught (except by the American Academy of Environmental
Medicine). And besides, what would you do with all those
fake eggs, and "low cholesterol" sausages and cheeses, not
to mention all those drugs to lower cholesterol? It would
just upset everything. Of course all of these synthetic
products are also free-radical initiators.

Needless to say, it would require a vast re-education
and restructuring of many institutions, so we'll probably
ease into it gradually over the next 50 years. The problem
is that in the meantime, someone near and dear to you may
needlessly and prematurely succumb.

Chromium is a well-known nutrient for its beneficial
effects on glucose (sugar) and cholesterol metabolism. In
other words we must have enough of it for these to be
handled properly in the body. It is particularly important
in regulating insulin and correcting hypoglycemia and diabetes (which also eventually accelerate arteriosclerosis).
Many people who are overweight because of hypoglycemia and
sugar cravings are actually chromium deficient and cannot
break the cycle until an rbc chromium is measured.

Researchers have shown that 70% of people over age 77
are chromium deficient. In line with that, the incidence of
diabetes rises with age. In fact, 40% of the people over 40
(without diabetes) have abnormal glucose tolerance tests and
50% of these improved with chromium.

Furthermore, whole grain wheat contains 1.75 mcg/gm of chromium while white flour only contains 0.23 and white bread contains 0.14. Likewise, many processed foods contain very little chromium, so people are gradually becoming progressively more deficient. When we did a mineral analysis of hundreds of patients, chromium was one of the leading deficiencies. Why is this important? Because it is often an overlooked fact that exposure of the arterial wall to insulin (because of high sugar diets and lack of chromium) initiates the course of events that causes arteriosclerosis {smooth muscle proliferation, inhibition of lipolysis and increase in cholesterol, phospholipids and triglycerides}. In fact, in one study, people who died of arteriosclerosis had lower chromium content of their aortas (the major artery from the heart) compared with normal people.

Likewise, diabetic children have significantly lower levels of hair chromium than normal children (concentration of chromium in the hair of normal children and children with juvenile diabetes mellitus, Hambridge, KM, Rogerson, DD, O'Brien, D, Diabetes, 17; 8 517-518, 1968), yet how many diabetics have been checked for the chromium since 1968?

What does all this mean? It means just what we have observed. High cholesterol and arteriosclerotic plaques that plug up brain and heart vessels are not a simplistic result of a high cholesterol diet. Instead, they are the result of multiple proven deficiencies like chromium, magnesium, vitamin B6, Omega-3 essential fatty acids, and the many more nutrients found only in whole food diets. The levels are too low in processed food diets and only become progressively worse with time. No chemist can hope to scoop mother nature. We can correct some blatant deficiencies, but maintenance of health requires that the true balance of nutrients should come predominantly from organic whole grains and vegetables.

Studies show that platelets (blood clotting cells floating in the blood stream) play a significant role in creating blood clots, especially in people with elevated lipids (blood fats) and arteriosclerosis. It has been shown that moderate amounts of dietary Omega-3 fatty acid supplementation in humans can significantly effect the platelet activity in patients at risk (Levine, PH, et al, Dietary supplementation with omega-3 fatty acids prolongs platelet survival in hyperlipidemic patients with arteriosclerosis, Arch. Intern. Med., 149, 1113-1116, May 1989).

In essence, chromium regulates the metabolism of sugars, lipids (cholesterol), and amino acids. All of these are crucial factors in the genesis of arteriosclerosis, not to mention diabetes, cataracts, and heart disease. Yet we do not measure rbc chromium and change the diet; instead we prescribe drugs because it's quicker, easier, makes more money, and the compliance is probably greater. Yet studies abound showing 17.6% of major tissues in American subjects lack chromium, compared with 1.57% of the same tissues from individuals from other parts of the world (Schroeder, HA, Am. J. Clin. Nutr., 21:230, 1968). Clearly the land of plenty offers too much of the wrong foods.

Among millions of U.S. diabetics, how many have had an rbc chromium checked? I never met one. Yet experimental chromium deficiency in animals causes diabetes and is reversible with chromium (Schroeder, HA, J. Nutr., 88:439, 1966). And when chromium was administered to diabetic people, 50% had reversion of their glucose tolerance tests to normal within 4 months (Glinsmann, WH, Metabolism, 15:510, 1966). The other 50% most likely had other deficiencies as would be expected and would not improve until they were all found. Bear in mind that this study is nearly a quarter of a century old and many have followed it.

Clearly we have been remiss in not assaying rbc chromium levels in all cardiac patients. In many studies the groups with coronary artery disease have significantly lower chromium levels than the normal group with unobstructed arteries. And this eleven year old study used serum which isn't as sensitive. (Newman, et al, Serum chromium and angiographically determined coronary artery disease, Clin. Chem., 24, 4, 541-544, 1978). And their study showed persons dying of coronary artery heart disease to have virtually no chromium in their arteries (Abraham, AS, et al, Serum chromium in patients with recent and old myocardial

infarction, Am. Heart. J., 99, 5, 604-606, May 1980). There
is no doubt that chromium deficiency is one of the mineral
deficiencies causing diabetes and arteriosclerosis (Boyle,
E, et al, Chromium depletion in the pathogenesis of diabetes
and arteriosclerosis, Southern Med. J., 70, 12, 1449-1453,
Dec. 1977).

Besides being important in glucose and cholesterol
metabolism, chromium is necessary for energy and membrane
synthesis for the detoxication system (Chromium In Nutrition
and Disease, G. Saner, Alan R. Liss, Inc., NY, 1980). As
well, the digestive enzyme typsin requires chromium. Since
chromium is concentrated in hair, it makes a good assay
(Doctors Data, Chicago, IL), especially since the plasma
level (as with many other minerals) is useless. An rbc (red
blood cell) chromium is looking promising, however.
    The absorption of chromium is depressed by calcium,
zinc, iron, manganese, and phytates (undercooked grains).
So a deficiency is easy to cause. And like other minerals,
the diet is the major cause of deficiency since it is vastly
reduced in processed foods so that they last longer. Severe
deficiency states rarely exist, only marginal or "subclinical" states do. Which translates into symptoms that are
impossible to diagnose. There is no symptom that will tell
you that you absolutely lack chromium. Besides that, if you
lack chromium, most assuredly you lack many other nutrients,
for it would be unusual to get a singular deficiency. Like
cancer, the symptoms take years to insidiously amount to
anything diagnosable. Then when you finally have end organ
failure (hypertension, diabetes, cardiac arrhythmia, heart
attack, stroke), the acute care medical team takes over and
drugs are used.

    Meanwhile, advertising, the food industry, and pharma-
ceutical companies rake in huge profits as you guzzle plastic foods and medications in attempt to control arteriosclerosis. When in fact, even though the return to normal
of your blood test for cholesterol may help you breathe a
sigh of relief, it's an "ignorance is bliss" sigh. For
lowering your dietary cholesterol is only a small part of
the problem. Without adequate nutrients (vitamins, minerals, amino acids, essential fatty acids, and accessory

nutrients), the body can't even convert your cholesterol into the adrenal, testosterone and progesterone hormones that it must have. It cannot make adequate bile acids for Phase II conjugation or lipid membranes for the endoplasmic reticulum where Phase I detox takes place. And without these nutrients, cholesterol wanders about and appears more excessive than it may actually be, merely because the body doesn't have the mechanism to process it. So it gets deposited in the garbage heap: the inflamed, chromium deficient vessel wall.

Even if you didn't want to investigate the biochemical glitch that keeps you from properly metabolizing your cholesterol you could evaluate a trial of niacin (vitamin B3), for this handles the level nicely in many (Luria, M, Effect of low-dose niacin on high-density lipoprotein cholesterol and total cholesterol/high-density lipoprotein cholesterol ratio. Arch. Int. Med., 148, 2493-2495, 1988). And for those who flush from niacin, an aspirin prevents this (and is an anti-coagulant to boot!).

In essence, the body needs cholesterol and cannot live without it. It becomes elevated only partly because we eat high cholesterol foods. It also is elevated because we lack the nutrients to properly metabolize it. Finally when the detox mechanism of blood vessel walls fails, and the body lacks the nutrients to properly metabolize cholesterol, then cholesterol is pathologically deposited in blood vessel walls.

The same thing happens with people taking calcium. Their doctors tell them to take it to prevent osteoporosis. But without boron, magnesium, zinc, silica, copper, and other necessary nutrients, the body cannot incorporate it into the bone matrix. So what does it do with this excess trash floating in the blood? Sends it to the dump. So people taking calcium without good nutritional biochemical direction are actually laying calcium down inside (chromium deficient) blood vessels and raising their potential for senile arteriosclerosis or their first heart attack.

The Cholesterol Controversy

Furthermore certain aldehyde dehydrogenase isoenzymes (one of the biochemical bottlenecks) metabolize intermediaries of cholesterol metabolism (Vol 114, Enzymology of Carbonyl Metabolism, Alan R. Liss, Inc. New York, 1982). What does this translate into? If the aldehyde enzymes are busy metabolizing excess.....

sugars	(Americans are hung up on sweets and alcohol),
alcohols	(alcohols go through the aldehyde path),
antibiotics	(they foster Candida overgrowth that synthesizes acetaldehyde),
chemicals	(in home, office, and outside air, food and water),
cigarette smoke	(from yourself or second hand smoke from others)

and

neurotransmitters (mental stress causes formation of brain stress hormones which get metabolized via monoamine oxidase through aldehyde pathways),

...then there won't be enough aldehyde metabolizing enzymes to go around and something suffers. When cholesterol metabolism suffers, we tell people to eat less of it. The fallacy of that is they need cholesterol in order to make important hormones and membranes. Eating less of it does not solve the problem of the biochemical block leading to impaired utilization. You can easily see that what you should eat less of is sugars, alcohol, antibiotics, chemicals, cigarette smoke and stress! It's all so simple when you understand the chemistry.

Ironically, when eating less cholesterol doesn't help, physicians prescribe drugs to lower the cholesterol. Now you're in deeper trouble, because not only does this further overload the aldehyde path with another chemical so that you're bound to get other symptoms and/or diseases, but it

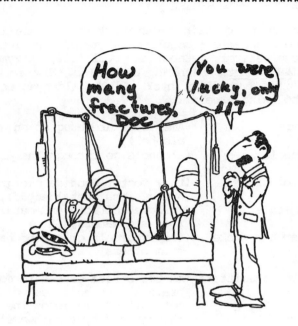

```
***********************************************************
*                                                         *
*                                                         *
*                                                         *
*                                                         *
*                                                         *
*                                                         *
*                                                         *
*                                                         *
*                                                         *
*                                                         *
*                                                         *
*                                                         *
*                                                         *
*                                                         *
*                                                         *
*                                                         *
*                                                         *
*                                                         *
*                                                         *
*                                                         *
*                                                         *
*                                                         *
*                                                         *
*                                                         *
*     Before you succumb to osteoporosis, make sure you   *
*     have sufficient magnesium, zinc, manganese, boron,  *
*      nd other trace minerals so that the calcium you    *
*     take can be deposited in the bones, not in your     *
*     brain and coronary blood vessels.                   *
*                                                         *
***********************************************************
```

dangerously interferes with the amount of cholesterol available to the body. This will cause very serious deficits in hormones and functional membranes necessary for energy, detox, etc. Some of these membrane deficits are bound to be in the brain and eventually contribute to senility.

And it's not just an overloaded detox path from daily 20th century chemical exposure that interferes with cholesterol metabolism. It's not just an unrecognized chromium deficiency from years of sweets that interferes with cholesterol metabolism. It's not just a magnesium deficiency from years of processed food and prescription medications that interferes with cholesterol metabolism. It's not just manganese, zinc, vanadium, and vitamin E and B6 deficiencies that promote arteriosclerosis. It's not just being over-stressed, causing the metabolism of the brain neurotransmitters or stress hormones to overload the aldehyde bottle-necks of the detoxication scheme. It's all of these factors and many more. But the most exciting fact of all of this, is that, IF YOU CHOOSE, you can have total control.

You see now why the ball is in your court. You can be as healthy as you choose. The price you will need to pay is spending time to get smart. The price you need to pay is making time to educate yourself, to change your diet, life-style, and attitude. But look at the rewards. Are you going to wait 20 years when this knowledge about health will be in vogue, or do it now?

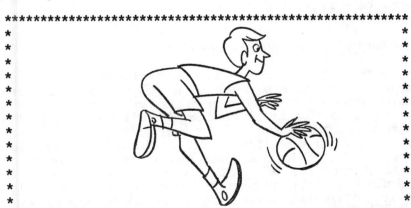

****

The ball is in your court now. You are armed with enough facts to appreciate that you are the major determining factor of how healthy you will be.

****

The Myth Of The Calcium Craze

Now-a-days we're not even waiting for the sick to get sicker. We're taking the well ones and teaching them how to make themselves sick.

How many physicians who recommend calcium go to the trouble to be sure that the other nutrients that are depended upon for calcium to be laid down in the bone where it belongs are also adequate? Do they remind patients to cut sugars way down to reduce the inflammation in the wall of the vessel so that it doesn't become the dumping ground for excess unmetabolized calcium? Do they remind them that nearly all processed foods (especially sodas) contain high amounts of phosphates that inhibit absorption of calcium? Or that 2 cups of organic greens a day can supply more calcium than a glass of milk and provide many of the missing trace minerals as well? These are the very minerals that many people are lacking and without which the calcium will never be incorporated into the bone.

The Myth Of Osteoporosis Prevention

The way osteoporosis is taught to physicians and subsequently to their patients boils down to estrogen, exercise, sometime fluoride (which is an aging factor) and plenty of calcium in the diet and in pill form. Many recommend the carbonate form which actually doubles as a antacid, in spite of studies showing that sufficient gastric acidity must be present for the first step of assimilation of calcium (Nicar, MJ, Pak, CYC, Calcium bioavailability from calcium carbonate and calcium citrate, J. Clin. Endocrinol. Metab., 61:39-393, 1985; Recker, RR, Calcium absorption and achlorhydria, N. Engl. J. Med., 313, 70-73, 1985; Brechner, J, Armstrong, WD, Relation of gastric acidity to alveolar bone resorption, Prov. Soc. Exp. Biol. Med., 44:98, 1941).

The field of nutritional biochemistry understandably changes the cookbook of medicine where we expect one disease to have one treatment, and another disease to have a different one. For example, papers cite the lowering of cholesterol by correcting deficiencies in copper, essential fatty acids, and vitamins B5 and B3. It depends on where the biochemical glitch is for the particular individual. On the flip side, one singular nutrient can improve diverse conditions. Reports show, for example, that vitamin B6 has improved PMS, carpal tunnel syndrome, depression, exhaustion, hyperemesis gravidarum, arteriosclerosis, Chinese restaurant syndrome (MSG sensitivity), abnormal glucose tolerance test, asthma, renal stones, schizophrenia, and stocking and glove type neuropathies (numbness and tingling) (Buist, R, Intern. Clin. Nutr. Rev., 4, 1, Jan. 1984). It all depends on the individual's needs and target organ vulnerability. Our biochemistry is very individually unique.

But the reasons medicine is so frustrated with its results in treating osteoporosis are many:
1. It may take 10-50 years to find out if what was recommended worked, since there is not yet any fully adequate blood test or X-ray to detect early stages.
2. They have concentrated on calcium and estrogen to the neglect of multiple trace minerals, like zinc (Frithrof, L, et al, The relationship between marginal bone loss and serum zinc levels, Acta. Med. Scand., 207:67-70, 1980), manganese (Leach, RM, et al, Studies in the role of manganese in bone formation, J. Nutr., 78, 51-56, 1962), silicon (Carlisle, EM, Silicon localization and calcification in developing bone, Fed. Proc., 28:374, 1969), and boron (Nielsen, FH, et al, Effect of dietary boron on mineral, estrogen, and testosterone metabolism in postmenopausal women. Found. Adv. Sci. Exp. Biol. J., 1:394-397, 1987).

This latter element is particularly exciting because it not only decreased the urinary excretion of calcium by

44%, but increased the natural estrogen in the subjects so that their levels were comparable to those of women on estrogen. The only difference is they were not subject to the potentially dangerous side effects of women on exogenous estrogens. The list of complementary nutrients required for proper bone formation goes on. The fact that they are deficient in modern diets leads us to the third reason why current osteoporosis treatment fails:

3.   The diets are progressively more mineral depleted because of depleted soils, food processing, and poor food choices or selection by the individual. Over one-half the manganese is lost going from a whole grain wheat to a refined flour (Wenloch, RW, et al, Trace nutrients. 2. Manganese in British food, Br. J. Nutr., 41:253-261, 1979). And evidence for widespread deficiencies are scattered throughout the literature. For example one study reports 68% of adults consumed less than 2/3 of the RDA of zinc (Holde, et al, Zinc and copper in self-selected diets, J. Am. Diet. Assoc., 75:23-28, 1979).

4.   Phosphates (higher in processed foods) inhibit the absorption of calcium. But rarely are patients prescribed a whole foods diet, not to mention getting off (calcium-losing) sodas, sugared goodies and prepared foods. Also self-prescribed minerals can interfere as well.

5.   Rarely is the amount of gastric hydrochloric acid checked even though it is well-known that it decreases with age (N. Engl. J. Med., 1973) and a significant percent of the population is without teeth and has a host of other maladies that could be traced in part to hydrochlorhydria (low hydrochloric acid, or HCl for short, in the stomach). It's the stomach acid that allows minerals to begin the chemical changes necessary so they can be absorbed further on down in the small intestine. A test for adequate acid and a betaine-HCl supplementation may be necessary.

So osteoporosis prevention is far more than calcium. And to add estrogen with its increased risk of cancer is risky, especially when levels can be raised with nutrient balance. Besides calcium, zinc, manganese, silicon and boron, copper strontium and magnesium as well as B6, C, D, K, and folic acid are necessary. (One manufacturer puts all these in a preparation, Osteo-Prime Forte: 1-800-553-2370).

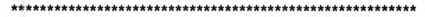

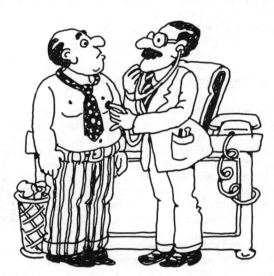

The calcium you take for your bones may well end up in your coronary or brain arteries, leading to an early heart attack or senility, if you choose to remain ignorant of your chromium and magnesium status. You are the major determining factor of the outcome.

Probably there are other factors missing and only time will tell. But the weight of the evidence suggests the balanced nutritional route makes a great deal more sense than calcium carbonate being recommended and prescriptions of estrogen. This should be the last resort because if the estrogen is insufficient, its production may be hampered by mineral deficiencies that have not been sought. And to add calcium, unaccompanied by the minerals that facilitate its uptake into bone, is to promote vascular calcification and arteriosclerosis (see magnesium section for references).

In essence, people advised to "take calcium to prevent osteoporosis" are actually accelerating the chemistry of aging, degenerative disease and death.

Magnesium Solves Many Medical Mysteries

We discussed magnesium earlier. Just remember several serious points. As with many minerals, the average diet is deficient, providing only 40% of the RDA. It is estimated by Dr. Mildred Seelig, a nationally recognized magnesium specialist, that over 80% of the population is low. And this is about what we saw in the first few hundred we studied. Since it is in over 300 enzymes, it can mimic virtually any symptom. It is not adequately diagnosable by blood test, but the urine magnesium loading test works.

The commonest symptoms to improve are any spastic (caused by muscle spasm or unopposed contraction) conditions like asthma, migraines, cystitis, colitis, angina, hypertension, vasculitis, Raynaud's, chronic back pain, and twitching. It is also nature's tranquilizer and results in a marked improvement in well-being, as well as irritability, depression, fatigue, panic, anxiety, and mood swings.

Suffice it to say that I have over 50 research papers on my desk just at this moment that suggest it is ludicrous to subject anyone to a lifetime of cardiac and blood pressure medications, not to mention tranquilizers, addicting pain medications and anti-depressants without first knowing the magnesium status {mag loading test is in the appendix}. Instead very expensive, high-tech medications are prescribed. Did you ever wonder why there are so many calcium channel blockers prescribed now? Calcium and magnesium must be in balance for the cell to function. When there is a deficiency of magnesium, then the calcium must be blocked so that they still balance and you do not get an over abundance of calcium with resultant muscle spasm. If the spasm is in the coronary arteries, it causes angina or arrhythmia. If it's in other arteries it causes hypertension (Iseri, LT, French, JH, Magnesium: Nature's physiologic calcium blocker, Amer. Heart Journal, 188-193, July, 1984).

```
*****************************************************
*                                                   *
*    Brand Names Of Calcium Channel Blockers        *
*                                                   *
*    Cardalate       Cardiezem                      *
*    Calan           Isoptin                        *
*    Cardene         Procardia                      *
*                                                   *
*****************************************************
```

The weight of the evidence would suggest that these should not be prescribed for long term use without first investigating the magnesium status. You might be aghast at how simply logical this is, but complete nutritional biochemistry just is not taught in medical schools to this day, because what is taught is controlled by what is researched. And what is researched is what makes money.

Now I ask you. Do you want to take $3 worth of magnesium a month or $100 worth of a calcium channel blocker? And which one contributes more to your total health and longevity?

Clearly, magnesium plays a major role in regulating the vascular tone (hypertension), electrical conductivity (cardiac arrhythmia), and calcium deposits in blood vessels (arteriosclerosis). (Rayssinguier, Y, Role of magnesium and potassium in the pathogenesis of arteriosclerosis, Magnesium, 3:226-238, 1984). It also can cause senility or the organic brain syndrome (Hall, RCW, Joffe, JR, Hypomagne-

242

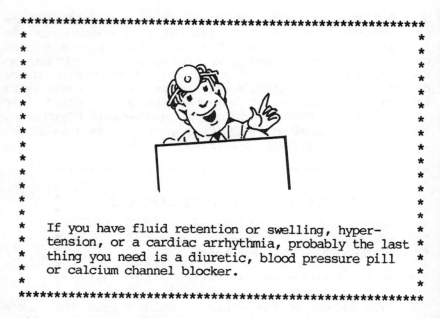

```
**********************************************************
*                                                        *
*                                                        *
*                                                        *
*                                                        *
*                                                        *
*                                                        *
*                                                        *
*                                                        *
*                                                        *
*                                                        *
*                                                        *
*                                                        *
*                                                        *
*   If you have fluid retention or swelling, hyper-      *
*   tension, or a cardiac arrhythmia, probably the last  *
*   thing you need is a diuretic, blood pressure pill    *
*   or calcium channel blocker.                          *
*                                                        *
**********************************************************
```

semia; physical and psychiatric symptoms, J. Amer. Med. Assoc., 224, #13, 1749- 1757, Hune 25, 1973).

Fortunately the importance of magnesium in asthma is just beginning to filter into the allergy literature (Rolla, G, et al, The effect of intravenous magnesium sulfate on airway obstruction of asthmatic patients, Ann. Allergy, 61, 388-390, Nov. 1988). But wide investigation and use still await. We have frequently witnessed many asthmatics who become less reactive to their triggers once the magnesium deficit is corrected. Magnesium deficiency is clearly one of many vulnerable aspects in the asthmatic.

The trek down the escalating magnesium-deficient path can begin with many roads. You know you had better investigate it if you have hypertension (Altura, BN, et al, Magnesium deficiency and hypertension: Correlation between magnesium deficient diet and microcirculatory changes in situ, Science, #223, 1315-1317, 1984). You know if you have chronic muscle spasms, cramps, or back pain you had better check it out.

And, if you have swelling, edema, or fluid retention, again do not leave it unchecked. For diuretics or fluid pills cause magnesium deficiency. They will only accelerate your problem so you'll inevitably develop new problems. For magnesium controls the sodium pump that diuretics mimic control of (Sacks, JR, Interaction of magnesium with the sodium pump of the human red cell, J. Physiology, 40, 575-591, 1988).

Most everyone knows diuretics cause potassium loss, so they are told to have fruit juice with their pills. But some have such severe loss they need potassium pills as well. Those cases are in even more severe probability of concomitant magnesium deficiency. And when it gets severe enough, the potassium becomes difficult to control. In many studies of potassium-deficient patients, over one third of them had a magnesium deficiency as well (Boyd, JC, Frequency of hypomagnesemia in hypokalemic states, Clin. Chem., 29; 1, 178-179, 1983).

I didn't intend to present so much information, but as you can see there is overwhelming evidence for not only one but every nutrient. Researchers have shown vast evidence, for example, that every hospitalized patient should be checked for hypomagnesemia, yet it is rarely done (Whang, R, Predictors of clinical hypomagnesemia, Arch. Int. Med., 144, 1290-1294, 1984). The nutritional evidence and information is staggering and I think that is one major hold-up to getting it organized, taught, and utilized. Meanwhile diabetics and hypertensives die every day.

Permit me one last example: The end-stage for many organs and tissues occurs when they begin to harden from accumulated calcium. Calcification of blood vessels makes them hard and brittle, as opposed to their natural rubbery state. So hypertension results, but what is worse is when they finally crack and rupture. Strokes and aneurysms result. But sufficient magnesium can deter this calcification (Boskey, AC, Pasner, AS, Effect of magnesium on lipid-induced calcification, Calcif. Tissue Int., 32, 139-143, 1980). And the magnesium sparing of calcium deposits has been known a long time (Leonard, F, Initiation and inhibition of subcutaneous calcification, Calc. Tiss. Res., 10, 269-279, 1972).

Medicine is hooked on medicines. We need to get hooked on finding the biochemical defects and correcting them. And as we begin, it is self-evident that environmental chemicals influence pathology as well. Clearly, it becomes impossible to separate nutritional biochemistry from environmental medicine as they both dovetail to contribute greatly in providing us with the explanation of the cause of many undiagnosable and untreatable diseases.

With our current era of molecular medicine, it's absolutely exciting how many illnesses become ancient history when you start looking for the biochemical cause. For the physician interested in entering this field, I'd suggest he first study one element, magnesium. For once he understands this one, he'll be able to treat over 30 "incurable" and very common conditions. And by the time he understands how it works in over 300 enzymes, he'll have a good foundation of biochemical knowledge on which he can build as he grows. For magnesium has solved many a medical mystery for me.

Many people, for example, were much less chemically sensitive, felt markedly more energetic, slept deeply and well through the night, and stopped all sorts of spastic conditions after correcting their magnesium deficiencies.

****

Are You Wearing A Time Bomb In Your Gut?

Actually, there's enough material for 6 volumes of books on current medical blunders, but let's just hit one more before we move on to how to get well.

You know that mold is everywhere. Lay a piece of bread in your desk drawer and check it in 2 weeks. It will be covered with mold: And like housedust, because it is everywhere, you can't escape it. We published 3 papers in the _Annals of Allergy_ (1982, 1983, 1984) on our mold research and discovered there were many molds in the air that doctors were not testing patients to.

When we did test to these molds we could clear a tremendous number of people who had resisted all the conventional medical and allergy therapies of internationally reputed medical schools. (_Clinical Ecology_, volume 5, p. 115- 120 1988). This included exhaustion, depression, "foggy headedness", migraines, chronic ear and throat infections, chronic sinusitis, bronchitis, laryngitis, asthma, eczema, colitis, and more. As you have learned, it doesn't matter what label has been placed on a symptom. What does matter is what causes it. And the cause is different or individually unique for everyone.

You also know that the stool is about 80% dry weight of bacteria and yeasts (molds, fungi). These organisms literally rot or digest our food in the intestine so it can be broken down into small enough molecules to be absorbed across the intestinal wall.

```
*****************************************************************
*                                                               *
*          Examples of Detoxication Reactions                   *
*                  Carried Out By Gut Flora                     *
*      *   hydrolysis of glucuronides, sulfates, oxides,        *
*          and esters                                           *
*      *   dehydroxylation of C-hydroxy and N-hydroxy           *
*          compounds                                            *
*      *   decarboxylation                                      *
*      *   dehalogenation                                       *
*      *   reduction of nitro and azo groups, aldehydes,        *
*          ketones, alcohols and N-oxides                       *
*      *   aromatization                                        *
*      *   nitrosamine formation                                *
*                                                               *
*****************************************************************
```

These bacteria and fungi also produce some of our vitamins. And last but never least, they also carry out a huge detoxication program of their own to help us with our total load. And as you have seen, in this era we need all the help we can get.

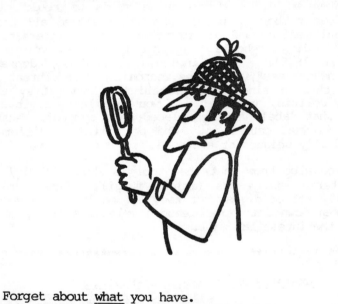

Forget about <u>what</u> you have.
Ask <u>why</u> you have it and how you're going to find out.
Avoid rushing into drugs to mask symptoms forever.
Use them judiciously for a temporary crutch while you find the cause.

Also the gut wall cells have their own detox {cytochrome P-450 monooxygenase} system. But when the wall becomes inflamed from chronic yeast infestation, the function of this system declines.

For in many people, the good bugs have been killed off
by prescription antibiotics (penicillin, ampicillin, sulfa
drugs, tetracycline, erythromycin and scores more). To make
matters worse, the not so desirable bugs have taken over and
grown in huge numbers. How do you get your bad bugs to
multiply like crazy? Easily, have a lot of soda, sweets,
chocolate, yeast breads and donuts, cookies, alcohol, or
use drugs like birth control pills, corticosteroids (prednisone), and more antibiotics. These are just a few of the
items that will foster this.

What are the effects of these abnormal bugs? Many:
1. You get poor digestion with gas, bloating,
    alternating diarrhea and constipation, cramps,
    foul smelling stools and breath, and toxic
    blood. The digestion is poor because the good
    bacteria needed to adequately break down the
    foods are crowded out by the bad. The bloating
    partly comes from the gas that yeasts produce as
    they have a growth spurt when you feed them
    sugars.
2. Because you have poor breakdown, the absorption
    of nutrients from your food suffers.
3. The gut wall can become irritated and inflamed
    by the presence of these yeast bugs. It then
    lets larger molecules of food across its border
    than it normally does. The body is startled by
    these "foreign" big molecules and, never having
    seen them before, does not recognize them.
    Anything foreign is attacked as an enemy.
    Antibodies are made and we have the start of
    food allergies.
4. The good bugs are not around in plentiful enough
    numbers to make the vitamins they should, like
    vitamin K that is synthesized in the gut.
5. Some yeasts like Candida krusei and Candida
    parapsilosis produce a substance called
    thiaminase that actually destroys thiamine
    (vitamin B1) before you have a chance to absorb
    it.
6. The detox system suffers badly since its

right-hand man (the gut flora you recall carry out a lot of detox) is out of commission. So it gets backed up and chemical allergies appear.

7. Since many yeasts (molds, fungi) have grown in huge numbers (their competing bacteria were killed off by antibiotics taken for that sore throat or root canal, and their growth was stimulated by a diet high in sugars or alcohol), the body sees them as foreign invaders.

The body makes antibodies against these gut yeasts in attempt to defend itself and control the yeasts. Hence when you have antibodies to a yeast or mold, you often behave toward it as though you are allergic to it, because these antibodies do bad things like cause the release of histamine and can create any symptom you can think of. One of the first rules of allergy treatment is to get rid of the thing you are allergic to. The problem is that he is wearing in his gut the very antigen to which he is allergic. It's like wearing a cat around your neck if you have cat-induced asthma! You never get away from the very thing that is causing your allergy.

And one can be sensitive to the Candida or other organisms, by a variety of mechanisms (Marone, G, et al, Activation of human basophils by bacterial products, Int. Achs. Allergy Appl. Immunol., 77: 213-215, 1985; Ray, TL, et al, Activation of the alternative (properdin) pathway of complement by Candida albicans and related species, The J. Investig. Dermatol., 67: 700-703, 1976; Chattaway, FW, et al, An examination of the production of hydrolytic enzymes and toxins by pathogenic species of Candida albicans, J. Gen. Microbiol., 67, 255-263, 1971).

You can return the numbers of good, beneficial gut bugs to normal with Vital-Plex (Klaire Laboratories) and Nystatin pure powder (4 million units per teaspoon, see The E.I. Syndrome for details), but then you risk growing the form that is resistant to the Nystatin treatment, Candida tropicalis. Then you have a really serious problem because there is no antifungal to easily kill this type. So resist getting hooked into the old drug routine. There is a better way to get well.

8.   Furthermore, some yeasts, like Candida albicans, make acetaldehyde!

Yes, the biochemical bottleneck. So now every little thing --- food, chemical, mold, and bad thought, makes you worse: food, because the inflamed gut fosters food allergy; chemicals, because the bad ratio of organisms lowers the detoxication efficiency so chemical allergies arise; molds, because you're wearing the very thing you're allergic to; and emotional influences, because even the neurotransmitters or brain hormones must funnel through the aldehyde bottleneck to get metabolized.

That's why when some people clear the Candida from their gut, they suddenly become less sensitive to foods and chemicals and they become happier and more energetic. This baffles physicians who know nothing about the chemistry of

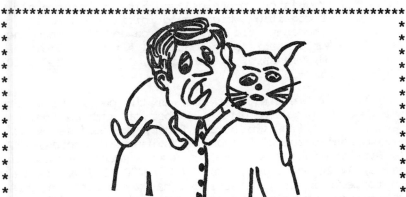

```
******************************************************
*                                                    *
*                                                    *
*                                                    *
*                                                    *
*                                                    *
*                                                    *
*                                                    *
*                                                    *
*                                                    *
*                                                    *
*                                                    *
*                                                    *
*    Being allergic to the yeast (mold, fungus) Candida,  *
*    and wearing it in your gut 24 hours a day, is like   *
*    being a cat-allergic asthmatic and wearing a cat     *
*    around your neck. You'll never get better until      *
*    you get rid of it.                                   *
*                                                    *
******************************************************
```

detox nor even one of the 10 mechanisms of the Candida-related complex of symptoms, that you now know. But it's exciting to help people get well when this is understood.

9. Candida organisms can raise havoc by producing hormones that mimic human hormones and even receptors for our hormones on their surfaces! They produce estrogens and steroids (Fungal Metabolites, Vol. II, Turner, WB, Academic Press, 1983) to which we can react or which can cause feedback inhibition of our own hormones.

10. Many "Candida victims", feel remarkably better with just getting off sugars. There are many biochemical explanations for this, including the fact that sugar (glucose) actually attaches to the body regulatory proteins and nucleic acids and can inactivate enzymes, cause abnormal function of nucleic acids (genetic material and regulatory proteins) and alter macromolecule recognition which could initiate allergies (Nonenzymatic glycosylation and the pathogenesis of diabetic complications, A review, Brownlee, M, Vlassaro, H, Cerami, A, Ann. Int. Med., 101: 527-537, 1984).

It's interesting that most of the people with potential Candida problems have a number of nutrient deficiencies. I don't know which came first, the deficiency or the disease, and suspect it's highly individual (Montes, LF, et al, Hypovitaminosis A in patients with mucocutaneous Candidiasis, J. Infect. Dis., 128, 2, 227-230, 1973). Certainly the numbers of drugs prescribed has a bearing on this as most drugs cause loss of many nutrients and it is rarely monitored (Roe, DA, Nutrient and drug interactions, Nutrit. Reviews, 42, 4, 141-154, Apr. 1984).

How do you diagnose whether you have this 10-pronged Candida problem? One way is to see what a month trial of

the yeast program (detailed in The E.I. Syndrome) does.
Another is to follow the detox program in the next chapter.

Case Example:

O.P. was a 31 year old business man with extreme
exhaustion, depression, acne, spastic colon, chronic sinusitis, and arthritis.   In less than one week on the yeast
program (as described in The E.I. Syndrome), he felt better
than he had in 10 years.   But many people get hung up here
and risk growing the resistant Candida tropicalis by staying
on Nystatin for over 6 months. In order to get off the program and still progress to new levels of wellness, continue
to Chapter 8.

```
******************************************
*     24 Hour Urine Amino Acid          *
*     Findings That Suggest The         *
*     Presence Of Foreign Flora         *
*                                       *
*     decreased tryptophan              *
*     increased ethanolamine            *
*     increased gamma butyric acid      *
*     increased beta-alanine            *
*     abnormal proteolysis              *
*     increased anserine, carnosine     *
******************************************
```

        There are many ways to suspect foreign flora in the
gut. Laboratory tests can measure antibody titers to Candida (blood tests to see if you have antibodies to Candida and
other species), proctoscopic (rectal) cultures will identify
foreign bacteria and protozoa, and even a 24 hour urine
amino acid analysis will hint at the existence of foreign
flora.

        None of these diagnostic tests is as fool-proof as a
therapeutic trial because we're dealing with so many variables. Not only are there many types of organisms that may
be responsible for the symptoms, but even among one organism

like the yeast, Candida, there are many mechanisms to cause the symptoms, as you saw. That is one of the main reasons why there are so many adversaries to the yeast problem. They have no concept of the 10 mechanisms and are waiting until a solo explanation emerges: just as they are waiting for a solo cause for arthritis, high cholesterol, cancer, arteriosclerosis, and osteoporosis.

That will be a long wait, for you see Candida (and many other intestinal organisms that grow out of control) can create symptoms through allergy (via IgG, IgE, IgM antibodies, or even immune complexes). It can also function on a metabolic basis, as with the elaboration of acetaldehyde (Truss, Intern. Clin. Nutr. Rev., 5; 2, 61-66, 1988), or mediate through a nutritional basis by elaborating thiaminases; remember some species of Candida produces thiaminase, an enzyme that destroys thiamine or vitamin B1 before it ever gets absorbed. And, of course, any foreign flora can steal precious nutrients for its own growth. And it can interfere with the detox pathways or hormones, receptors, and much more.

And the yeast Candida is just the tip of the iceberg. There are many other yeasts, bacteria, and protozoa that can cause similar and even worse problems for the body by taking over in the intestinal tract. Camphylobactei pylori, for example, is an abnormal stomach bacterium that can make you think you have an ulcer.

One note of caution. Rule out Candida before you try to rev up the detox system. Taking cysteine stimulates Candida growth in the budding stage. When this excessively stimulated growth becomes invasive, it is much more difficult to get control.

It's all so logical and extremely dramatic when you treat someone who has Candida or any other abnormal intestinal flora overgrowth.

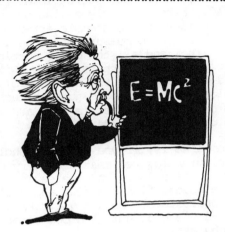

```
*************************************************************
*                                                           *
*                                                           *
*                                                           *
*                                                           *
*                                                           *
*                                                           *
*                                                           *
*                                                           *
*                                                           *
*                                                           *
*                                                           *
*                                                           *
*                                                           *
*                                                           *
*                                                           *
*                                                           *
*     You don't have to be a genius to clearly see that     *
*     we now have the biochemical explanation of how a      *
*     Candida overgrowth, a magnesium or zinc deficiency,   *
*     for example, can mimic all the symptoms of E.I.       *
*     with multiple food, chemical and mold intolerances.   *
*                                                           *
*************************************************************
```

QUICK STOP SUMMARY

(1)   Cholesterol lowering drugs put extra xenobiotic load
      on detoxication systems, bind important nutrients so
      they cannot get absorbed through the intestine, and
      put extra strain on the liver which still has to
      synthesize cholesterol for membrane function, sex
      hormones and adrenal hormones. Life itself cannot go
      on without cholesterol. These cholesterol-lowering
      drugs also interfere with the monooxygenase xenobiotic
      detoxication system of the gastrointestinal tract.
      There are enzymes in the intestinal wall that are a
      major part of detoxication, and which are interfered
      with by cholesterol-lowering medications.

Unfortunately, when cholesterol lowering drugs are prescribed, there is rarely advise on cutting out sugar, that is known to promote arteriosclerosis. Likewise there is no measure of magnesium, B6, EFA's, chromium, zinc, and all the other nutrients necessary to properly metabolize cholesterol. Without these nutrients to metabolize the cholesterol, it hangs up in the blood, until there's just so much that it deposits out in blood vessels that are inflamed and grab the cholesterol to patch it up.

The bottom line is, if you have cut cholesterol levels down by eliminating red meat and dairy products as well as processed foods and are eating whole grains, fresh vegetables, fish and fowl and still have an elevated cholesterol, do not yet take drugs. First try to find the biochemical block to proper metabolism of your cholesterol.

(2) Voluminous biochemical evidence exists for correct amounts and sources of Omega 3 and Omega 6 essential fatty acids, as well as the need for avoidance of free radical generators and harmful "trans" fatty acids in margarines. Once this is understood and practiced, high cholesterol usually corrects itself.

(3) Calcium is recommended by doctors without measurement of, and regard for, the balance with other minerals such as magnesium, zinc, manganese, and boron that are essential for its incorporation into the boney matrix. We even see a startling number of people for whom calcium was prescribed who have subnormal vitamin D3 levels. Also one must eliminate processed foods and soft drinks which are high in phosphates and compete with the absorption of calcium, or there will be inferior calcium uptake in spite of supplements. And the excess calcium, unbalanced by complementary minerals, is unable to lay down in the bone, and thus deposits in vessel walls, instead. We call this arteriosclerosis.

Therefore the current recommendation to "take a

calcium supplement" without sound biochemical guidance and monitoring is actually promoting arteriosclerosis, chronic disease, and aging.

(4) Furthermore, tests like indicies of red blood cells are useless, contrary to what we were taught in medical school (New England Journal of Medicine, 1988). Many studies show that iron deficiency, B12 deficiency, and folic acid deficiencies occur without macro- and microcytoses. Translation: It is taught that a doctor usually need not concern himself with B vitamin deficiencies if the size of the red blood cell on a standard blood count is normal. This is simply not true.

(5) Additionally, a deficiency of a mineral may be present when the intracellular assay is normal. This has been borne out in many studies where a therapeutic trial of intravenous magnesium has cleared asthma attacks and the rbc magnesium was normal, for example. Homeostasis (the body's attempt to make the blood look normal even if the rest of the body is sorely lacking) interferes with recognition of nutrient deficiencies in blood tests and we need more sensitive tests, like intra-cellular levels (measurements in red and white blood cells).

(6) Hypertension is treated with drugs instead of looking for common causes like magnesium deficiency, or food and chemical intolerances (Motayama, T, Hypertension, 13: 222-232, 1989).

(7) Single nutrient deficiencies like magnesium are known to be epidemic, but are rarely checked. They can cause any symptom. A whole foods diet could correct this in millions (Juan, DR, Clinical review: The clinical importance of hypomagnesemia, Surgery, 91, #5, 510-517, 1982).

The key is......

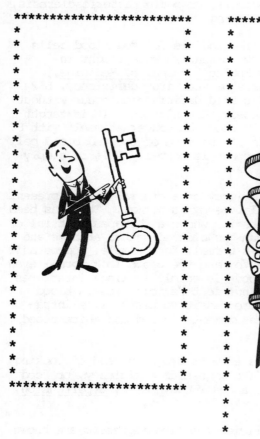

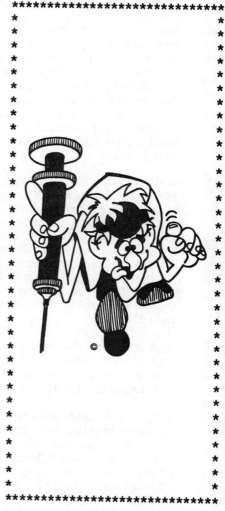

to find the cause of symptoms,
not mask them with drugs.

(8)   Single nutrient deficiencies, like chromium, can
        proceed to propagate degenerative decline in mental
        function through arteriosclerosis. A whole foods diet
        could correct this in millions of people.

(9)   An overgrowth of intestinal organisms, like Candida,
        because of over use of antibiotics and high sugar
        diets can cause an avalanche of problems leading to
        the full blown universal reactor. This person is
        sensitive to foods, chemicals, molds, and usually has
        multiple nutritional deficiencies. This person has
        over a dozen symptoms and usually all medications make
        him worse. We have the knowledge to make these people
        well, but not enough trained physicians to carry it
        out. Many improve just on the diets (The E.I.
        Syndrome).

(10)   We have a health care system that has ignored the
        biochemistry of detoxication, nutrition, and
        environmental illness. Meanwhile it continues to
        pigeon hole every symptom into a computer-based
        treatment program, most of which eventuate in drug
        treatments to merely mask symptoms. And it consti-
        tutes 11% of the G.N.P.

        Every diagnosis (which usually represents end stage
target organ damage, like colitis, asthma, hypertension,
diabetes, arthritis) has been reduced to a coded number.
Insurance companies then have a list of pre-determined acceptable treatments (usually drugs and surgery) for each
one. If your treatment doesn't fall into one of those categories, guess what? You don't get reimbursed for your medical care. It doesn't matter if it was the only treatment
out of thousands of wasted dollars that got you well.

        With people all being biochemically unique, how do we
begin to sort out this mess? Do we do thousands of dollars
of vitamin, mineral, amino acid and essential fatty acid
tests on everyone? No. There's a better solution.

```
*********************************************************
*                                                       *
*                                                       *
*                                                       *
*                                                       *
*                                                       *
*                                                       *
*                                                       *
*                                                       *
*                                                       *
*                                                       *
*                                                       *
*                                                       *
*                                                       *
*                                                       *
*                                                       *
*                                                       *
*                                                       *
*                                                       *
*                                                       *
*                                                       *
*                                                       *
*                                                       *
*                                                       *
*                                                       *
*                                                       *
*                                                       *
*                                                       *
*                                                       *
*                                                       *
*                                                       *
*                                                       *
*                                                       *
*                                                       *
*                                                       *
*                                                       *
```

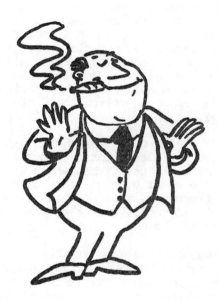

```
*                                                       *
*   Congratulations!  Your mind has just taken a giant  *
*   step into the future.  You have released yourself   *
*   from the bonds of antiquated medical concepts and   *
*   are able now to begin to learn how to soar to new   *
*   levels of wellness.                                 *
*                                                       *
*********************************************************
```

Chapter 8: THE TRANSITION INTO DETOX

So you now are aware of more 21st century medicine
than many physicians. How are you going to use this to get
yourself well? And how are you going to bring this about
without a culture shock? After all, I don't want you saying, "I'd rather die happy than healthy!"

Getting started always appears overwhelming, but bear
in mind that if you're going to put to use what you've begun
to learn, it will require some major lifestyle changes.
Obviously you're not going to accomplish it all in a day or
a week. And people are tremendously variable, so the following is a general outline and you can work at it at your
own pace. There are also other references to help you,
depending upon your individual needs.

Some will actually have it all accomplished in a week,
because they're sick enough and smart enough. Others will
have a variety of obstacles to overcome from doubting
spouses, commitments which you choose to put ahead of your
own health, or just plain procrastination and laziness, etc.

The journey to wellness is outlined in 5 phases:
(1)   Get organized.
(2)   Detox your diet.
(3)   Detox your person.
(4)   Detox your bedroom.
(5)   Detox your mind.

Phase I: GETTING ORGANIZED

Read all the material, digest it, get a notebook and
map out your plan. Set your goals and set periodic evaluation times when you will re-evaluate what you have accomplished and whether your goals require any modification.
Just bear in mind that this is a learning experience and a

potentially therapeutic trial. YOU ARE NOT PERFECT, AND YOU WILL NEVER BE PERFECT. NEITHER WILL ANYONE YOU EVER MEET.

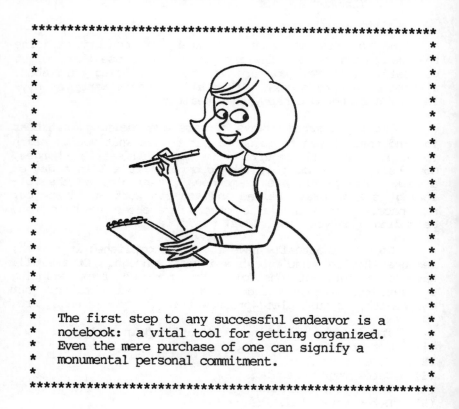

The first step to any successful endeavor is a notebook: a vital tool for getting organized. Even the mere purchase of one can signify a monumental personal commitment.

If you can just remember that, you won't get discouraged if you find the going tough. Instead you'll take it for what you can learn from it, pick yourself up and dig in again.

Phase II: DETOX YOUR DIET

It's obvious that most people are eating a diet high in processed grocery store foods, laced with chemical additives and pesticides. They have the wrong oils in their membranes and a host of nutrient deficiencies. How can the detoxication system function optimally when it's operating at such a disadvantage?

Because changing life styles is difficult, we'll take you through 5 levels which can be separated by as many days or weeks as you need. Myself and many people that I see did all 5 levels cold turkey on day one. But we had no choice: we were too sick to do otherwise. Regardless of which route you choose, remember this is a trial, not a life sentence. You will see what you learn from it and then make your final decision of what is the best diet for you. And even then it will change with time as your total package of needs changes. After all, to be alive is to be constantly changing, adapting to your environment. So nothing is static; even when you're dead you're decomposing.

Two cautions: As you go through these levels with your health professional, your high blood pressure or diabetes may normalize. But when you're still on medication to bring them down, the net effect is you will feel horrible when your pressure/sugar becomes too low. Also you could get dangerously low levels of these, so work closely with your doctor. Second, you may have a hidden addiction to some foods and may go through withdrawal symptoms beginning somewhere in the first week. It will usually end in the second week. It's not fun, but necessary (see The E.I. Syndrome). But be aware of the need to have not only professional guidance, but a partner at home. Infrequently, the withdrawal can be so severe as to precipitate a suicidal depression or psychotic behavior. No one knows how addicted you are.

Level I   Omit all alcohol. If this is a problem, you have a problem. See your local AA; they have a great track record. If you are blocked here, you'd better find out what you are escaping from and fix that area of your life first.

             Omit all sweets, cookies, cakes, pies, candy bars, sodas, fruit juice, chocolate, gum,

```
*********************************************************
*                                                       *
*                                                       *
*                                                       *
*                                                       *
*                                                       *
*                                                       *
*                                                       *
*                                                       *
*                                                       *
*                                                       *
*                                                       *
*                                                       *
*                                                       *
```

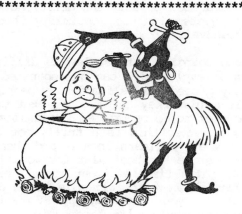

```
*                                                       *
*   One man's meat is another man's poison.  There are  *
*   no 2 people who have the exact same food intoler-   *
*   ances nor mold and chemical sensitivities.          *
*   Detoxing your diet is the only way to determine     *
*   which sensitivities you have.                       *
*                                                       *
*********************************************************
```

candies, ice cream, sugar, honey, maple syrup.
Often trouble here stems from not enough love in
your life to satisfy your needs for pleasurable
feelings. Also ingesting too much salt, makes
you crave sugar for balance.

Substitute: glass bottled spring water, nuts,
two fruits a day, 1/2 cup dried fruits* a day,
carrots, squash, popcorn.

Reason: Many people with early stage Candida
feel wonderfully revitalized merely by eating at
this level. Between the first and 3rd week of
this level their energy level triples, their
brain fog lifts, they feel reborn.

Remember you can stay at this level days, weeks or
months. The sicker you are the quicker you'll need to move
on to the more progressive levels.

Level II   Omit all mold foods, commonly called Ferments.
This includes any food with mold: cheese, yeast
breads (muffins and pasta* have no yeast so are
fine), all processed foods, coffee, tea,
vinegar, commercial salad dressing (cold pressed
sesame or flax oils with lemon/lime is OK),
ketchup, mayonnaise, mustard.

Substitute more vegetables like kale, collards,
Brussel sprouts, cauliflower, cabbage, onions,
squash, carrots, turnips.

Reason: People with tougher cases of Candida
need to be more strict. In fact they cannot
tolerate even a trace of the foods in this
chapter that are marked with the asterisk*.
Also coffee is a common cause of headaches, mood
swings, anxiety, and bowel and
bladder spasm.

Level III   Omit all dairy and wheat. This means all milk
products. You're already off ice cream in Level
I and cheese for Level II, so what the heck!
As for wheat, this means wheat muffins, wheat
pasta, and wheat cereals go. Level I omitted
pastries, Level II omitted yeast breads, so
you've been wearing down anyway.

Substitute: Whole grains: brown rice, whole
or steel cut oats, rye flakes, buckwheat, teff
quinoa, millet, barley, etc. Whole means
unbroken. Flour products are from ground or
broken grains. You're getting rid of them
temporarily here and having only unadulterated
whole grains that need to be cooked for about
45 minutes. Whole grains are also alive. They
still have the precious life force in them. You

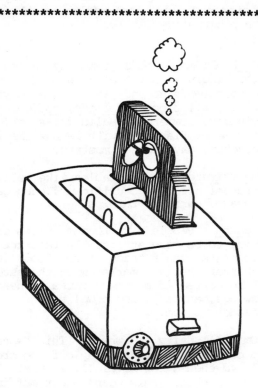

****
One of the first things you can dispense with is
all white sugar and white flour products. By the
time they grind, blend and store it, there's
barely any nutrition left anyway.
****

could put organic brown rice in a little saucer
of water on your window sill and it would grow
green rice plants. Flour will only mold.

Most of these can be purchased in an organic
form (grown without pesticide) at your local

health food store. If you're in a remote area or do not have time to shop, they can be mail ordered from N.E.E.D.S., Syracuse, New York, or Mountain Ark Trading Co., Fayetteville, AR.

Reason: Milk and wheat are the backbone of the American diet. For that reason they are the commonest causes of hidden food allergy. Many people stop having chronic nasal and chest mucous as soon as they do this level. Also, much of the world has a lactase deficiency. They don't make enough of an enzyme in the gut to break down milk. The result is gas, bloating, indigestion, and alternating diarrhea and constipation.

Furthermore there's a population of people who are gluten sensitive. When they have grains containing gluten (wheat, rye, barley, and triticale) it causes a reaction in the intestinal wall (villous atrophy) where it becomes incapable of absorbing nutrients well and causes a host of gastrointestinal complaints. This gluten enteropathy is called celiac disease and can be likened to a severe form of wheat allergy. Sometimes even the slightest amount of wheat can set off a chain of events causing such severe malabsorption that these people look like they just came from concentration camps. Even a trace of wheat flour in a food can damage the intestinal lining for months! This makes it a serious reason to avoid all processed foods, for "modified food starch" (or simply food starch), malt, MSG, and vegetable protein hydrolysate are ubiquitous and are even found in some prescription tablets. And of course these grains are also in many alcohols. And whole grains, like brown rice, contain three times the magnesium, for example, as does white bleached instant rice.

We have been educated to think that milk is

necessary. Yet many healthy cultures do not
have milk and cheese. When I lectured for a
month in six cities in China with Drs. Rea and
Randolph (1985), we never saw any milk or
cheese. A study of 250 women with breast cancer
(Feb. 15, 1989, Journal of the National Cancer
Institute) revealed they consumed much more milk
and high-fat cheese and butter than 499 healthy
women of similar age.

Other studies show that some milk sensitive
children and adults have the stomach as an
allergic target organ. Milk caused atrophic
changes in the lining within days (observed with
a gastroscope). This left them with poor
gastric acid for weeks. This in turn caused
poor digestion which in turn can produce
behavior and learning problems due to lack of
neurotransmittor precursor amino acids and
complementary minerals. So one "tiny" indiscretion, as with the wheat sensitivity, can secretly produce changes that affect assimilation and
digestion for weeks. So when you do a trial try

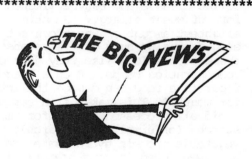

```
**********************************************************
*                                                        *
*                                                        *
*                                                        *
*                                                        *
*                                                        *
*                                                        *
*                                                        *
*                                                        *
*                                                        *
*                                                        *
*                                                        *
*   The best news is that most people can feel 50%       *
*   better in just a few weeks of changing their diet.   *
*   Isn't it worth a few weeks' trial to you?            *
*                                                        *
**********************************************************
```

to do it whole-heartedly, or it may fail to improve symptoms and you'll draw the wrong conclusions.

Level IV   By now I know you're wondering what's left to cut out? You guessed it.

Omit red meats and eggs. That includes beef, pork, and lamb. Wild venison or rabbit could be had once a week. Also poultry or fish are OK.

Omit the deadly night shade family: This includes potatoes, tomatoes, peppers, chili, eggplant and tobacco.

Substitute: beans like tofu, lentils, chickpeas, navy, pinto, aduki, split pea, etc.

Reason: many people just plain stop the stiffness, aching, and hurting of their muscles and joints when at this level.

Caution: avoid getting stuck in the same monotonous foods. Vary your diet daily. Don't have any one food every day.

The reasons given for each are merely the commonest improvements noted in thousands of patients. But because of individual variation, any symptom relief is possible. The more you can substitute organic foods for pesticided, the more chance you have of feeling better quicker, also.

Many people will protest that this is impossible to do, but I've eaten at Level IV for 2 years. I had to. it's the only thing that brought me back to total health. As I lecture around the world, I have a hot plate in my suitcase and have taken my meals to 5-Star restaurants when I was in the strict healing phase. If you're determined enough to get well, you'll figure out what you need to do. And don't try to force this on the rest of your family. I cook "regular" meals for my husband. Not everyone is ready for, or needs this at the same moment in time that you do.

Before starting this program with your medical guide, you may want to get some nutrient levels drawn. It may be up to 4 weeks before these are processed (some labs have a turn around time of up to 4 weeks for tests that are infrequently ordered. It's more economical to run their tests in batches, so they only do the specific tests a few days a month). In the meantime, after having had your nutrient levels drawn, the two of you may decide to start you on a simple trial of a yeast (ferment) free B vitamin and a multiple mineral (Allergy Research Group, Klaire Laboratories, Cardio Vascular Research, Neesby, Thorne, Twin Labs, DaVinci, are just a few of many reliable companies).

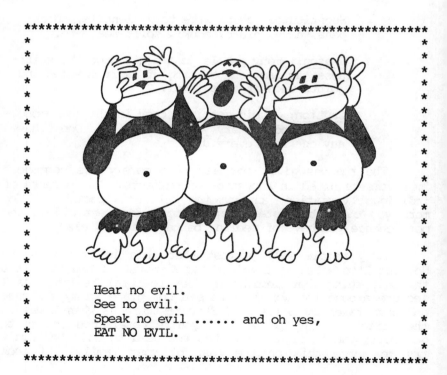

```
*****************************************************************
*                                                               *
*                                                               *
*                                                               *
*                                                               *
*                                                               *
*                                                               *
*                                                               *
*                                                               *
*                                                               *
*                                                               *
*                                                               *
*                                                               *
*                                                               *
*                                                               *
*                                                               *
*                                                               *
*                                                               *
*          Hear no evil.                                        *
*          See no evil.                                         *
*          Speak no evil ...... and oh yes,                     *
*          EAT NO EVIL.                                         *
*                                                               *
*****************************************************************
```

And now could be a good time to initiate your oil change with 1-2 tablespoons of organic cold pressed flaxseed oil a day. Then later after you know your status, you can add your antioxidants (vitamin A, C, E), cysteine or taurine, phosphatidyl choline, etc. and correct your deficiencies.

Some like to move in stages to evaluate each part of the process. Others of us had so much wrong we just wanted to unload as fast as possible and start feeling well. Which ever you elect is fine. Some are so sensitive they must rotate foods (see The E.I. Syndrome). Actually varying the diet from day to day so that you never repeat the same food (or any food related to it) more often than every few days, also serves to assure more variety of trace nutrients as well as staving off further food allergies. And remember to eat as fresh and organic as possible. It will come with time as you work at it.

Most people's initial reaction to the loss of processed foods is denial. Immediately they are not so sick as to need to go to such drastic measures as eating real live whole foods. So let me give you just a glimmer of what's going on.

You already know processed foods are loaded with phosphates that inhibit the absorption of calcium. And you're no longer naive enough to think that that's all that is bad for you in them.

Let's look at another example. Alzheimer's presenile dementia is on the rise in this country. What are the early signs? For this disease must be caught early since by the time you suddenly diagnose it, it is usually too late for significant reversal. So what are soft signs that the mind is going? First short term memory starts to suffer. You can't remember what you had for breakfast. But because you remember the past in intimate detail, others are lulled into a false security assuming the memory must be good if you can remember trivia from years ago. You may stop sentences in mid-stream, be frequently at a loss for a particular word, have unexplained mood swings, stop learning, stop bathing, suddenly turn on a loved one, or have blunted emotions.

Of the many nutritional factors contributing to the pathology of Alzheimer's is excess aluminum in the brain. How does it get there? We have laced our lives with it. Prolonged cooking of acid tomato sauce in an aluminum pot, aluminum cans for food, soda and beer, factory effluents, aluminum absorbed from under arm deodorants, aluminum in baking powder, salt (yes, check the label, that's what makes it pour when it rains), antacids and as an anti-flocculant in drinking water are just a few of the sources. Some of the highest levels I've seen are ulcer and stomach problem patients who have ingested years of over the counter aluminum-containing antacids.

In many areas of the world where aluminum is high in the soil (Guam, Japan, New Guinea), they have a higher than normal incidence of neurologic diseases like amyotrophic lateral sclerosis (Lou Gehrig's ALS), Parkinsonism, and pre-senile dementia (losing one's mind before the rest of the body shows a comparable rate of decline). In the U.S., high aluminum in the soil displaces magnesium and calcium, and comes from acid rain, auto and industrial exhausts. Consequently, the produce grown in these soils is deficient as well, as are the bodies which consume it.

Other problems seen in brain biopsies of dementia patients are loss of phosphatidyl choline (PC) from cell membranes and nerve sheaths. Researchers have discovered that an "auto-cannabalism" occurs as the body "eats" its own PC from brain tissues in order to supply it to other tissues (endoplasmic reticulum, and other cell membranes that are being destroyed by chemicals for lack of protective vitamin E, etc.) that are in more immediate danger. Why do we have a shortage of PC? Because we eat very few beans (a good source of lecithin) and more processed foods (a poor source). The analogies could go on and on. We cannot pollute the earth, oceans and atmosphere without also altering the contents of the body. We are all one.

As you detox your diet, you eventually get so cleaned out that when you eat a wrong food, you know it right away. Don't think you're developing a food allergy; you're really unmasking a food intolerance you've had all along. In your current state of addiction, you have lost many of your instincts, but they can recover.

For example, you rarely see an animal in the wild that is diabetic, overweight or arthritic. He eats from his instincts. If he doesn't feel good he doesn't eat. If he's thirsty he drinks. But you don't see him "feeding his cold" in front of the T.V. with a bowl of ice cream, or sucking down five cokes in a day. And when he's sick, he doesn't run to the drug store, he stops eating. But our processed foods not only lead to nutritional deficiencies, but distort our tastes to the point where our instincts have been suppressed.

In essence, you want to make every mouth full of food really count. And no processed food can hold a candle to a whole food that mother nature has made on good soil.

```
***************************************************************
*      As you can see, the goal of the diet is to progres-   *
*      sively unload the most common food problems first.    *
*      And you should continue down the line until you are   *
*      symptom-free. For changing the diet has a profound    *
*      effect on the detoxication scheme.                    *
***************************************************************
```

QUICK STOP SUMMARY:

Just Tell Me What To Eat

If the preceding seems overwhelming, back off and try this.

Breakfast: (* means these foods may have to be limited by the more severely affected individual)

Cereal   No sugars, no names you cannot explain, no chemicals, no bleached, no "enriched" flour.

	Should contain whole grains (like oats, barley, brown rice, quinoa, teff, amaranth), millet, nuts, seeds, dried* or cooked fruits*.
Pancakes	From whole grains, freshly ground into flour by you, no wheat.
Muffins	Non-aluminum baking powder (use Rumford)
Vegetables	Unlimited, but no tomatoes, potatoes, peppers, chili, eggplant.
Beans	Unlimited.
Fruits	1-2 a day if needed.

Lunch:
50/50 whole grains and vegetables.
Bring your own food or gang up on a local eatery and tell them where to buy organic whole grains. Teach them to vary your menu and give you something simple, like the following:

Mondays:	Brown rice, kale and parsnips
Tuesdays:	Millet, carrots, mustard greens
Wednesday:	Barley, bok choy, and onions
Thursday:	Quinoa, broccoli, and hard winter squash
Friday:	Am___ :h and cauliflower

Then they could learn to add some extras like:
   Raw watercress and red radish salad with tofu, tamari, umeboshi paste, scallion dressing
   Gomashio or roasted sunflower seeds for grains
   Miso soup (any leftover cooked grains and vegetables can be added)
   Bean dishes, like hummus on whole grain bread or celery sticks
(See our third book, **The Macro Almanac**, for details and recipes that are infinitely more delicious than the above bare-bones start.)

Dinner:
Cut out all processed foods.
Basically omit any white flour, white sugar, and red meat to once a week while you attempt to increase whole grains and vegetables to a proportion of roughly 50/50.

Beans, seafood, fowl, nuts, limited seasonal fruits, should
    be worked in as you learn a new way of life.
Give yourself a "junk day" every Saturday for a while if you
    need. This will be your day to have your favorites.

Red meats: Reduce to once or twice a week, maximum;
                eventually phase out for a one month trial,
                for many arthritics, for example, never clear
                until they are off a month.
White flour: Omit. Substitute whole grains or grind fresh
                flour from them
White sugar: Omit. Substitute limited amounts of
                unrefined natural sweets, like real maple
                syrup, barley malt syrup, yinnie rice syrup,
                molasses, dates
Butter: OK to use. Never use margarine. Tofu mayon-
                naise is a substitute (recipe in The Macro
                Almanac).
Oils: Cook with olive oil or unrefined, dark brown
                sesame oil. For uncooked foods, use 1-2 tbs
                of linseed (flax seed oil) daily. Be sure it
                comes in a hard plastic or opaque glass dated
                bottle. Or use cold pressed walnut or saf-
                flower oil.
                Use only cold pressed oils. Never use
                hydrogenated, polyunsaturated oils from the
                regular grocer. These are refined to be
                totally colorless and in bottles that permit
                light to further destroy any vestiges of
                nutrition. Think about it. You never see
                fine oils in a clear bottle. People who are
                proud of the nutritional value of their prod-
                ucts know better.
No fruit drinks, soda, coffee, tea, alcohol:
                Substitute herb teas, grain coffees (Inka),
                spring water in glass containers, macrobiotic
                teas. (Anyone who puts spring water in
                plastic containers just plain doesn't under-
                stand or care that phthalates leach into the
                water and into your brain and deposit in your
                tissues.) Limit alcohol and coffee to one
                day a week. If you can't limit alcohol, you
                had better ask yourself if you are not hooked

and check with your local Alcoholics
Anonymous. Fruit juices just load you with
mold antigens and sugar and do not contain
the balance of fiber and nutrients that were
lost in the pressing and storage.

****
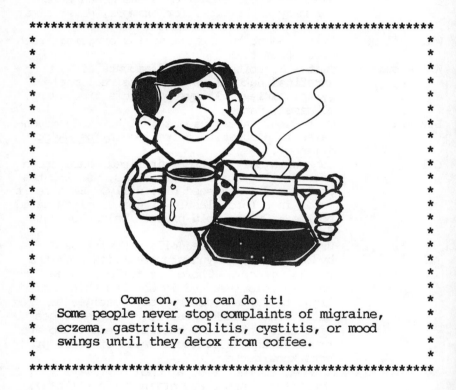

Come on, you can do it!
Some people never stop complaints of migraine,
eczema, gastritis, colitis, cystitis, or mood
swings until they detox from coffee.

****

Snacks: Any raw seeds (like sunflower), or nuts (like
                 almonds), but be sure they are not roasted in
                 oils or salted. You can roast your own in a
                 skillet (The Macro Almanac).
                 Popcorn
                 Any vegetables, raw or cooked.
                 Limited amounts of fruits*, raw, cooked or

dried (1-2 cups of fruits per day).
Any whole grains
Use limited amounts of broken grain foods
(made from freshly ground flours, cold
pressed oils, with substitutes for cane, corn
or processed sugars like yinnie rice syrup
and aluminum-free baking powders like
Rumford).

Always opt for organic food.
Always opt for as fresh food as possible, but organic should
take precedence over this.
Try to rotate or vary the diet so you do not have monotony,
which leads to food allergy and nutrient deficiencies.
Always avoid irradiated food, since it reduces the average
vitamin content about 25% for many nutrients, fosters
the growth of undetectable mycotoxins that are capable
of causing cancer years down the road, and contain
unique radiolytic products (URP's) which have been
untested yet by the government and have potential
carcinogenicity.

Avoid foods from foreign countries as much as possible,
since they are the benefactors of our banned
pesticides.

Remember:
Rotate, or vary your diet on a day to day basis so you
get a wide range of foods. Do not eat in a monotonous rut;
by eating more variety:
1. You'll stave off boredom and not be driven to
eat things that are not right for you now.
2. You will increase your chances of getting more
trace minerals which are rarely measured or for
which we have no current measures, but which
nevertheless are critical to detox function.
3. By rotating you'll decrease your chances of
developing food allergies.

Phase III: DETOX YOUR PERSON

You've learned how overburdened your detox system can get from 21st century chemicals. But like the asthmatic wearing a cat around his neck, have you ever considered how many chemicals you wear on your body each day?

The average person uses a fragrant shampoo with petrocarbon additives (all those names you can't pronounce on the ingredients label), conditioner, hair spray or mousse, shaving cream, toothpaste, skin toner, makeup, after shave (perfume), deodorant, skin lotions, and powder.

Then the clothes contain odors (and other odorless chemicals) from detergents, fabric softeners, not to mention formaldehyde and other chemicals to make them color fast and wrinkle resistant. And you've learned what the chemicals in dry cleaning fluid, moth balls and shoe polishes can do to the brain.

So what are you waiting for? From now on when you buy new, only get unscented products. (Brand names are found in The E.I. Syndrome.) And you'll save money. For example, baking soda makes an inexpensive dentrifice and deodorant powder (and when you really detox, you won't need a deodorant).

Detox your body and pretty soon you'll be able to notice how bad everyone else smells and how good you feel.

QUICK STOP SUMMARY

How Do I Make My Grooming Less Toxic?

Use nothing scented: There are progressively more products on the market in health stores and health oriented pharmacies, and numerous books on substitute products (D.L. Dadd, Non-Toxic and Natural).

As you get less toxic you will find that you do not need deodorant. However in the beginning as you are getting yourself detoxified, you may have even worse odors that no amount of perfume can cover up, as you sweat out old toxins. If you do, rejoice. You are eliminating toxins. If it isn't self-limited in 2-4 weeks, see your doctor.

```
*******************************************************
*                                                     *
*                                                     *
*                                                     *
*                                                     *
*                                                     *
*                                                     *
*                                                     *
*                                                     *
*                                                     *
*                                                     *
*                                                     *
*                                                     *
*                                                     *
*                                                     *
*                                                     *
*                                                     *
*                                                     *
*                                                     *
*      Avoid scented fabric softeners and polyester or *
*      acrylic clothes for they add to the burden you  *
*      must eventually detoxify.                       *
*                                                     *
*******************************************************
```

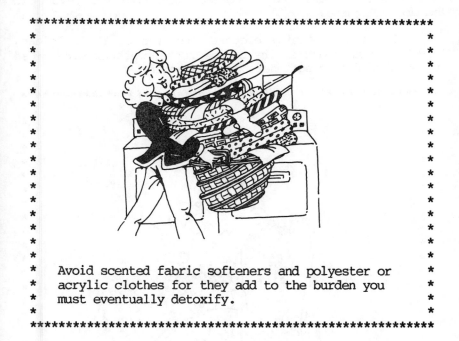

Clothing: Gradually replace with cottons and silks and things that can be washed and not dry cleaned. Also gradually replace polyesters and other synthetics with natural fibers that feel good on your skin, do not cause burning, heat, prickling, itching, spaciness, weakness, or other reactions and that allow your skin to breathe.

As you get cleaned out, many of you will notice that you are unable to tolerate polyesters touching your skin, that you feel an unusually warm or burning or tingling sensation, or have flu-like achiness. These are common

symptoms, but, most people are unable to appreciate them
because they are so overloaded that this is a drop in the
bucket compared with their total load.   As you get unloaded
however, these environmental insults will be more like being
hit with a brick.   You'll notice them like you never did
before. Rejoice.

For the remaining clothes that you still dry clean,
try to air them out in the garage for a month or more.   Use
no scented fabric softeners in the laundry.

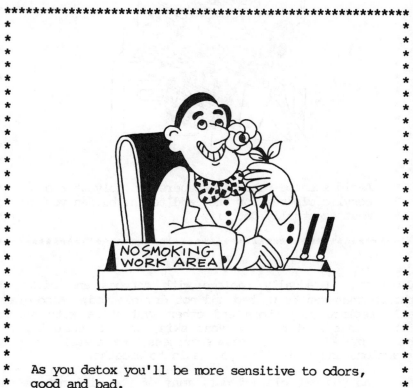

As you detox you'll be more sensitive to odors,
good and bad.

Stop Smoking: You may find some smoke-permeated clothes that you just can't stand because you can't get the smell out of them. These will have to be discarded.

Phase IV: <u>DETOX YOUR BEDROOM</u>

Do you wake up feeling great? Can you recall your dreams? And were they nonstressful? Do you awaken without stiffness or achiness, without tiredness? Are you happy, playful, and alive with anticipation for the day? If so you can skip this phase.

If not, why not? After all there are only four reasons why you wouldn't wake up feeling great:
1. Something is very wrong with your diet.
2. You have a toxic bedroom.
3. Something is wrong with your psycho-social life.
4. You have chronic disease.

For many, one problem is that they have a toxic bedroom and they wake up exhausted and symptomatic because the detox pathways have not had a rest, much less a chance to catch up all night long.

Here are the commonest sources of toxicity in the bedroom: Carpeting outgases formaldehyde, benzene, toluene, xylene, methacrylates, and more. The newer it is, the worse it is, generally. Some do not finish outgassing, even for 20 years. And by then it is a trade off, of whether to keep it since so much dust and mold has accumulated underneath it. Some of the same chemicals can outgas from glues and particleboard, lacquers, and laminates in night stands, dresser drawers, chairs, dressing tables, and headboards. The younger they are, the more glued joints, the the more pressed board or particleboard, then the more xenobiotics they tend to outgas.

The mattress itself, is often one of the most toxic objects in the bedroom, as it is made from foam (formaldehyde), and contains not only pesticides, but fire retardants. Did you know you can get one pesticide-free, fire retardant-free (<u>The E.I. Syndrome</u> has sources)? If it is a waterbed, it will be outgassing vinyl and phenol until it dries and cracks. Vinyl wall papers, glues, and panelings add even more chemicals. Polyester draperies with plasticized thermal linings, polyester filled comforters, permanent pressed and polyester sheets, mattress pads, and pillows, as well as scented detergents and fabric softeners, add a plethora more. And we haven't even gotten to the closet where leathers, shoe polishes, and dry cleaned clothes outgas trichloroethylene and other chemicals to your blood stream. And who knows what precious treasures might be stored under the bed?

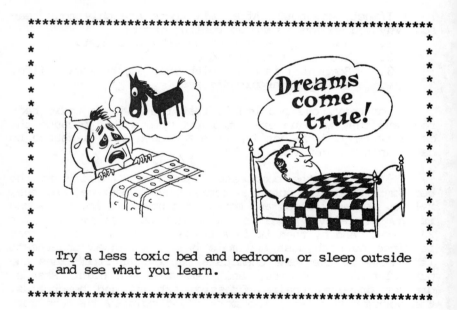

Try a less toxic bed and bedroom, or sleep outside and see what you learn.

To determine if it is the bedroom, you could sleep on the porch one night. If you have a great sleep you know the bedroom is toxic. So reduce the chemicals as best you can. Obviously, the best bedroom would have only the bed in it. No other furnishings, carpeting, closets, or dressers laden with perfumes and sachets. Use only non-scented cleansers and polishes. A prescription cotton mattress free of fire retardent and pesticide is the best, but many do very well with several layers of extra heavy duty restaurant grade aluminum foil (shiney side up) covered by several cotton flannel sheets and blankets. How much you need to do will be governed by how well you feel when you awaken. An air cleaner can cover a host of sins, but it is best to rent one on a trial basis before purchasing it (details in The E.I. Syndrome). Whether the windows get opened will depend on what is coming in. If it is highway traffic exhausts, with diesel fumes, or nearby industrial effluents from some paper or plastic factory, you had better not open them, but get a

```
******************************************************
*                                                    *
*                                                    *
*                                                    *
*                                                    *
*                                                    *
*                                                    *
*                                                    *
*                                                    *
*                                                    *
*                                                    *
*                                                    *
*                                                    *
*                                                    *
*                                                    *
*                                                    *
*                                                    *
*                                                    *
*                                                    *
*                                                    *
*                                                    *
*   Never use smelly cleansers in your home, especially *
*   in your bedroom.  If you lie there inhaling toxic   *
*   chemicals all night you'll awaken with a fatigued   *
*   detox system.                                       *
*                                                    *
******************************************************
```

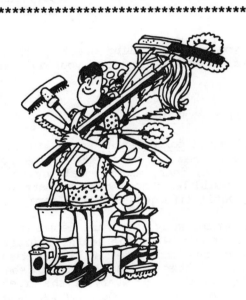

room air depollution device (Allermed, Puri-dyne, Clean-air, Dust-Free, etc.).

The only way to determine if mold is a problem is to get a mold plate and expose it in the room for one hour (see Appendix for details). Return it by mail and the lab will identify and quantify the fungi and mail the report to you. If there is too much mold, you will need to identify the source and correct it. Frequent sources are heavy shade trees about the house, lack of gutters to carry water away from the foundation, and too tight of a house, so that it holds in too much moisture. Also, house plants, an adjacent poorly ventilated bathroom, moldy carpet, lack of storm windows and lack of good window seals can add to the high mold count.

When you awaken feeling great, with no symptoms and enthusiastic to tackle the day, you will have come a long way.

Phase V: DETOX YOUR MIND

We all store toxic mental wastes in our minds, just as we store toxic chemical overloads in the fat and tissues. What toxic guilt, fear, anger, jealousy, or sadness do you bear? When would be a good time to part with it? Or are you waiting until life gets a little more perfect?

For example, many women are depressed. When a little girl falls from her bike, she learns quickly that it's considered precocious and cute if her brother kicks it and calls it four letter words. But if she does, she is instantly reprimanded. However, if she cries, she gets comfort from Daddy's lap. Consequently, women, especially, learn early to stifle their anger and turn it into depression. Do you have repressed anger masquerading as depression? What are you going to do about it? Get mad or stay sad?

There are professionals galore to help. The answers are as varied as people. Religion, meditation, acupuncture, energy balancing, shiatsu, massage, kinesiology, balancing exercise, yoga, etc. You'll notice that because the mind is known to be part of the body that some people devise just as much mind benefit from physical therapies (like shiatsu, chiropractic adjustments, or exercise) as others do from meditation, gestalt psychotherapy, or religion.

Exercise is doubly important, not only for the release of mental strain that it provides, but sweat is one of the ways through which the body discharges toxic wastes, you'll recall.

One prescription you should follow is to bring some happiness to yourself each day. It's not called selfish, it's called smart. Because if you're an unhappy SOB who doesn't have time for themselves, just how much happiness do you think you bring to those that you supposedly love (or are secretly trying to punish)? The second part of the prescription is to also bring some happiness to someone else each day. It doesn't have to be much, but it should be con-

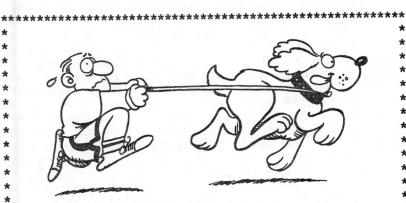

If you can't force yourself to get some exercise, how about a pet? They not only provide an excuse to exercise, but also unconditional love.

sistent so that it develops into a healthful habit. Make sure you hug someone each day, and preferably not the same someone each day.

The attitude you bring to your new endeavor will make or break its success. Some people will find any excuse to be unsuccessful: (1) they don't believe they deserve to be happier and healthier, (2) they are not ready to be happier and healthier; it has become a way of life and they don't know any other way. But if you believe you're worth it, and you're sick of feeling sick, you know what has to be done.

The moment you awaken, count your blessings, get into your song or dance routine, even if it's just mentally. Meditate or creatively visualize being successful at what lies ahead for the day. Do whatever it takes to energize your psyche, for remember, once the bad chemicals, foods, mold allergies, and gut organisms are conquered and nutrient deficiencies are corrected, all the chemistry that goes on inside that skull is of your own creation.

And through the day, practice whatever it takes to keep you up. It's very soothing to the immune system to give/get hugs. If we treated more adults as warmly as we treat babies, this would be a better world. Have you ever watched people around a baby? They immediately become compassionate, complimentary, smiling, considerate, and loving. Why can't they carry those feelings into their relationships with adults? Most babies get more love than they know what to do with while most adults are starved. Why not treat people as though they were adorable and cuddly? For after all that's how many would like to be. Just because they're fat and ugly doesn't mean they are not crying out to be loved, appreciated, respected, nurtured and admired for what they do well. You'll find some miraculous changes in your life (and theirs) when you start understanding this.

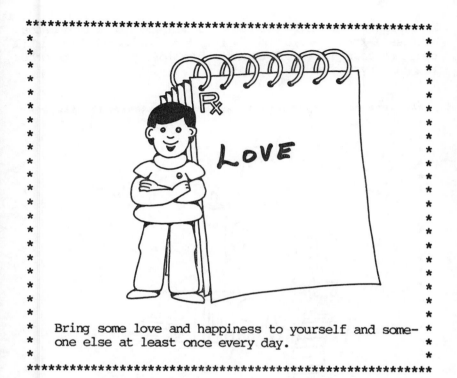

```
*************************************************************
*                                                         *
*                                                         *
*                                                         *
*                                                         *
*                                                         *
*                                                         *
*                                                         *
*                                                         *
*                                                         *
*                                                         *
*                                                         *
*                                                         *
*                                                         *
*                                                         *
*                                                         *
*                                                         *
*                                                         *
*                                                         *
*                                                         *
*  Bring some love and happiness to yourself and some-   *
*  one else at least once every day.                     *
*                                                         *
*************************************************************
```

Case example: A 35 year old doctor came to see me for treatment of his asthma. He didn't want to test many of the items that I knew asthmatics needed. I was content to let him run the show, because what usually happens is that as people start feeling better, they realize they can feel even better than this. By then they have read our books and understand the method to my madness, and want to go all the way to wellness.

But one statement stopped me dead in my tracks. "Listen, I can't get completely well. My body provides me with a form of catharsis. I need this spitting up of mucous to help me get rid of other things. I just want to take the edge off the severity of my asthma, not clear it entirely."

I couldn't, in all fairness, acquiesce to his demands, because I knew I would be feeding his psychopathology until the day that it would consume him (or me, or some other innocent bystander).

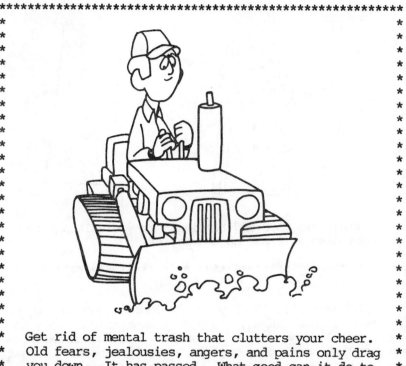

```
************************************************************
*                                                          *
*                                                          *
*                                                          *
*                                                          *
*                                                          *
*                                                          *
*                                                          *
*                                                          *
*                                                          *
*                                                          *
*                                                          *
*                                                          *
*                                                          *
*                                                          *
*                                                          *
*                                                          *
*                                                          *
*                                                          *
*                                                          *
*                                                          *
*                                                          *
*    Get rid of mental trash that clutters your cheer.     *
*    Old fears, jealousies, angers, and pains only drag    *
*    you down.  It has passed.  What good can it do to     *
*    keep it around?  Replace it with powerful, healing    *
*    love.                                                 *
*                                                          *
************************************************************
```

What I'm trying to point out is that you should make sure you're honestly ready to get well. Can you close your eyes and visualize what life would be like with boundless energy? If not, why not? Are you punishing yourself or someone else? If you are eager to get well but have just been ill so long that you can't conceive of any other way, start visual imagery of how you will be, how you will feel, what you will do. Practice imagining, for it often turns out to be a rehearsal for the real thing that materializes.

```
*************************************************************
*                                                           *
*                                                           *
*                                                           *
*                                                           *
*                                                           *
*                                                           *
*                                                           *
*                                                           *
*                                                           *
*                                                           *
*                                                           *
*                                                           *
*                                                           *
*                                                           *
*                                                           *
*                                                           *
*                                                           *
*                                                           *
*                                                           *
*                                                           *
*                                                           *
*                                                           *
*     The attitude and enthusiasm you bring to this         *
*     endeavor will make or break your success.  If you     *
*     fail to make the effort this time, how successful     *
*     do you think you'll be with future endeavors?         *
*                                                           *
*************************************************************
```

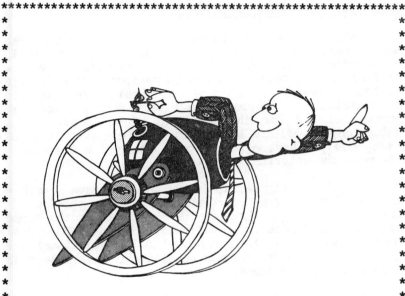

Hugs

Remember one thing about hugs; if you do not give any, you rarely will get any. If you want to remain a stone, that is your choice.

Evaluating Your 5 Phases of Detox

Once you have gone through the program to the best of your current ability, it will be time for you to evaluate your progress. And again do not be too harsh on yourself. The first time through will not be perfect, and neither will the last. Remember, many are too tired to do the program well initially. Do your best, learn from it, and as you improve, dig in for higher levels of wellness. At your evaluation, if you are less tired, you were certainly toxic. And by now you have a pretty good idea which areas of your life were the culprits.

If you're only partially better, you have a much more serious problem; get your nutrient levels checked. Our first book, The E.I. Syndrome is 650 pages on the scope of environmental illness. It will show you how to diagnose and treat symptoms that have resisted all conventional thera-pies. It will teach you how to diagnose the cause of many of your chronic symptoms.

The second book, You Are What You Ate is a special program that has cleared people who have markedly improved but were not 100% well through the use of the techniques in the first book.

It is a very difficult change for many, however, and so a book to ease one into a transition diet is The Macro Almanac.

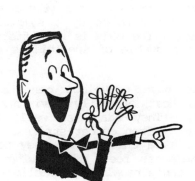

```
***********************************************************
*                                                         *
*                                                         *
*                                                         *
*                                                         *
*                                                         *
*                                                         *
*                                                         *
*                                                         *
*                                                         *
*                                                         *
*                                                         *
*                                                         *
*                                                         *
*                                                         *
*                                                         *
*                                                         *
*                                                         *
*                                                         *
*                                                         *
*                                                         *
*                                                         *
*                                                         *
*                                                         *
*                                                         *
*                                                         *
*                                                         *
*                                                         *
*  Periodically Evaluate ....                             *
*                                                         *
*  The 5 phases of detox:  organization, diet, person,    *
*  bedroom, mind.  How strict were you?  What symptoms     *
*  improved?  What did it teach you?  Now what do you      *
*  have to do to get to a yet higher level of wellness?    *
*                                                         *
***********************************************************
```

More On Masking

Remember the masking phenomenon, where the body adapts or "gets used to" certain chemicals and symptoms go underground for a while? The same effect can be created with medications to hide or cover-up or mask symptoms. Eventually other symptoms will surface instead, because you have failed to heed the alarm of nature and make a change in your lifestyle. That's why when a person finally gets his back problem covered, he starts going to the urologist or gastroenterologist or sinus doctor. It's like any piece of machinery. Ignore or poorly patch up a symptom and it breaks down somewhere else. The body is no different. Before you know it, you have a stable of specialists and cabinet full of drugs.

Some people have marvelous genetics. They adapt beautifully to a host of daily environmental, including dietary, insults. They adapt so well, that they never notice any symptoms. Then cancer strikes. Others have had so many illnesses as a child, that they never even got to know what real wellness feels like. They think they are well because they can't recall ever feeling any differently.

These people consider themselves well, and are shocked when they do the detox program. "I never knew I felt so bad until I got well" is what we hear frequently. So even if you think you are well, detox yourself for a month and see what you learn. You may be in for a pleasant surprise that you're not as old as you thought.

The following was borrowed from our second book, You Are What You Ate. It's more sophisticated than many of you will need at this point, but it provides a good check list to help determine where your weak areas might be.

E.I. Checklist

Is your inhalant load covered?

_____ (1) Have you exposed mold plates in the bedroom
and other places you most commonly frequent?
If the mold count is high, have you
recultured until the plates show your
environmental controls are good? (Anyone can
send for petri dishes or mold plates to
expose in the home. Directions are included
plus a return mailer. A list of the types
and numbers of molds identified by a Ph.D.
mycologist will be mailed to you as soon as
the last mold has stopped growing. This is
usually within 4-7 weeks. Petri dishes or
mold plates, as they are called, are
available from Mold Survey Service, 2800 W.
Genesee St. Syracuse, NY 13219, $15 each).

_____ (2) Is there an air cleaner in the bedroom,
regularly serviced?

_____ (3) Is the carpet out of the bedroom?

_____ (4) Is there an air conditioner in the bedroom?

_____ (5) Has there been removal of all objects except
the bed if you are very sensitive (especially
bureaus and closet contents)?

_____ (6) Has there been cutting of nearby trees,
installing gutters, trenches, and dry wells
about the house to reduce dampness; correction of leaks, removal of old wallpaper,
bathroom tiles and other hidden sources of
mold?

_____ (7) Test titrated inhalants (pollens, dust,
molds, mites) and receive injections twice
weekly until symptoms are clear. Return to
twice weekly interval if symptoms recur.

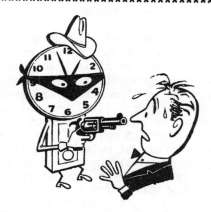

****
If time is the hold-up, get some help with time
management. The most concise book I ever saw was
a little paperback by Alan Lakein, How To Get
Control Of Your Time And Your Life.
****

_____ ___ (8) Break down mixes (trees, grasses, molds) and
test to individual components of mixes that
are especially allergenic.

_____ (9) Test newer molds.

_____ ___ (10) Retest phenol and glycerine if injections
cause a problem.

_____ (11) Do you have cotton mattress covers and bed-
ding, regularly washed? Did you evaluate an
old foil covered mattress?

_____ (12) Is there regular wet dusting to remove and
not merely redistribute the dust?

_____ (13) Did you remove allergenic animals?

Has food allergy been ruled out?

_____ (1) Use glass bottled spring water for a one month trial.

_____ (2) Did you evaluate the rare food, rotated diet for one month?

_____ (3) If there was no difference, a different rare food diet, not necessarily rotated of extremely rare foods and as organic as possible should be evaluated on the chance that your initial one contained hidden food allergies.

_____ (4) Have you fasted five days?

_____ (5) Did you evaluate food testing and daily injections for at least 6 months?

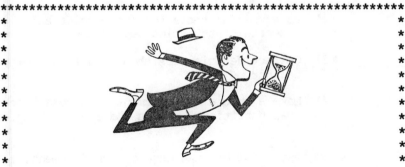

```
**********************************************************
*                                                        *
*                                                        *
*                                                        *
*                                                        *
*                                                        *
*                                                        *
*                                                        *
*                                                        *
*                                                        *
*                                                        *
*                                                        *
*       If you're waiting for a time when things slow    *
*   down and life is less hectic before you make some    *
*   diet changes, you'll probably die first.             *
*                                                        *
**********************************************************
```

Is Candida a problem?

_____ (1) Did you do a ferment-free (bread, cheese, alcohol, vinegar, catsup, mayonnaise, salad dressing, packaged foods) and sugar-free (anything with corn syrup, maple syrup, cane sugar, dextrose, maltose, malt, honey) diet for two months?

_____ (2) Use a known viable source of acidophilus such as Vital Dophilus used for 6 months?

_____ (3) Did you evaluate a trial of Nystatin with all of the above for 2 months?

_____ (4) And the addition of a 2-4 week trial of ketoconazole (Nizoral)?

Is there a hidden nutritional deficiency?

_____ (1) Have all the latest vitamin and mineral assays been drawn? There are new tests available every few months, that we didn't have before.

_____ (2) Have special tests for amino acids and essential fatty acids been drawn?

_____ (3) Correct deficiencies then re-assess the balance.

_____ (4) Make a special appointment to assess biochemical nutritional status and diet quality.

The toughest problem: the chemical environment.

_____ (1) Create an oasis (preferably bedroom) where you can clear.

_____ (2) If you can't clear, stay outdoors in a safe area like near the ocean or go to the Dallas environmental unit. (If you are considering this, you would be wise to read Dr. Rea's book first on how to build an ecologically

```
***********************************************************
*                                                         *
*                                                         *
*                                                         *
*                                                         *
*                                                         *
*                                                         *
*                                                         *
*                                                         *
*                                                         *
*                                                         *
*                                                         *
*                                                         *
*                                                         *
*                                                         *
*                                                         *
*                                                         *
*   What will it take to get yourself motivated to get    *
*   truly well?                                           *
*                                                         *
***********************************************************
```

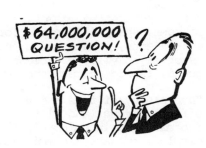

safe house. <u>Your Home and Your Health</u> is available from Environmental Health Center, Suite 200, 8345 Walnut Hill Ln. Dallas, TX 75231, $24.)

____ (3) Go on oxygen temporarily.

____ (4) Only after you are clear can you re-enter environments to identify the culprits. Some of the worst triggers are urea foam formaldehyde insulated buildings, tight buildings, traffic and industrial exhausts, gas heating systems and appliances, glues and adhesives (carpet, tiles, cupboards, furnishings), gasoline (benzene) and oils (pumps, furnaces, machines), plastics and synthetic materials (xylene, formaldehyde, toluene, acrylics, vinyls, benzene, phenol), cleaning solutions and air fresheners (xylene, benzene, tri-chloroethylene, phenol), pesticides, and municipal water (chlorine, chloroform).

(5) Chemically-free personal grooming is manda-tory: no scented cosmetics, deodorants, mousses, shampoos, soaps, lotions, sprays, astringents, conditioners, new fabrics, poly-ester or acrylic, dry cleaned items, deter-gents, fabric softeners or cigarette smoke.

(6) Have plenty of fans and vents in the home and office: fresh (and filtered if in contam-inated area) incoming air, adequate enough to displace outgassed chemicals.

(7) Allow 1/2-2 years in a chemically clean environment (on a sound ecologic program with periodic monitoring) for healing to occur. It takes time. Only drugs give responses overnight.

(8) Remove yourself from contaminants as soon as possible, shower, cleanse the bowel, take antioxidants and recover as quickly as possible.

(9) Do you need to test chemicals? (We published the protocol in the National Institutes of Health medical journal, Environmental Health Perspectives, volume 76, pp 195-198, 1987.)

(10) Do you need a detoxification program?

(11) Have you reread The E.I. Syndrome?

IS YOUR BRAIN IN A HEALING MODE?

(1) Do you need to be ill? Are you more comfort-able being ill than well? If so, you need a professional counselor.

_____ (2) Do you practice positive imagery and not just wishful thinking?

_____ (3) Have you reduced your personal stress to show your body that you respect and love it? Are you making a commitment to lifestyle changes and wellness?

_____ (4) Have you changed your schedule to purposely make time for exercise, meditation and healing? Or are you still clinging to the excuse that you don't have time to make yourself well?

```
****************************************************
*                                                  *
*            LET'S FACE IT!                         *
*                                                  *
*                                                  *
*                                                  *
*                                                  *
*                                                  *
*                                                  *
*                                                  *
*                                                  *
*                                                  *
*                                                  *
*                                                  *
* Let's face it.  Only the guy in the mirror has the *
* power to determine how healthy you're going to be. *
* What are you going to do about it?                *
*                                                  *
****************************************************
```

_____ (5) Do you frequently involve yourself with "up", happy, positive people?

_____ (6) Do you make sure you sing and laugh several times a day?

_____ (7) Do you set realistic goals and periodically assess your progress?

_____ (8) Do you feel optimistic and believe you are worth the effort, and that you will get well?

Have you ruled out special problems? For example:

_____ (1) The need to have another thorough medical exam? There are constant new nutrient levels available.

_____ (2) Special tests of hormones and neurotransmitters.

_____ (3) Test ionization and electromagnetic field effects.

_____ (4) A non-supportive spouse.

_____ (5) Consider phenolics, macrobiotics.

Note: The above areas (2,3,5) are so new your only recourse will be to see the doctor for an explanation of these. They are not written up yet.

Go For It!

Chapter 9:   HEALTH IS NOT AN ABSENCE OF DISEASE

Ask any doctor, "What is health?"   The majority will erroneously tell you it is the absence of disease.

Why does an asthmatic patient, for example, have to be cared for by a nurse bathed in perfume, have the cleaning people use strong hydrocarbon floor washes in her room, and eat red dyed sugar water (jello) for lunch? When I see E.I. patients who have just been released from the hospital, they are aghast at how little the medical profession understands the triggers to their disease and the relationship to the environment.

We are one of the few medical cultures that considers man and health to be independent of the environment. This is a life-sentence to obsoletism, for in the end <u>what is health, but balance or equilibrium with our total environment?</u> Balance internally and externally, with micro- and macrocosm. That nightly martini has to be balanced, or you'll get cirrhosis and brain damage. One way the body has of balancing is through the detox system. But balance is also external, with the environment, with nature. You saw how chemicals in your environment can dangerously overload your detox paths and make the alcohol toxic to you. Hence balance with nature is just as important to health as is one's own internal balance. Not all drinkers get cirrhosis of the liver. You have to have the right genetics (be missing some enzymes for detox), and overload yourself in other ways (paint cars all day and go home to new carpeting).

The old Chinese yin and yang hasn't survived thousands of years by being based on anything less substantial. Western medicine, by being infatuated with its own progress, has egocentrically lost sight of the cosmic nature of health. Instead man has tried to bend, twist, and shape nature into a form that he considers smarter for his well-being. In the process he has become entangled in the web of

financial gain and now feels locked into a fight with
nature, instead of a marriage. A fight he cannot win. For
even if he wins, he pays for it with his health.

On the other hand, disease is a loss of equilibrium
which extends far beyond the boundaries of the body. As
people become sicker their decision making processes become
impaired. I can't help but wonder each time I leave
Washington, having been there to give a lecture, how much of
the decision making is influenced by the way people feel.
The pollution level is high and I get further symptoms upon
leaving my contaminated hotel to take a walk. It's interesting to evaluate the pollutant level as I stand gazing at
the White House. Then I recall how each new tenant completely repaints and renovates to his tastes. And as I
board my plane, I say a little prayer in hopes that my pilot
knows enough to suck on his oxygen if he starts to get
spacey from his cabin filling up with exhaust fumes as he
taxis to the runway, nose pointed directly into the tail of
the leading plane.

And this fact, that health is balance, explains why it
is never static. You can destroy it in one second --- if
you don't believe it, walk in front of a truck. This will
compromise the balance between the environment and you. Or
get exposed to a massive radiation leak, chemical spill, or
touch a high voltage line. Or you can destroy it slowly, by
eating and living out of balance with nature.

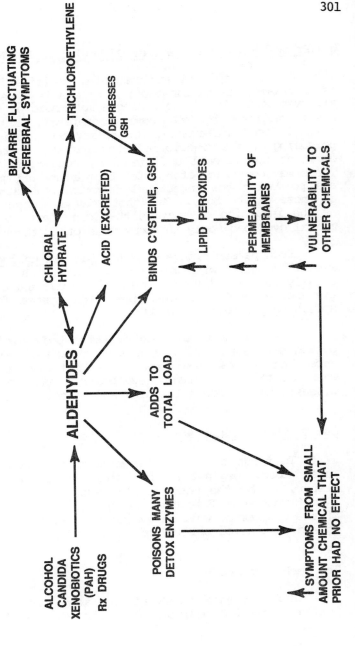

HEIGHTENED SENSITIVITY AND SPREADING PHENOMENON

The Principles And Procedures Of Environmental Medicine

One principle of environmental medicine is that there is a reason, an explanation, a treatable cause for nearly all symptoms. It may be a single IgE mediated allergy or it may be mediated by IgG, immune complexes, or the pH mechanism of food intolerance. Or it may be a toxic overload or poisoning of the xenobiotic detox system. There may be concomitant nutritional deficiencies, congenital or acquired. There may be toxic metabolites from uninvited gut flora that are poisoning the intestinal detoxication pathways as well as those in the body. And there may be enzyme deficiencies or the induction of enzymes that can adapt to the environmental overload, only to compromise other functions.

Each person brings with him his own unique biochemical way of dealing with his surroundings. He also has his totally individual target organ selection and toxicity. And his own unique time when his detox system fails and the spreading phenomenon begins.

There is a total load or total body burden that each person can bear. And beyond that threshold, symptoms start appearing. These symptoms are mild early warnings, which when masked with drugs, eventually lead to degenerative disease, target organ failure, and cancer.

Use Of These Principles In Diagnosis

To treat these people we merely whittle through the total load, beginning with what is perceived from the history to be the most likely cause (as described in The E.I. Syndrome). Extensive patient education is also a part of the program as well as evaluating the psychological make-up and adaptation ability of the person.

The Mechanisms of E.I.

E.I. mechanisms vary as much as do the symptoms. Some patients are IgE mediated in their sensitivities (pollen, dust, mold, sometimes food, sometimes chemicals). This is the type of allergy that most allergists restrict themselves to treating. But other people react by different immunologic mechanisms and many allergists chose not to deal with this type, usually because they are not yet trained in the biochemistry of nutrition and detoxication. When you choose not to treat the whole person, you understandably rely more on medications. But I wonder how many know, for example, that a common asthma medication, terbutaline causes increased loss of magnesium in the urine? This is dangerous when you realize many asthmatics are already magnesium deficient. Furthermore, studies have been done on people reporting to the emergency room with heart attacks. One of the determining factors of whether they lived or died was their magnesium status. All hypomagnesemic patients died (Cannon, LA, et al, Magnesium levels in cardiac arrest victims: relationship between magnesium levels and successful resuscitation, Ann. Emer. Med., 16: 11, 1195-1199, Nov. 1987). Similar results occur when stroke victims are studied.

But as you have learned, some reactors are a product of a damaged xenobiotic detoxication system. For example, some people with E.I. will often have excessive blood levels of xenobiotics (high formaldehyde, xylene, toluene, or pesticides, for example), compared with other people exposed to the same environments. There is such an incredible array of detoxication pathway distortions alone, that that chemistry by itself, could explain most symptoms. But beyond that, deficient nutrient levels contribute even further to an abnormal detoxication scheme. For example, a zinc deficiency (zinc is in 90 different enzymes) can explain the entire spreading phenomenon that we see in E.I. (This has been described in our book You Are What You Ate).

Last, but not least, chemicals the body cannot handle go on to damage other systems: immune, endocrine, nervous, cardiovascular, metabolic, and more.

```
**************************************************************
*                                                            *
*     THE 5 PRINCIPLES OF ENVIRONMENTAL MEDICINE             *
*                                                            *
*     1.    Total body burden or load (explains why          *
*           reactions from day to day are never the same).   *
*     2.    Adaptation or masking (acute toxicological       *
*           tolerance where the body "gets used to" a        *
*           toxin and adjusts to a new set point; mean-      *
*           while due to chronic exposure, bioaccumulation   *
*           and depletion of detox nutrients, the system     *
*           is stressed to where it appears that there is    *
*           sudden deterioration).                           *
*     3.    Bipolarity (the stimulatory phase is often       *
*           misinterpreted as health. Because it is          *
*           followed by a depressive phase, the victim       *
*           quickly learns what he must keep doing to        *
*           feel good, hence addiction to food, etc.         *
*           The alcoholic is a good example. At first        *
*           he feels high and aggressive, then he's          *
*           depressed. He keeps drinking until the end       *
*           organ damage appears. Chemicals like             *
*           toluene can be the same thing).                  *
*     4.    Biochemical individuality and individual         *
*           susceptibility (so that no two people get        *
*           the same symptoms from an exposure, likewise     *
*           people with the same symptoms all have a         *
*           different set of causes).                        *
*     5.    Spreading phenomenon or cascade (where as        *
*           the detox path becomes simultaneously more       *
*           depleted and overloaded, the individual          *
*           starts reacting to more chemicals, foods,        *
*           dusts, molds, and it takes progressively         *
*           less of the triggers to cause a reaction).       *
*                                                            *
**************************************************************
```

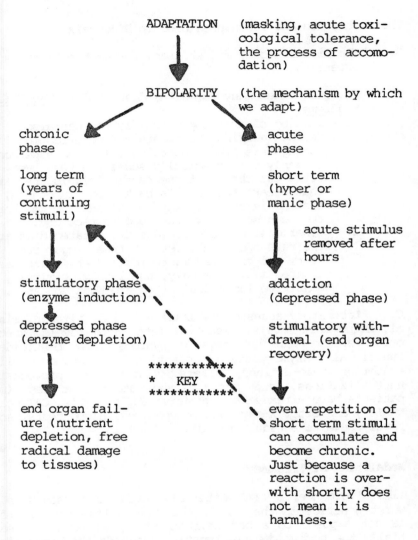

ADAPTATION (masking, acute toxi-
cological tolerance,
the process of accomo-
dation)

BIPOLARITY (the mechanism by which
we adapt)

chronic   acute
phase   phase

long term   short term
(years of   (hyper or
continuing   manic phase)
stimuli)
                                          acute stimulus
                                          removed after
                                          hours

stimulatory phase   addiction
(enzyme induction)   (depressed phase)

depressed phase   stimulatory with-
(enzyme depletion)   drawal (end organ
                                 recovery)

            ****
            *   KEY   *
            ****

end organ fail-   even repetition of
ure (nutrient   short term stimuli
depletion, free   can accumulate and
radical damage   become chronic.
to tissues)   Just because a
                                 reaction is over-
                                 with shortly does
                                 not mean it is
                                 harmless.

*   The above scheme is courtesy of Dr. William J. Rea.

The Techniques and Procedures Used in Diagnosis

A.   The history, oral and written, for each patient is extensive.

B.   The diet takes many forms (as described in The E.I. Syndrome).
1.   Fasting clears people rapidly but can also deplete marginal nutrients and detoxication conjugaters like glutathione, leaving a person suddenly more chemically sensitive than ever. It turns out that in these people this is the straw that breaks the camel's back. But in others, fasting is the only way to unload them to where they can start down the road to recovery.
2.   Other diet methods besides the rotated diet are the rare food diet, ferment free, sugar free diet, and modified macrobiotic diet, which has cleared many seemingly, hopelessly chemically sensitive individuals (You Are What You Ate).

C.   Laboratory assessments usually include vitamin, mineral, amino acid levels, essential fatty acid levels, xenobiotic levels (volatile organic hydrocarbons, pesticides), functional enzyme assays, quantitative immunoglobulins, endocrine auto-antibody titers, single-blind provocation-neutralizations, and gastric and stool analyses (most patients have already had extensive EKG's, EEG's, CAT scans, NMRI's, and other x-rays and conventional blood tests, so we rarely have to schedule these).

Modalities of Treatment

(1)   Avoidance is key. After all, even the person with the worst genetics in the world, will have little problem if he is not exposed to a bad environment. Avoidance is essentially the number one treatment; it unloads the biochemistry and allows healing; treatment is rarely successful without it.

(2) Nutrition: At least the more common vitamin and mineral levels readily available in the average commercial hospital and office laboratory should be looked at. It's amazing to me how many people are low in B1, folic acid, B6, A, rbc zinc, magnesium, copper, or iron. These tests are available in every doctor's office. Over 50% of the people are deficient in one or more nutrients (or high in formic acid). As more people are tested, it will show us whether this is a general trend, or we are just seeing the sicker patients by the process of elimination.

(3) Biological detoxication many include exercise, referral to a place with saunas or the personally tailored modified macrobiotic plan.

(4) Antigens include pollens, dust, molds, mites, biologics, hormones, neurotransmitters, and sometimes chemicals (described in The E.I. Syndrome).

(5) The acutely ill person is sometimes referred to an environmental unit; occasionally we will temporarily resort to medications, sometimes we will fast them, other times we will just carry on with testing and treat with injection therapy as well as environmental and dietary controls.

(6) The chronically ill person is our forte; the end-of-the-road, undiagnosed, incurable, hopeless person who has been told there is nothing more that can be done. He is the type of person that we address every day.

Air and water pollution are so important that some people will never recover unless they move from their town. For example, one dentist became so chemically sensitized by formaldehyde in the cold sterilization trays at work that he could no longer tolerate his home and ended up sleeping in the garage for a year, because he now became deathly ill every time he entered the house. It was not until he moved out of the city, into the country miles away, that he could start to recover more fully. Likewise many people will never clear until they find a glass-bottled, chemically less-contaminated water. Drinking the small amount of the hundreds of chemicals found in the average U.S. city water

supply is the final part of the total load that keeps some
from getting well.

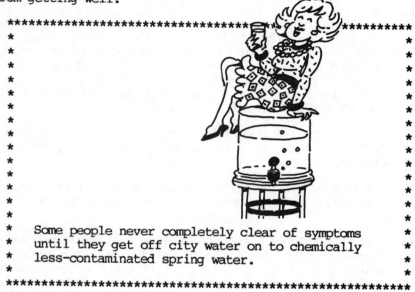

```
***********************************         *********
*                                                   *
*                                                   *
*                                                   *
*                                                   *
*                                                   *
*                                                   *
*                                                   *
*                                                   *
*                                                   *
*                                                   *
*                                                   *
*                                                   *
*                                                   *
*   Some people never completely clear of symptoms  *
*   until they get off city water on to chemically  *
*   less-contaminated spring water.                 *
*                                                   *
*****************************************************
```

In the same vein, food must be organic for many people
to clear. There are just too many chemicals that overload
an already ailing system otherwise.

Medico-legal: Proof for disability comes in two ways
and we usually use both ways so that it is more convincing.
We use before and after blood levels of the suspected xenobiotic, coupled with single-blind, provocation-neutralization. For example, a lady suffering from intense headaches
for 11 years has a much higher level of trichloroethylene
after a day at work than she does after a day at home. And
single-blind testing to it provokes her symptoms.

In terms of any other medico-legal work, I have put
everything I possibly can, in terms of warnings about ill
effects, in the book given to all of our patients, The E.I.
Syndrome. Many people would like to blame work environments
for their ills. Unfortunately, it's often not that simple.

For the diet and home environments have a major bearing on their health and vulnerability. This makes the legal aspects very tricky.

****
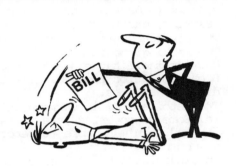

It's far too expensive to merely go chasing symptoms with medications. And in the end you pay the biggest price in 2 ways!
****

Why Is There A Need For A New Medical Specialty?

I. Modern man is exposed to more chemicals than any other generation in our history.
    A. The brain is the primary target organ for many.
    B. The detoxication system is the other primary target organ that is damaged. This leads to:
        1. The spreading phenomenon.
        2. Resetting of the body's thermostat.
        3. Symptoms fluctuate due to total load.
        4. Individual biochemical variation and target organ response.
        5. Individual susceptibility.
        6. Genetic change.
            (a) Faulty gene repair, ushering in

allergies.
(b) Xenobiotic adducts, initiating cancers.
7. Osmols penetrate the blood stream, blood-brain barrier, mitochondria, and endoplasmic reticulum.
8. The damaged detox system affects all other systems (endocrine, neurologic, cardio-vascular, gastrointestinal, etc.).
9. The environment is constantly changing.
10. The masking phenomenon or induction of enzymes facilitates adaptation.
11. Bioaccumulation proceeds silently until disaster strikes.
12. The detox system is unknown and undervalued.
(a) Some discoveries take years to study and and then many more to report on and change.
(b) Individuality of biochemical response, target organ and total load.
(c) There are no adequate non-human research models. For example, the laboratory rat does not have the same chemistry as a human and is not as easily poisoned by formaldehyde (or Thalidomide and many other xenobiotics) as the human, so they are erroneously assumed to be less harm-ful than they actually are for man.
C. Nutritional deficiencies.
1. Processing, irradiation, hooked on sweets, salts and fats, depleted soils, medication, abnormal intestinal flora causing inflam-matory malabsorption, chemical pollutants damaging and depleting nutrients of the detox system, individual metabolic abnormal-ities, and chronic disease all serve to com-promise the nutritional status.
2. Dysfunctional detoxication is not easily recognized because of lack of biochemical knowledge, and inadequacy of current medical tests.
3. Examples of a serious lack of nutritional biochemical knowledge that are currently

occurring (regarding calcium, magnesium,
chromium, essential fatty acids and their
role in hypercholesterolemia and
cardiovascular disease, for example).

Example of biochemical individuality: A family with a
recently urea foam formaldehyde insulated (U.F.F.I.) or
paneled home might have five members, for example. Even
though the exposure was clear cut, the onset of symptoms
varies, as do the target organs and the intensity. Some
individuals may not be affected, others will have different
symptoms, and different target organs. The one who is worst
affected will develop other sensitivities and slip down hill
and will gradually react quicker and more severely with each

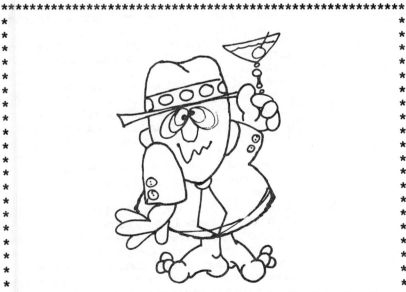

****

The commonest symptom of dysfunctional detoxication
is feeling spacey, dopey, dizzy, unable to concentrate ---- often as though you had had too many
drinks (but without the euphoria).

****

exposure and to exposures that never before bothered him.
The symptoms will fluctuate unpredictably but the brain is
usually always involved as well as the energy metabolism
system.

Dozens of specialists and thousands of dollars later,
these people are left doubting their own sanity. Some had
nutrient deficiencies when we studied them and sensitivities
to molds, foods, and many chemicals. They were improved, but
forever changed in that they could not abandon the chemically less contaminated lifestyle and tolerate all of the foods
and chemicals that they had tolerated before the formaldehyde exposure.

II. Two forms of medicine: Illness- or sickness-oriented
   medicine, and wellness-oriented medicine.
   A. Sickness-oriented medicine concerns itself right-
      ly so with acute care and inappropriately with
      chronic care.
   B. Wellness-oriented medicine has different
      principles:
      1. The patient shares the responsibility.
      2. Intensive patient education is necessary.
         The patient is not just an innocent bystand-
         er.
      3. The patient learns to listen to and
         appreciate symptoms as early warning
         devices.
      4. The specialty is not specialist oriented,
         nor organ oriented, but body oriented.
      5. It is not laboratory test oriented because
         the symptoms are too early to produce major
         enzyme changes as are seen in end stage
         degeneration (chronic) or vastly decompen-
         sated (acute) stages that are commonly
         treated by illness-oriented physicians.
      6. It is not a cookbook science with a single
         symptom that is universally treated with a
         single drug.

```
*************************************************************
*                                                           *
*   A mind is a lot like an umbrella:  it works better      *
*   when it is open.                                        *
*                                                           *
*************************************************************
```

III. Other issues:
   A. Bizarre psychiatric symptoms are due to acetaldehyde and chloral hydrate and other metabolites of xenobiotics.
   B. Thoughts produce chemical changes and contribute to the total chemical load, since neurotransmitters share common detox pathways.
   C. Candida albicans is a symptom, not a disease. And it is not the only intestinal imbalance to contribute to the total load.
   D. Provocation-neutralization is evidenced throughout biology and is a documentable fact, invaluable for diagnosis and treatment.
   E. Serial dilution endpoint titration is infinitely more individualized and safer than conventional testing.
   F. Also more cost effective in the grand scheme.
   G. Life quality effective. There is no comparison between the quality of life of someone who depends upon drugs and eats and lives willy-nilly versus someone who clears all their symptoms without suppressive medications.
   H. Outdated practices of merely drugging people with treatable chronic symptoms.

Digging Our Graves With Our Teeth

I may not sound it, but I have great admiration and respect for the 'old guard" of medicine. For we all owe them our lives. They got us to where we are (or at least where you are). What I do resent is their attempt to suppress progress because it interferes with the status quo. There are more than enough sick (and lazy) people to go around. The only ones I choose to concern myself with are those who, as I was, are on a steady downhill course getting more ailments every month, but who pass all physicals with flying colors, but realize that there must be a way to feel vibrant.

Meanwhile we corner the market on every prescription drug sold trying to find the one magic bullet that will make us feel whole again. And if you had ever told me that I could heal myself of all my complaints by changing my diet and environment, I would never have believed it.

But it's true. As one of my handsomest and oldest patients put it, we are digging our graves with our teeth. But once you get your nutrient deficiencies corrected, clean up your mold and chemical environment and go on the ultimate diet for wellness (You Are What You Ate, a macrobiotic diet modified for people with E.I.), you'll know when you are eating wrong for your system.

I went on the diet with my migraines, chronic sinusitis, asthma, and eczema already cleared (as long as I took my allergy injections). My back pain in an area of an old break 20 years prior was clear as long as I avoided beef, alcohol, formaldehyde, and natural gas. This is in spite of x-rays showing total loss of a disc (over the years I just ground it up), arthritic spurs and collapsed vertebrae bodies. And I had corrected my vitamins A and B6, magnesium and zinc deficiencies.

My depression was nonexistent as long as I avoided wheat, sugar, and chemical overload. My exhaustion was clear with the total program that controlled everything else.

I was walking on air. I felt so grateful to be that well, I was beyond words. But I still had problems: a cracked molar into the root, abdominal pain, warts that regrew every time they were removed over 2 years, and a painfully immobile shoulder for half a year.

Within the first month of the diet everything cleared. In four months I no longer needed any injections for
the first time in 20 years, and no supplements.

I am now, healthier, stronger, and sleep less than
ever before in my life. But I'm not naive enough to think
that just because it's good for me, it's good for you. It's
not for everyone. We have hundreds of patients who have
accomplished many more impossible feats than this with this
same program.

I was on the program for over a year when I decided to
see what would happen if I ate "regular" food again. It was
the perfect opportunity, for my husband had won an all-
expense paid trip to Nassau for his accomplishments in his

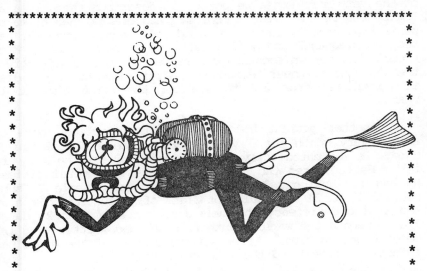

I was happy scuba diving, petting six-foot sting
rays at 80 feet below the surface. But within four
days I was bedridden and had to be carried to the
bathroom.

business. For four days I had a ball. I was scuba diving, petting live stingrays at 80 feet, and eating "normal" foods again. Then it hit. Within four days I was bedridden with severe back spasm (and I hadn't even done anything physical to precipitate it). Needless to say, I got right back on the program and was amazed to see I got out of trouble faster than I ever had before when I had gotten that bad. Now, a year later, I am wiser and healthier. If I have a one night indiscretion, I'll have minor symptoms the next day until I clear out again. If I space my treats to a couple a month, I have no symptoms. You also can find your level of tolerance, and it improves with time.

Rheumatoid arthritis of even over 10 years' duration responds beautifully to the diet in many. Seven out of nine of the very first ones we put on it described themselves as 80% better in the first 3 months. And one gal had a leuko-penia (dangerously low white blood cell count) since she had been on plaquenil and gold injections 16 years prior. Even though they were discontinued because they were ineffective, the white count never responded. After 3 months on the diet it normalized from 2.2 to 4.8 for the first time in 16 years.

Another patient had severe sinus infections once or twice every month for 3 years, ever since a dental proce-dure. He was chronically on antibiotics or else he was very ill. He consulted the best specialists in several cities. He had low antibody levels (hypoimmunoglobulinemia G, sub-classes 1 and 2) and could not fight off infection. He also had a zinc deficiency that was uncorrectable over 2 years. I even phoned the world's authority who had written over 1/2 dozen books on zinc. After several months of the diet, the infections ceased and the zinc was normal.

Many people who were devastatingly chemically sensi-tive, and who were prisoners in their homes, or ventured out for only short periods wearing a mask, were finally liber-ated, as the diet helped them get so healthy that they were no longer as chemically sensitive.

In fact, that was one of the main reasons we set out to investigate the diet. We hoped that since it had had such a miraculous track record of helping to clear cancers, that it could help ailing detox systems. With considerable modification, it did.

It is so healing, that people go through periods of "discharge" where the body gets rid of old chemicals in the process of healing and regeneration.

One 41 year old hair dresser oozed the color purple from her palms and neck for two weeks. It also stained her sheets where she had placed healing compresses over the liver and eczema sites. Purple was the color of the permanent wave solution she had used on patrons for 18 years. After 2 weeks it ceased and she was at a new level of wellness.

Another gal had sudden onset of depression, body aches, recurrence of eczema, and diarrhea with liver pain. Her liver enzymes were elevated during this crisis or discharge, and within a few days all was back to normal, except that, as is the case, she was at a higher level of wellness and tolerance.

On a global level this modified macrobiotic or detox diet of grains, greens, and beans makes more sense than our present one. One report claims that the world population is around 4000 million. There are about 500 million who are underfed. The amount of plant foods that we feed our farm animals would feed 15,000 million people; almost four times the world population. In other words, it takes many acres of grazing land and of grain products to grow a hamburger. In the meantime these grains could have fed many, while the grazing land could be saved for the trees we need to help balance the earth's carbon dioxide. And, in addition, we all would be healthier.

I've heard every excuse in the world why people can't be on a diet of grains, greens, and beans. Just let me remind you that where you decide to put your priorities is what will determine your present and future health.

I lecture all over the world. I have a hot plate in my suitcase for every country's current. I have one extra suitcase for all my cooking utensils and organic grains. The veggies I buy when I arrive. I cook in my hotel room much of the time. When I go out with my husband I take my food or select carefully (unless I'm on an infrequent splurge). I've taken my food to four star restaurants from Stockholm to Australia. We just hand a little container to the Maitre d' and ask him to serve a little of it to me whenever he brings my husband another course. I have a wonderful time. I'm with the person I idolize and adore most in life, it's a romantic setting, he's eating what makes him feel good, and I'm eating what makes me feel good. What else could we want?

Biochemical Mechanisms Of Macrobiotics

To a physician it seems incredible that any diet could be so powerful (read how Anthony Satillaro, M.D., who was given 6 months to live, cleared his own cancer of the prostate that had metastasized or spread to the skull in Recalled By Life, or Elaine Nussbaum, who was given 2 months to live with ovarian cancer metastasized to the liver, lung and back bones, cleared hers in Recovery). Yet when one understands the biochemistry of the detox system, it is not at all mysterious. For macrobiotics, the diet these two people and many others used to help clear their cancers is:

(1) a diet low in sugars, which are notorious for depleting the B vitamins {and you know how B1 (thiamine) helps metabolize aldehydes, drive GGPD to regenerate glutathione, and supply energy via the pentose pathway for synthesis of detox conjugates}. This in part explains the improved energy most experienced in the first month.

(2) It unloads the body of the biochemical work of buffering or balancing the pH (acid/alkali) by avoiding very acid meats (amino acids), sugars, and processed foods with all their chemical

additives. Often the end stage of Phase I is an acid. With the left over energy from not having so much buffer work, the body is able to actually heal (instead of merely keep up as most people do). Clearly chemicals compete with foods to stress the pH buffer (acid base balance) system all the more (Forncizzari, L, Internal Medicine, 9:6, 99-109, June 1988). This explains how people start turning off long-standing symptoms in the first few months.

(3) As well as being a major buffer for acid, carbonic anhydrase also creates hydrochloric acid for the first phase of gastric assimilation of minerals and amino acids. So if it is not used up by balancing cokes, coffee, meats, and sweets, there is more available for these functions. Many report better digestion in the first few months.

(4) By avoiding red meats, it frees up xanthine oxidase {a molybdenum requiring-enzyme, that not only metabolizes purines (meat) but aldehydes (to carboxylic acid) by doubling for aldehyde dehydrogenase when needed}. So it unloads the aldehyde bottleneck. With emphasis on beans, the molybdenum enzymes (aldehyde oxidase, xanthine oxidase, and sulfite oxidase) improve. Many report improved chemical tolerance in the first few months.

(5) As more beans are consumed more phosphatidyl choline is available for the endoplasmic reticulum, (it loses phosphatidyl choline when overloaded with detox work). Also, lecithin is the precursor to choline and acetyl choline in the hippocampus of the brain where new memory is formed. Lecithin can render new long-term memories less susceptible to destruction following training (Mizumori, SJY, et al, Effects of dietary choline on memory and brain chemistry in aged mice, Neurobiology of Aging, 6, 51-56,

1985). This many explain in part the improved memory that patients on the diet usually report within the first half year.

(6) With fresh organic ferments from products like miso, the bowel flora normalizes to promote biotin, and vitamins B12 and K synthesis. We don't have 3 1/2 pounds of bacterial flora in our guts without reason. They serve many beneficial functions. There is a decrease in the "good bugs" (Lactobacilli) and and increase in the "bad bugs" (like <u>Clostridrium welchii</u>, a cousin of the tetanus or lock-jaw bacteria) with high meat diets. Low meat, high grain (cereal) diets reverse this (Scheline, RR, Metabolism of foreign compounds by gastrointestinal organisms, <u>Pharmacol. Rev.</u>, 24: 4, 451-523, 1973). As well, there's a decrease in the flora that produces thiaminase, an enzyme that destroys vitamin B, before it ever gets absorbed.

(7) By eating less meat and concentrating on plants, we eat foods that have synthesized nutrients that mammals are biochemically incapable of, thus replenishing out stores (for example, plants make vitamin C, while man does not). No vitamin pill can ever come close to duplicating nature. By eating whole grains, you get the minerals and vitamins that processing removes. So B6, magnesium, zinc, vitamin C, and many other levels self correct without supplements. This is because the nutrient gradient of the whole foods is much higher. So mouthful for mouthful you get more nutrition to metabolize the calories. As the nutrition improves, people seem to lose cravings and so frequently weight (part of the weight loss is the reduced oils in the healing phase as you diet off all your bad fats with years of stored chemicals, so that you can later put it back with good clean healthy fat). Cravings are the body's only way of communicating that something is missing. Our problem is in what we

choose to grab to satiate that craving. We have
too many handy wrong choices available to us.
Anyway, reducing obesity and improving nutrition
have very favorable effects on the immune system
and resistance to disease (Chandra, RK, Nutrition
and immune responses, Can. J. Physiol.
Pharmocol., 61: 290-294, 1983).

(8) By eating as many organic foods as possible this
also boosts the nutrient level: studies show that
organic foods have higher intrinsic nutrient content than commercially grown (Rutgers Univ., NJ).

(9) By not eating devitalized (processed) foods that
slow peristalsis and sit in the gut and rot, and
by increasing foods with more bulk and fiber,
there's faster bowel transit time and less
putrefaction. Bowel movements become daily and
non-odorous and easy. As well, this helps the
bowel wall heal and restores its detox contri-
bution. There isn't the formation of as many
bowel toxins like putrescine and cadaverine to
compete with neurotransmitters like serotonin and
histamine for detoxication by diamine oxidase.
Under normal anaerobic conditions, the gut monooxygenase system can reduce potentially highly
reactive and carcinogenic arene oxides back to
the parent hydrocarbon. This translates into
better detoxication of cancer causing chemicals.

(10) Being off processed foods has a multitude of
unimagined advantages. For example baby foods
often contain MSG (mono sodium glutamate) as a
flavor enhancer. Striking irreversible degenerative changes in the infant mouse retina can be
observed with low doses of MSG (Olney, JW, HO,
OL, Nature, 227, 609-610, August 8, 1970).

(11) By making the body pH more alkaline (less acidic)
this pH also is optimally favorable to many detox
enzymes like aldehyde dehydrogenase. {Also
carcinogenic aromatic amines and amides react

with tissue nucleophiles at acid pH.} Many body
reactions proceed more adversely at acid pH's,
which is one reason we give I.V. bicarbonate in
the emergency room (Hess, ML, et al, Free radical
mediation of the effects of acidosis in calcium
transport by cardiac sarcoplasmic reticulum in
whole heart homogenate, Cardiovasc. Res., 18,
149-157, 1984; Tate, T, et al, Stimulation of
erythrocyte transketolase by added thiamin
diphosphate is pH dependent, Clinica Chimica Acta
137, 81-86, 1984.

(12) By trading milk for greens (2 cups of cooked
greens provides more calcium than a cup of milk),
there is not only more calcium, but more of the
trace minerals needed for incorporation of this
calcium into the bone matrix. Also by avoiding
milk products there is often dramatic cooling off
of many symptoms, bowel and otherwise, either
from a lactase deficiency standpoint or food
allergy or intolerance (Wilson, NW, et al,
Severe cow's milk-induced colitis in a 4 day old
exclusively breast-fed neonate, Ann. Allerg., 61,
207 (abstract), 1988). Basically, macrobiotics
is an oligoantigenic (very few foods in it that
people are allergic to) diet. (If you are too
sensitive to do it, read You Are What You Ate).
This serves to turn off many reactions that are
food induced.

(13) Low meat diets decrease the B-glucuronidase of
intestinal flora, and hence further protects us
from chemical overload. {The effect of this is
to decrease the enterohepatic circulation of
xenobiotics. For B-glucuronidase in the gut
splits glutathione off the xenobiotic, allowing
the xenobiotic which the body just worked so hard
at excreting to be reabsorbed into the body.}
Western high meat diets were compared with non-
meat diets in human volunteers. In a high meat
diet, intestinal bacterial B-glucuronidase
activity was higher. This translates into

"deconjugation" of intestinal xenobiotics, leaving these people at higher risk of colon cancer, since they have unprotected or unconjugated cancer-promoting chemicals in prolonged contact with the gut lining (Reddy, BS, et al, Fecal bacterial B-glucuronidase: Control by diet, Science, 183, 416-417, Feb. 1974).

(14) Also, a prolonged dietary protein restriction has a sustained beneficial effect on decreasing the rate of decline in diabetic renal function (Evanoff, G, et al, Prolonged dietary protein restriction in diabetic nephropathy, Arch. Intern. Med., 149, 1129-1135, May 1989).

(15) By restoring the nutrient balance, stimulating lymphatics with skin brushing, exercise, and relaxing muscles (that tighten and block normal flow of energies) through meditation, there is more aerobic body metabolism, as evidenced by the rosy glow and sparkling eyes that invariably appear in the first month. (If they don't, the program needs closer scrutiny and modification.) Translation: stimulating lymphatics unblocks them and allows more life-giving oxygen to reach tissues.

(16) Also during the first month there's a tremendously noticeable calming. Things don't set people off like they used to. I call these people "macro mellow". It's obviously partly due to the fact that the neurotransmitters can get properly metabolized through the aldehyde bottleneck now instead of hanging up and creating symptoms of irritability, etc.

It's also probably from an increase in nature's tranquilizer, magnesium, which is pivotal in chlorophyll. Lots of greens are the best source of magnesium; it's the best choice for a vast majority. We have witnessed it repeatedly in unsolicited reports on the effect of the magnesium loading test, "Oh, I can't believe how relaxed and calm I feel". It mimics what we hear in the early months of macro, which, of course doesn't build it up as fast.

Many factors facilitate or enhance the aldehyde path per above (less acid from diet for body to buffer, molybdenum from beans, restoration of other nutrients as some people rarely eat greens and are sorely lacking in B vitamins, decrease in toxins absorbed from stagnated bowel, avoiding meat frees up xanthine oxidase and reduces enterohepatic circulation, more sulfur from cruciferous vegetables is available for conjugation, with organic foods fewer xeno-biotics competing). This all serves to unload a highly stressed system and also adds to the relaxed state, possibly.

There is only one type of carrier molecule that transports six neutral charge amino acids across the blood brain barrier. Since tryptophan is in much lower ratio in most proteins than are tyrosine, phenylalamine, leucine, isoleucine, and valine, there's too much competition. With a high carbohydrate meal, the resultant increased insulin secretion reduces the plasma level of competing amino acids more than it does tryptophan. Consequently, after a carbohydrate meal there is a rise in tryptophan reaching the neurons (Fernstrom, JD, Wurtman, RJ, Nutrition and the brain, Scientific American, Feb. 1974; Wurtman, RJ, Effects of dietary amino acids, carbohydrates, and choline on neurotransmitter synthesis, The Mount Sinai Journal of Medicine, 55; 1, January 1988). So a meal low in protein and high in carbohydrates generates serotonin synthesis. Hence, another reason for the mellow tranquillity, in part, that is experienced in the first few weeks of a macrobiotic diet.

(17) Again by cutting down meat, there's another

explanation for the macro mellowness. The B2 requiring enzyme, monoamine oxidase (MAO), has many roles. One is to inactivate gut amines from bacterial putrifaction from tyramine (cheeses, for example). If there is sufficient MAO, it is also supposed to metabolize neurotransmitters like noradrenalin and adrenalin. Patients taking MAO inhibitors (some anti-depressants and blood pressure medications) can get a severe headache and even hypertensive crisis from tyramine-containing foods (mature cheeses, yogurt, chocolate, red wine). But what happens to the person not on prescribed drugs but who has marginal functions of this enzyme? (Jarroth, B, et al, The current status of monoamine oxidase and its inhibitors, The Med. J. of Austral., 146, 634-638, June 15, 1987). They will be sufficiently unloaded to clear symptoms and enjoy what I call, the macro mellowness.

(18) Children should not be eating the large amounts of meat that they commonly do in the American diet. The carnosine enzyme matures slowly between ages 7-11 (girls mature faster in this respect). The result is in some, insufficient carnosine to break down anserine from meat/fowl and an elevated B-alanine. This in turn has a lowering effect on taurine. Taurine deficiency is known to cause seizure disorders, cardiac arrhythmia, decreased ability to fight off infections (it gobbles up the OCl- generated by white blood cell phagocytosis). Also children have immature sulfotransferases, and meats are high in sulfur. The result could be increased incident of infections.

(19) As explained earlier, a Swedish study (European J. Pediatrics) showed via gastric biopsy that there was lymphocytic infiltration and decreased hydrochloric acid in the stomach of some milk allergic children for months after ingestion. This means that for months after they had

inferior assimilation of proteins and minerals.

This is also well documented in celiac disease.
One tiny indiscretion with wheat and the villi
of the intestine undergo severe and dangerous
atrophy (deterioration, faulty absorption) for
weeks and months secondary to the reactions. The
problem for them is the minute antigens that they
unknowingly get when eating out or having
processed foods. They must know precisely what
is in their foods. So for people who have
symptoms brought on by foods, the macrobiotic diet can be free of common antigens, milk
and wheat being the top two in the U.S.

(20) Cancer of the breast is positively correlated
with total fat intake, whether it's saturated
(beef, coconut) or unsaturated (polyunsaturated
safflower oil). Probably the dieting off of fat
deposits that inhibit lymphatic drainage is one
of the mechanisms of helping to clear cancer.
(Carroll, KK, Hopkins, GJ, Dietary polyunsaturated fat versus saturated fat in relation to
mammary carcinogenesis, Lipids, 14, 2, 155-158,
1978).

(21) By stressing organic foods, you avoid pesticides
and the "inert vehicle" solvents that carry them
and the barrage of "idiopathic" symptoms that
stem from them (Marsh, et al, Acute pancreatitis
following cutaneous exposure to an organophosphate pesticide, Am. J. Gastroenterol, 83, 1158-
1160, 1988; Lockey, JE, et al, Progressive
systemic sclerosis associated with exposure to
trichloroethylene, J. Occup. Med., 29:6, 493-496,
1987).

(22) There are many other benefits from reduced meat
ingestion. Some of them include the fact that it
reduces the ammonia load to the detox system,
leaving more glutathione to handle xenobiotics
(Takahashi, S, et al, Ammonia production by

IMR-90 fibroblast cultures: Effects of ammonia on glutathione, gamma-glutanyl transpeptidase, lysosomal enzymes and cell division, J. Cell, Physiol., 125, 107-114, 1985). Even low methionine diets have decreased tumor metastases (Breillout, F, et al, Decreased rat rhabdomyosarcoma pulmonary metastases in response to a low methionine diet, Anticancer Research, 7:861-868, 1987).

(23) There's no question now that man sequesters many chemicals. But through macrobiotics he has depurated many substances: Our hairdresser friend whose hands, neck and liver area oozed purple (the color of the permanent wave solution she used for 18 years on patrons) for 2 weeks, tumor (benign or malignant) patients often ooze black under compresses (my own baby sister) or urinate black when depurating or discharging accumulated substances.

Indeed there are many routes through which man can discharge: the skin, sebaceous glands, urine, saliva (that's how we measure some drug levels), bowel, and more (Root, DE, et al, Excretion of a lipophilic toxicant through the sebaceous glands: A case report, J. Toxicol - Cutan. and Ocular Toxicol., 6:1, 13-17, 1987; Schwartz, et al, Effects of heat and exercise on the elimination of pralidoxime in man, Clin. Pharmacol. Ther., 14, 83-89, 1972; Imamura, M, et al, A trial of fasting cure for PCB-poisoned patients in Taiwan, Am. J. Indust. Med., 5:147-153, 1984).

(24) Aside from the obvious cholesterol-lowering effect of a macrobiotic diet, the increased use of onions is effective in increasing fibiolytic (anti-clotting) activity in the blood. They also lower cholesterol and triglycerides and even raise high density (the "good" ones that are associated with longevity) lipoproteins

(Constant, J, Nutritional management of diet-
induced hyperlipidemias and atherosclerosis;
Part IX, Int. Med., 9:6, 125-131, June, 1988).

(25) And a macrobiotic diet is in harmony with the
current and progressively evolving National
Research Council's recommendations. They concluded that "the American public could substantially reduce its risk of heart disease, cancer,
and many other chronic diseases through widespread adoption of specific changes in eating
habits. This could be done by such simple
measures as roughly doubling the daily per capita
consumption of fruits, vegetables and starches"
(Fanning, O, National Research Council issues new
recommendations on diet and health, Internal
Medicine World Report, pg 2, April 15-30, 1989).
This is what we call a transition diet in macrobiotics. It's such a culture shock for many to
cut down fats, butter, processed foods, sugars,
coffee, and meat, that they must be eased into
it. Unfortunately many stay on this type of
diet. You can always tell who is a fruit-freak.
They have that bloated full face from eating lots
of watery sweet fruits. It eventually drives
them to crave salts and they yo-yo back and
forth, actually believing that a high fruit diet
is a healthy diet.

(26) By advocating meditation and a more peaceful and
organized life, macrobiotics unloads the adrenal.
Remember the adrenal does not store its hormones.
It has to make them fresh at the moment the body
demands them. Not only do many adrenals lack
nutrients, but they have been poisoned by
pesticides and other xenobiotics. In fact many
organochloride pesticides are concentrated in the
adrenal (EPA: Recognition and Management of
Pesticide Poisonings, 4th ed, Morgan, DP, 19,
1986, EPA, Washington DC 20460) and have an
inhibitory effect on corticosteroid synthesis. A
macrobiotic lifestyle tends to favor allowing the

adrenal to rest (see Cortrosyn Stimulation test for office assessment of adrenal reserve).

(27) In terms of preventive medicine and the future of the individual, there are myriads of benefits. For example, people eating high protein diets have more acidic blood (proteins are metabolized to amino acids) which requires extra buffering when the buffer becomes depleted, calcium is pulled out of bones to act as a buffer. Osteoporosis can result. This is partly why there is far more osteoporosis in Eskimos versus Japanese.

By being a diet low in cholesterol, the blood is not as sluggish. Through improved blood flow in small vessels there is less likelihood of calcium precipitation and platelet aggregation, which contribute to arteriosclerosis and strokes.

(28) Coffee (or caffeine), causes a pronounced and prolonged increase of plasma free fatty acids in man. This is because caffeine inhibits the proper metabolism of fats. {The enzyme cyclic 3',5'-nucleotide phosphodiesterase which degrades cyclic AMP (from ATP) to 5'-AMP is inhibited by caffeine. Lipolysis is controlled largely by the amount of cyclic AMP.} When there is a prolonged rise in the level due to frequent coffee ingestion, for example, you have prolonged free fatty acids floating in the blood, looking for a home to lay down and rest in (Feuer, G, de la Iglesia, FA, Molecular Biochemistry of Human Disease, Vol.I, Chap. 3, 111-153, CRC Press, Boca Raton, FL, 1985). The avoidance of coffee is one of many mechanisms of macrobiotics that decreases arteriosclerosis.

(29) Macrobiotics is not a "canned" or "cookbook" approach. It is individualized to the person, because it recognizes that there is sometimes extreme biochemical individuality between people

(Scriver, CR, et al, Eds., The Metabolic Basis of Inherited Disease, 6th ed, Vol I+II, McGraw-Hill, NY, 1989). It also recognizes that any imbalance, like acidosis, effects the body mentally as well as physically. It pays close attention to small changes in mood as important clues to imbalance.

(30) Many people brag about the fact that they eat a large quantity of fruits, thinking it's healthful. They are shocked to learn that macrobiotics limits them. But fruit sugar, fructose, has damaging effects on the body chemistry: it provokes an elevation in uric acid (known to cause gout and raise the risk of heart attacks), it reduces UDP-glucose (needed for Phase II detox), decreases ATP in the liver (the main chemical energy source for all of its functions), interferes with detoxication of ammonia (from meats), inhibits protein and RNA synthesis, and is slowly damaging to the endoplasmic reticulum (where detox Phase I occurs) (reference: ibid Chap. 11, 399-424).

As a doctor starts learning macrobiotics, he is apt to be turned off by the macrobiotic concept of disease, as I was. They assert such notions, for example, that fruits are too yin and expansive. They cause swelling of organs like the liver, and bog down the function by making it too watery.

You can imagine my surprise as I accidentally stumbled across pathophysiologic evidence for this truth in the medical literature (Pathogenesis of fructose hepatotoxicity, Yu, DT, Burch, HB, Phillips, MJ, Laboratory Investigations, 30, 1, 85-92, 1974). Fruit sugar (fructose) does actually cause liver cells, and in particular the endoplasmic reticulum (where detox occurs) to take up water and swell; it thereby disturbs and compromises the normal functions. So this is one more way in which macrobiotics' restriction of fruit is so healing to the body's detox function.

(31) Macrobiotics emphasizes chewing. To reduce allergies and other symptoms, they recommend chewing each mouthful one hundred times, at least (two hundred times to increase one's spirituality). There are many benefits to this. First, remember one of the reasons people with Candida develop food allergies and intolerances is that Candida infection inflames the gut wall. Consequently, large food molecules are allowed to cross the intestinal wall into the blood stream. Since the body has not seen these before, it recognizes them as foreign, makes antibodies so it can attack them; hence, food allergy.

In the same fashion, many people chew their food a couple of times and then bolt it down. This not only fosters food allergy, but poor digestion, so nutrient deficiency results. With prolonged chewing, you get physical breakdown as well as chemical. When the food becomes liquid and mixes in the mouth with salivary enzymes for 2-3 minutes, it is of the smallest possible particle size, and digested to a size that promotes optimum assimilation of the nutrients. This helps stop indigestion, food allergy, and promotes faster healing.

Often one will ask how we get so many chews from a mouthful. You must keep pushing the food forward in your mouth with the back of your tongue rather than letting it slip down the hatch. After all, if you are going to only feed your high-performance machinery high octane (nutrient dense) fuel, you'll want to make every mouthful count and be as good for you as possible. So it's only logical to be sure you can get the maximum nutrition from it.

(32) Getting off sugars plays a major role in healing. Glucose chemically attaches to proteins and nucleic acids {forming nonenzymatic glycosylation products}. This sugar-body protein combination is capable of multiple adverse and major biological effects which include:

(1) Inactivation of enzymes (stops enzymes from working; they could be pivotal in the energy, detox, endocrine or any path).

(2) Inhibition of regulatory molecular binding (which translates into the ability of axing the body chemistry at any crucial point.

(3) Fostering abnormal nucleic acid function (which could include genetic change, or synthesis of faulty regulatory proteins).

(4) Altered macromolecular recognition (formation of auto-immune diseases or collogen vascular diseases, or allergies of any sort).

In essence, excessive sugars can cause just about any disease or symptom (Nonenzymatic glycosylation and the pathogenesis of diabetic complications, A review, Brownlee M, Vlassara H, Cerami A, Ann. Int. Med., 101:527-537, 1984; and Advanced glycosylation end products in tissue and the biochemical basis of diabetic complications, Brownlee M, Cerami A, Vlassara H, NEJM, 318, 20, 1315-1321, May 19, 1988).

The list could go on, but you get the idea. I am forced to reflect now how much of this startles, offends and threatens our belief system. When Dr. Frank Oski wrote "Don't Drink Your Milk" (Molica Press Ltd., 1914 Teall Ave., Syracuse, NY 13206), I was enraged. I wondered how anyone could be so stupid. It took me ten years to learn that he was right. There are undoubtedly many other biases I hold that I have yet to correct. So if anger comes your way, try researching the facts to help you decide on the truth.

If I hadn't seen the utterly impossible occur right before my eyes time and again, I would not be writing this. But when you've done family practice medicine for 15 years and suddenly see alopecia areata, bedridden rheumatoid arthritis, recurrent infections with hypogammaglobulinenemia G, uncorrectable nutrient deficiencies, leukopenia of 16 years, or severe chemical sensitivity clear with the help of a diet, it gets your attention......and gets you researching the biochemical mechanisms. During only 6 days at a residential macrobiotic seminar (Kushi Institute, Brookline, Massachusetts), I saw a young man who was bedridden with a brain tumor and given no hope by medicine, actually healing his neurologic status. Now these are things one cannot fake!

My first day there I spotted him in the dining room. He could barely walk with a cane (I was told it was his first week out of bed). One side of the face had an obvious palsy, and when he removed his eye patch and closed his good eye to say grace, the defective eye was wide open, with no pupil in sight......just a huge white globe that dysfunctional muscles had rolled into an abnormal position.

When he tried to eat, due to chewing and swallowing muscle dysfunction, he coughed and sputtered all over. At that point I wasn't sure I was exactly cut out for this.

By the sixth day, the eye patch was off, facial palsy gone, both eyes conjugate and focused. He was talking, smiling, eating and walking (no cane) normally. Now in neurosurgery I never recall having seen our patients respond that quickly. And remember, he was given up on and told to go home and die in the next month by his doctor (his words).

It's ironic, but when these people go back to their doctor, hoping they would like to know about it to help others, I've seen and heard the most ridiculous responses, from their "initial diagnosis must have been wrong", to "it was a miracle and couldn't work for anyone else".

I often play a game when I sit next to a stranger on a plane. I casually ask if they ever heard of macrobiotics.

So far 50% of the time the answer is "Huh? Come to think of it, I had a neighbor (friend, relative) once who had cancer and was given only a few months to live. He ate this strange diet." "And.......?" "Oh, he's still alive. Won't eat anything else. Strange." I sincerely hope my scientific curiosity doesn't die that soon.

In essence, the seemingly unbelievable improvements that occur with a macrobiotic diet are easily explained by events that would affect the detoxication scheme. It is incredibly logical why it is so healing once we understand the biochemistry of detox. One of the macro guidelines says, "The bigger the front, the bigger the back". As you see, the demise of the detox system creates an avalanche of disordered metabolic steps which leads to the resultant symptoms. But fortunately when you make a serious effort to reverse that, the reactivation of the beneficial chemistry is also multi-faceted: it's like playing a video of dominoes falling in reverse. The house of cards is restored. The biochemical explanations above are only a few of the reasons why macrobiotics has been so successful with end-stage cancers. You can't continually poison a system that is down and out (chemotherapy). The only hope is to help it heal (macrobiotics).

****

ARE YOU DIGGING YOUR GRAVE WITH YOUR TEETH?

Chapter 10: WHEN A MEDICAL EVOLUTION BECOMES A REVOLUTION

"All politics are based on
the indifference of the majority."
James Reston

Counter Point

In this chapter I will try to communicate an air of
the political problems that abound today. All establish-
ments are resistant to change, as are E.I. physicians to
some treatment modalities. The conclusion of the chapter is
that the patient must take hold of his life and pursue a
treatment style that simultaneously embraces a strong biochemical knowledge and reliance on the individual as the
ultimate decision-maker.

****

Through the history of science, man has fought tooth
and nail to resist change. Especially when it has threaten-
ed his ego, finances and power. And the medical man has
been no exception. Semmelweiss merely suggested they wash
their hands in between autopsies and childbirth deliveries.
He said he thought that the reason 9 out of 10 of his
patients didn't die of child birth fever as his colleagues'
patients did, was that he was washing some microscopic bacteria from the dead bodies off his hands. Rather than try
it themselves, the jealous, unthinking lot ostracized him,
saw to it that he lost his license, and he died a pauper of
suicide.

When the EEG (electroencephalograph or brain wave
machine) came to the United States, again scientific curiosity took a back seat to power and the AMA banned it. And
look how they smeared the chiropractor ----- without whom
many of us would not be walking today (not to mention the

fact that we would have succumbed to needless surgery in effort to escape our pain).

This power play gets to be absurd after awhile. The medical establishment has tried to put environmental medicine in a medical straight jacket for years. They want us subservient to the drug industry like the rest of the pack. But it's more difficult to squash success. They don't just pick on us, however. There are 150 medical specialties, but only 20 of which the AMA officially recognizes.

And this medical establishment is the one that helps make most of the rules governing insurance reimbursement. For example, did you know that some insurances pay for patients to rent a nebulizer for $60 a month, but they won't pay for him to own it for $100. I've personally seen patients who rented one under these conditions for 2 years, all the time begging for ownership. Likewise they pay for a drunk driver who mutilates himself in an auto accident, and they pay for a chronic smoker with emphysema and lung cancer, but they won't pay for a father of six who has chemical sensitivity or a hyperactive child with food allergies.

Likewise, they won't pay for a documented B6 and rbc zinc deficiency correction in an arthritic, but they pay for all the indocin he can consume........and they don't even require a blood test to show he has an indocin deficiency!

Furthermore they pay for coronary bypass surgery when the patients who refused it had the same mortality. And they pay for particular cancer therapies where it is known that the remission rate is almost non-existent, yet ignore studying alternative therapies that appear to have:
1. An interesting rate of spontaneous remissions.
2. The return to good health explained away by the fact that the initial diagnosis of cancer must have been in error.

When he has an insulin deficiency they pay for his diabetes care, but not if you find the cause is a deficiency of essential fatty acids, B6, chromium, zinc, magnesium, and give instruction in a modified macrobiotic diet. And heaven forbid you should make him well. Then they maintain he must never have had diabetes in the first place, because everyone knows it doesn't go away. So you're not allowed to get over it, I guess.

```
*********************************************************
*                                                       *
*                                                       *
*                                                       *
*                                                       *
*                                                       *
*                                                       *
*                                                       *
*                                                       *
*                                                       *
*                                                       *
*                                                       *
*                                                       *
*                                                       *
*                                                       *
*                                                       *
*                                                       *
*                                                       *
*                                                       *
*     It's only human to resist changing ones habits.   *
*     And the hardest one of all is eating.             *
*                                                       *
*********************************************************
```

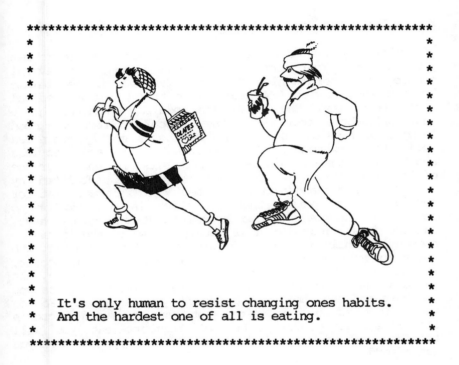

The American Academy of Environmental Medicine for years has invited many leaders in conventional allergy to come to our courses, free. They've even been invited as paid speakers. No takers. I guess their scientific curiosity died. If someone told me they could clear my failures and offered to show me how, I would beat a path to their doorway as fast as possible.

These are just a few of the reasons why you need to get educated and then involved, for your own protection.

And so it is that often evolution must, of necessity, become revolution when politics rears its head to retard scientific progress.

You've Never Met Your Real Doctor

You may not be aware of it, but you have never met your doctor. Your doctor is not one person, but several people. The demographics show that she is a married female between 20-55, with 0-4 years of college, and no medical school education. She smokes, has soda for lunch, and has a host of subtle complaints like chronic tiredness, mood swings, depression, back pain, PMS, eats mostly processed foods, knows extremely little about nutrition, and even less about environmental illness. She sits in an insurance office all day long and goes over forms submitted by doctors' offices and patients to decide on reimbursement for services. The person that you think is your doctor no longer has the power to decide what treatment you can have, but she does. Your doctor is merely a pawn of the insurance company's, while your real doctor is this unseen clerk who works for the insurance company. She is your real doctor, for although she never met you, and never examined you, she decides what diseases you can have, and what treatments you can have and even how much treatment you can have. For on the weight of her decision, not your presumed doctor's decisions, hangs the amount of reimbursement you will receive, and subsequently the amount and type of care you can afford.

One of the major goals these days of insurance companies seems to be to drive a wedge between the doctor and his patient. They use their self-awarded authority and confusing language to make you believe that your physician is practicing unnecessary medicine, or medicine not in keeping with the standard of medical care in the community. They love to say your doctor's charges were excessive and therefore disallowed. Sure we spend a much greater amount of time assessing nutritional deficiencies, and environmental triggers than the guy who just pops in the room for a few minutes, writes a prescription and leaves. The bottom line is that, in order to save time and money, insurance companies are still trying to cram everyone and their diseases into one easily computerized system, reducing every diagnosis and treatment into an alphabetized/numerical code. Meanwhile physicians interested in protecting the sanctity of their turf lobby and sit on government boards of these companies to make sure that unwanted progress does not invade their specialities.

So that the end result is, if you have arthritis, for example, the rheumatologist will do his blood test and x-rays. But he never checks for food or chemical sensitivity or nutrient deficiency. Meanwhile the insurance company has its computerized list of accepted therapies based on his diagnosis and any therapy falling outside of that list is disallowed. And the fact that you get well is irrelevant. You can go to 6 doctors and get the same medication that doesn't clear you, and that's covered. But get well with a treatment that is not sanctioned by the policy-makers and you are not reimbursed for your medical expenses.

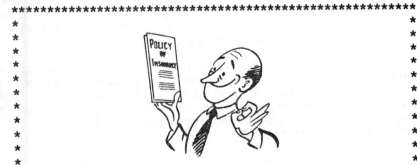

One of the major goals of insurance companies is to court you into their camp so that they can then dictate just what type of care and even how much of it your diagnosis deserves.

An example is Ray, crippled with rheumatoid arthritis for over 20 years. He had gone the gamut with life threatening drugs, to no avail. He couldn't even shake hands because of the pain. Once the food and mold allergies and vitamin/mineral deficiencies were corrected, he was free of pain and without medication, not only shaking hands, but climbing mountains. But the insurance company secretary let him know that they don't pay for food allergy treatment, nor do they pay for vitamins. Since they know nothing about it, the rheumatologists see to it that none of this new-fangled quackery invades their specialty. This is in spite of the fact that there are scientific papers in the literature demonstrating that food sensitivity is a cause of some people's arthritis. Now mind you, if Ray decides to return to a life of pain and drugs, this will all be paid for. But making him pain and drug-free is against the rules of the system. So he must pay out of his own pocket. Now if he were too poor to afford this, that clerk in the insurance company office becomes his real doctor, for she is indeed the final arbitrator of his medicine and his life. And of course she is only following the rules of her job. The sad part is that there is recourse to her supervisor and on up to a physician, but that Medical Director is even further away from treating real patients.

Whether or not all arthritics can find a cause, I don't know. But we have an over 80% success rate, so it certainly is worthwhile for each individual to look for hidden factors contributing to his suffering. You can't imagine what it's like to be imprisoned in a body of pain every moment of your life.

Following are just a few of the references in the scientific literature regarding food sensitivity as a cause of arthritis. You will note that some are over 70 years old, so this idea didn't just come about over night. Get the picture now? Thank you Dr. George Kroker of LaCrosse, Wisconsin for putting these together.

Food Sensitivity In Rheumatic Diseases

1. Talbot FB: Role of food idiosyncrasies in practice. New York State J. of Med. 17: 419-425, 1917.

2. Turnbull JA: The relation of anaphylactic disturbances to arthritis. JAMA 82: 1757-1759, 1924.

3. Rowe AH: Food Allergy. Lea & Febiger, Philadelphia, 1931.

4. Brown GT: Allergic phases of arthritis. J. Lab. Clin. Med. 247-249, 1934.

5. Lewin and Taub: Allergic Synovitis due to ingestion of English walnuts. JAMA 166: 2144, 1936.

6. Service WC: Hydroarthrosis of allergic origin. American J. of Surgery 37: 121-123, 1937.

7. Vaughn WT: Palindromic rheumatism among allergic persons. J. of Allergy 14: 256-263, 1943.

8. Turnbull JA: Changes in sensitivity to allergenic foods in arthritis. J. of Digestive Diseases 15: 182-190, 1944.

9. Creip LH: Allergy of joints. The J. of Bone and Joint Surgery, 276-278, 1946.

10. Zeller M: Rheumatoid arthritis: Food allergy as a factor. Ann. Allerg. 7: 200-239, 1949.

11. Zussman BM: Food hypersensitivity simulating rheumatoid arthritis. South Med. J. 59: 935-939, 1966.

12. Epstein S: Hypersensitivity to sodium nitrate: A major causative factor in a case of palindromic rheumatism. Ann. Allerg. 27: 343-349, 1969.

13. Randolph TG: Ecologically oriented rheumatoid arthritis. Chapt 17, pp 201-212 in Clinical Ecology, L.

Dickey Ed., Charles C. Thomas Publ, Springfield, Il.
1970.

14. Skoldstam L, Larsson L, and Lindstrom F: Effects of
     fasting and lactovegetarian diet on rheumatoid arthri-
     tis. Scand. J. Rheum. 8: 249-255, 1979.

15. Mandell M, Conte A: The role of allergy in arthritis,
     rheumatism and associated polysymptomatic
     cerebroviscero-somatic disorders: A double-blind
     provocation test study. Ann. Allerg. 44: 51, 1980.

16. Parke AL, Hughes GRV: Rheumatoid arthritis and food:
     A case study. Br. Med. J. 282: 2027-2029, 1981.

17. Little CH, Stewart AG, Fennessy MR: Platelet serotonin
     release in rheumatoid arthritis: A study in food-
     intolerant patients. Lancet 297-299, 1983.

18. Panush RS, Carter RL, Katz P, et al: Diet therapy for
     rheumatoid arthritis. Arthritis & Rheumatism 26: 462-
     471, 1983.

19. Kroker GF, Stroud RM, Marshall R, et al: Fasting and
     rheumatoid arthritis: A multicenter study. Clinical
     Ecology 2: 137-144, 1984.

20. Marshall RM, Stroud RM, Kroker GF: Food challenge
     effects on fasted rheumatoid arthritis patients: A
     multicenter study. Clinical Ecology 2: 181-190, 1984.

21. Kremer JM, Bigauoette J, Michalek AV, et al: Effects
     of manipulation of dietary fatty acids on clinical
     manifestations of rheumatoid arthritis. Lancet 184-
     187, 1985.

22. Ratner D, Eshel E, Vigder K: Juvenile rheumatoid
     arthritis and milk allergy. J. Roy. Soc. Med. 78:
     410-413, 1985.

23. Darlington LG, Ramsey NW, Mansfield JR: Placebo-
     controlled, blind study of dietary manipulation

therapy in rheumatoid arthritis. Lancet 236–238, 1986.

24. Panush RS, Stroud RM, Webster EM: Food induced (allergic) arthritis. Arthritis & Rheumatism 29: 220–226, 1986.

25. Kremer JM, Juviz W, Michalek A, et al: Fish oil fatty acid supplementation in active rheumatoid arthritis. Ann. Int. Med. 106: 497–502, 1987.

26. Malone DG, Metcalfe DD: Mast cells and arthritis. Ann. Allerg. 61 (part II): 27–30, 1988.

27. Brostoff J, Challacombe SJ, eds., Food Allergy And Intolerance, W.S. Saunders, 1987.

344

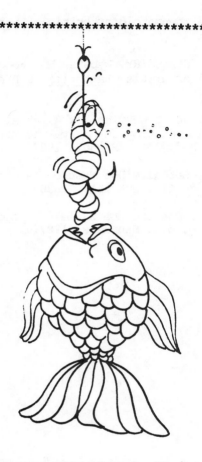

```
*********************************************************
*                                                       *
*                                                       *
*                                                       *
*                                                       *
*                                                       *
*                                                       *
*                                                       *
*                                                       *
*                                                       *
*                                                       *
*                                                       *
*                                                       *
*                                                       *
*                                                       *
*                                                       *
*                                                       *
*                                                       *
*                                                       *
*                                                       *
*                                                       *
*                                                       *
*                                                       *
*                                                       *
*                                                       *
*                                                       *
*                                                       *
*                                                       *
*                                                       *
*                                                       *
*                                                       *
*   Americans have swallowed hook, line, sinker, and    *
*   pole when it comes to medical insurance coverage,    *
*   only to later learn that the thrust is not in        *
*   promoting health, only drugs.  Furthermore, it's     *
*   rare to find a company that understands the cost     *
*   effectiveness and life-effectiveness of molecular    *
*   chemistry and environmental approaches.              *
*                                                       *
*********************************************************
```

It's Not A Battle Of Science, But Politics

This is one of the main reasons why you now have to learn so much science and medicine in order to make yourself well. Not only are you the only person that can heal yourself, but medicine has been taken out of yours and your doctor's hands by big business, namely the insurance companies and secondarily the pharmaceutical or drug companies.

Through the history of science man has resisted new ideas with a vengeance. Copernicus met with extreme hostility when he suggested that the earth was not the center of the universe. Harvey, likewise, as brilliant as he was, was blasted and denigrated for suggesting that blood flows through the body in vessels. You can imagine, if Semmelweis's washing of the hands was so threatening, what Pasteur or Jenner had to go through when, for example, Jenner wanted to actually inoculate people with the disfiguring and deadly material from the smallpox pustule to immunize them!

You might think, as I did for a long time, that these were signs of times gone by and that the world has changed. But these things are going on in this very day at an accelerated rate. And it doesn't matter how credentialed and respected the person is; once they cross over the line into the thinking realm of medicine, they are black balled. Dr. Coca is famous in many old allergy text books for having initiated many of the early ideas in allergy. Yet, he was denigrated once he started working on the simple pulse test as one of the parameters for judging food sensitivity. (Yes, your pulse often goes up 10 points a minute if you eat a food you're sensitive to. But you have to test in a special way to get this result - see The E.I. Syndrome.)

Dr. Linus Pauling is twice a Nobel Prize winner, first in biochemistry (he made some extremely important discoveries relating to chemical bonds that changed the world) and second in peace. But once he started talking about vitamin C, he was likewise black balled from the scientific, and especially medical, communities. Here is a man who knows more biochemistry than any 100 doctors pooled together. But let him explain some biochemistry that involves a non-prescription item and he is maliciously attacked for the rest of his life. Why? Because this non-prescription vitamin dilutes the power of the physician and the profits of the drug industry. I'm ashamed to admit that in my early days of family practice I recall parroting to patients what I had also learned in medical school: "No one in the United States needs vitamins if he eats a regular diet (of fast foods)". And I shudder to recall what I ate in those days and how horrid I felt. I was forever searching through thousands of dollars worth of my medical textbooks, always asking the same question, "Why isn't what I have in here?"

You might think that all we need to do in medicine is publish our facts and let the reigning scientific community decide. But there is a tremendous amount of deceit and corruptness in the scientific world. The Mayo Clinic published some studies supposedly proving that Dr. Pauling's vitamin C theories were wrong. However, their studies were flawed. But the same journal would not allow Dr. Pauling to publish a rebuttal letter on the faults of their study. (Details available through Insta-Tape, AAEM Annual Scientific Meeting at Clearwater, Florida, 1986.)

Likewise, Dr. Barbara McClintock received the Nobel Prize 30 years after her discoveries were published in several scientific journals. She was merely ignored because her theory of jumping genes just didn't fit with how they wanted the world to remain. And likewise, Dr. Jacques Benveniste has followed the same course. He is a brilliant French researcher with impeccable credentials. He discovered the platelet activating factor, which is one of the mechanisms of allergy. When he discovered that homeopathy actually works and that dilute solutions carry electromagnetic memory for antigens, his work was ludicrously denigrated. It's actually ridiculous when you get into the nitty gritty of what happened, because his methodology was so airtight and so perfect that his detractors could not find any fault with it. They therefore used vague, unscientific, self-contradictory terms to discredit and justify

ignoring it. And these were published throughout the
scientific and lay world. (The details of this are very
interesting, and available from Insta-Tape, AAEM Annual
Scientific Meeting, Lake Tahoe, 1988, and Man and His World,
Dallas, 1989.)

If I had not had many of these things happen to myself, I would have found it difficult to conceive of what
Dr. Pauling and Dr. Benveniste were telling me when I talked
with them. But I too have papers in my possession that I
have submitted to conventional allergy journals. They come
back with the most illogical reasons for not being published. For example, the physician/scientist reviewing the
paper said, "This paper cannot be published because it is
based on provocation-neutralization technique, and we know
that the provocation-neutralization technique does not
work". And yet there are no published papers in the world
literature showing that it does not work, even to this very
day. And my paper was explaining and demonstrating how it
does work. But the case was closed before the book was
opened.

Furthermore, these reviewers have never been to
courses to learn the techniques, and they have never witnessed the procedures and their results. They have merely
decided that they do not want to be scooped by outsiders in
what they consider their private turf. They are without
good scientific evidence that shows it doesn't work and yet
there are over half a dozen published papers showing that it
does work. They continue to this day to ignore all the
evidence and the double blind tests. Some of these self-
appointed "experts" sit on insurance boards and decide the
policy that affects your health.

Dr. Theron Randolph discovered chemical sensitivities
in 1951 and was even kicked off the staff of Northwestern
University because of his ideas. This is in spite of being
a brilliant internist and Harvard trained allergist, publishing over 200 papers, and over half a dozen books
(Environmental Medicine - Beginnings and Bibliographies of
Chemical Ecology, Randolph TG, Clinical Ecology Publ. Inc.
109 W. Olive St., Fort Collins, CO 80524, 1987). He is the

first man in history to publish the tight building or sick building syndrome. Yet now that it is being "rediscovered", you never see an honest reference to the man who deserves all the credit.

Dr. George Shambaugh is an 85 year old Harvard-trained ear, nose and throat surgeon, who is world famous for his fenestration operation which has saved the hearing of hundreds of people. But in his own town of Chicago, no one referred patients to him even though they came from all over the world to have this operation. This goes on everywhere in the country. And it wasn't a personality problem, for he is one of the sweetest and dearest people I know.

He recalls, in the early days of medicine, before antibiotics came along, how they were taught in medical school at Harvard to "shun those dangerous patent medications", but use vitamins and good nutrition. Then when the antibiotics came along, and drug companies began making megabucks, how things slowly changed, until today we have a 180 degree reversal. Now everyone is taught to prescribe patent medicine for nearly every condition, and to ignore nutrition. (Details of this available Insta-tape, AAEM, Dr. Shambaugh's lecture, Lake Tahoe, 1988.)

Dr. Rea was the cardiovascular surgeon called to operate on Governor Connelly. He never aspired to be the world's leading ecologist; it just happened that he developed severe E.I. after having his home pesticided. Likewise, he has been denigrated. Now he has been granted the first international chair (a prestigious position) in environmental medicine in Surrey, England. Some progress you just can't stifle.

The AMA has been notorious throughout its history for stifling any competition; homeopathy, acupuncture, chiropractic, etc., all of which have a beneficial role in medicine and for which there is much information substantiating their benefits. But the fact that American doctors have no training in these, is the one criteria that makes them useless. Look at the anesthesia complications and deaths that could be spared if we had our choice of acupuncture or surgical anesthesia, as they do in China. But too many people might opt for acupuncture, I guess.

Some will say that it isn't known how acupuncture works, but that never stopped them manufacturing and prescribing potent drugs that we use everyday. And there is an abundance of papers and books showing how acupuncture works (Strauss, S, The scientific basis of acupuncture, Austral. Fam. Phys., 16, 2, 166-169, Feb. 1987; Penzer, V, Malsumoto, K, Neuroanatomical and neurophysiological basis for use of acupuncture in dentistry, J. Mass. Dent. Soc., 36:2, 83-84, spring, 1987; Mann, F, Acupuncture: The Ancient Art of Healing and How It Works Scientifically, Vintage Books, Random House, NY, 1973; Toguchi, M, Warren FZ, Complete Guide to Acupuncture and Acupressure, Gramercy Publ. Co., NY).

Although the AMA did have power in the past, it appears that it is dwindling. The food industry appears to indirectly control the treatment of cardio-vascular disease now as cardiologists daily recommend hydrogenated trans vegetable oils and margarines, plastic eggs, and creamers, and other processed foods devoid of vitamin E, chromium and magnesium that are actually deleterious to health (and hearts!). The latest craze for high fiber has resulted in the appearance of breads actually containing methyl cellulose (sawdust!). Heaven forbid they should recommend whole grains like brown rice that contain fiber and vitamins and minerals. It's like a race to see how far away from nature and health we can really get. The cardiologists appear to be merely the pawns of big businesses: the food and chemical industries, insurance and pharmaceutical companies and HMO's. These health maintenance organizations are a riot. They come right out in print and tell the participating doctors not to order too many tests or they will be cutting into the profits of the company. It's business and profit first, appropriate medical care second.

It is obvious how much power the chemical companies have, for example, when one looks at the field of pesticides. Over 1,500 pesticides are on the market, most of which have not been adequately tested. Most of the ingredients are labeled as trade secrets. That means that a physician can't even get the exact ingredients even if a patient's life depended on it. I thought this was not true until I heard the lecture of Dr. Varner (Insta-tape, Man and His Environment World Conference, Dallas, 1987 and 1988).

Not only have the names been intentionally made extremely deceiving and confusing but the company responsible for safety data and testing is the manufacturer itself. No independent lab is required. Cases of fraud have been unveiled but not heavily punished. And the government just does not have the impetus to make it a priority to check for further suspected fraud.

Naturally no company looks at the synergistic effect of the real life exposure to multiple pesticides. The pesticides that have been banned here, have no government controls on them and are still made here (hopefully we won't have another Bhopal), but are sold to third world countries that sell us back their contaminated winter produce. Hence, most Americans have measurable levels of DDT in their blood streams (Insta-tape, Laseter, J.). The majority of these chemical companies also, are now into the business of making seeds, so that they can control the genetics of agriculture and further dependence upon pesticide companies. If you look down the list of the most predominant companies making pesticides, many of them are the same ones making the seeds and also the same companies that also make the majority of our prescription drugs. So that no matter which way you look at it, they have us coming and going, because when we get extremely sick, they are the ones who are going to profit even more.

In their book, The Bitter Truth About Artificial Sweeteners, Dr. Dennis Remington and Barbara Higa, of Provo, Utah, exposed much of the power and money used to cover up the harmful effects of aspartame. In subsequent lectures (Insta-tape, Monrovia, CA) they further detailed and documented, with the aid of legal investigations by the Senate Subcommittee and independent attorneys, the lengths that companies will go to get FDA approval for products that their own laboratory data proved harmful. Reading this shows clearly once more that it's a battle of politics and money, not science. Reading the gruesome details will leave you wondering how your best interests ever get served and will serve to convince you even more that you must educate yourself and be responsible for your own health, because bureaucracy cannot. There are just too many cooks in the kitchen, each with their own interests to serve.

I no longer use drugs as primary therapy. It means I'm intrigued by what could be the causes of symptoms. I look at vitamin and mineral levels to assess the biochemical machinery of the body and test to find environmental triggers to symptoms. I haven't had to sell out to an HMO and to insurance companies and let them tell me how to practice medicine. I am good enough to make it on my own, and because, in the end, results are what count.

The ethics and progress of science has been warped and held back and funneled off into chosen directions where drugs and surgery are the only acceptable treatments. This is far removed from anything that will be helpful, and will only serve to foster degenerative disease and profits for big companies. Not to mention, the continual pollution of the earth and devastation of its resources.

```
******************************************************
*  For every cross-roads to the future, there       *
*  are a thousand self-appointed guardians of        *
*  the past. (Just read any book on the history      *
*  of science or medicine.)                           *
******************************************************
```

But individuals have demanded change in medicine in the past and succeeded. And armed with enough knowledge and decisiveness, they can do it again. Look at obstetrics: they got husbands in the delivery room and PMS (premenstrual syndrome) to be recognized as an insurance reimbursable diagnosis, even though there are no blood tests or x-rays to prove its existence.

And where are some of the allied specialties when it comes to protecting our medical sanctity? Since toxicology is a part of environmental medicine, why haven't the toxicologists latched onto this information with more fervor? Like many specialties, it has developed a narrow focus, and in doing so lost the overall perspective which is so critical to the understanding of medicine in this century. Their focus is an overt overdose, not the insidious poisonings that are difficult to diagnose.

They are somewhat like the allergists who failed to jump on board. They got hung up with the IgE mechanism and couldn't believe any other form of allergy existed. So they fought the notion of foods and chemicals with a vengeance. Now that the average man on the street knows that foods and chemicals cause symptoms, the allergists are busy trying to prove the existence of these sensitivities with immunologic tests. They still are oblivious to the intricacies of the detoxication and nutrient biochemistry.

It is the same old story; if you go to a man to have something fixed and his only tool is a hammer, two to one he is going to use that hammer on it. The allergist is hung up on the immune system and thinks that all of allergy can be explained through the immune system. And so he tenaciously continues to ignore the heavy duty biochemistry that is necessary to understand environmental illness.

Likewise the nutritionists very seldom recommend blood tests to check vitamin, mineral, amino acid, and essential fatty acid deficiencies. They just assume the diet they learned to prescribe is best for you. There's no checking to see if it is correct as they recommend another processed food.

And so it is with many toxicologists. When they do toxicologic studies they look at the end point for their reactions in animals as death or cancer. But they never ask the rat how he feels when he wakes up in the morning. You cannot function with a headache all day, even if a chemical doesn't kill you. They can't ask the rat if he's depressed or tired or achey. They are not capable within the narrow scope that they work, of adequately recognizing the degree of toxic symptoms that man experiences, nor in recognizing the vast degree of biochemical individuality. For example, one inhaled chemical can be distributed 1% to the white matter of the brain, 1/2% to the gray matter, 15% to the liver, and the rest to the fat for storage. However, the distribution won't be the same for everyone in the room, nor for every chemical. It may not even be the same for the same person at another point in time, as you now know.

Medical specialties are still looking at gross parameters with the old gross tests, while we have evolved into a microscopic (and biochemical) era which requires (and possesses) very refined tools and techniques. These are some of the facts that make the phenomenon of chemical sensitivity so overwhelming to so many scientists, allied health professionals and physicians. Indeed environmental medicine pulls together not only allergy, toxicology, nutrition, but a science of adaptation, while keeping in mind the perspective of man with his environments. And it makes measurements at more sensitive levels out of necessity for what has transpired.

Once a chemical is inside a cell, the sequence of pollutant injury is just as varied. A chemical can cause dysregulation (interfere with the control) of an enzyme critical to detoxication, mineral metabolism, cell surface receptors and antigens, genetic information, energy synthesis, and much more. Acute disease results, then chronic, then end organ failure and death as the last end stage. Medical school teaches mainly the diagnosis of advanced end stage disease. Meanwhile, in this era, due to insidious chemical overload, and nutrient deficiencies, biological burn out is possible long before end organ failure. These people just plain feel lousy and have undiagnosable, "vague" symptoms by the old fashioned end organ system.

Alzheimer's Disease

Let's look at one nutrient you rarely think of, choline. A good source is eggs (but people have been scared off in the name of hypercholesterolemia) and beans (which are gassy if improperly prepared and considered a peasant food). Choline is essential for making phosphatidyl choline (PC), a key ingredient in all cell membranes (including the detox endoplasmic reticulum membranes). Choline also has 2 other crucial roles: it forms acetylcholine (responsible for nerve transmission and moods, a deficiency of which is one of the causes of Alzheimer's presenile dementia) and forms methionine (which is the essential amino acid from which cysteine is made. Cysteine is pivotal in many Phase II detox conjugations you recall).

As people get exposed to more chemicals that overload the detox system (and create free radicals, especially since many have "subclinical" levels of antioxidants, A, C, E, selenium, etc.) these chemicals chew holes in the cell wall, mitochondrial and detox membranes and phosphatidyl choline (PC) is destroyed. When the body needs more phosphatidyl choline and doesn't get it from the diet, it does an auto-cannibalism act: it takes PC from cells that have a great deal of it, namely the brain. This is part of the pathologic cause of Alzheimer's disease: when the body doesn't have enough choline, it eats it from its own brain tissue, causing eventual brain damage (Blasztajn, JK, Wurtman, RJ, Choline and cholinergic neurons, Science, 221, 614-620, 1983; Wurtman, RJ, Alzheimer's disease, Scientific American, 252: 62-75, 1985). Researchers have reversed early stages of senility with PC supplementation (Little, A, et al, A double-blind placebo controlled trial of high dose lecithin in Alzheimer's disease, J. Neurol. Neurosurg. Psych., 48: 736-742, 1985). But the problem is that a percentage of permanent damage occurs long before the symptoms are diagnosable by current means.

You can appreciate how important this information is in the long run and why this form of medicine is, and will continue to be, fought for about 50 more years. It is just too complicated and requires a total learning of biochemistry, and out-dates much of what is currently known. Furtermore it is urgent since we are on such an accelerated downhill course. Remember, we are not only the generation of man exposed to all these chemicals, but we are the first to

eat such a nutritionally inferior diet. This is a deadly
combination. Unfortunately, the time is now for those of
us who want to avoid Alzheimer's or any other disease, so we
need to step up the program.

```
***********************************************************
*                                                         *
*    The Cell Membrane  and  Endoplasmic Reticulum        *
*    (directs the function  (the location of Phase I      *
*    of the cell)           detox)                        *
*                                                         *
*                    both depend on                       *
*                    phosphatidyl choline,                *
*                    but it's low because it is...        *
*                                                         *
*              (1)    deficient in the diet               *
*              (2)    lost through chemical               *
*                     destruction                         *
*              (3)    lost through auto-                  *
*                     cannibalism                         *
*                                                         *
*    The result is the detox function suffers, chemicals  *
*  backlog, the cell gets further damaged, then disease   *
*  begins in multiple organs.                             *
*    The brain and nerves are the most severely affect-   *
*  ed because the choline is stolen from these areas when *
*  levels are low. This silently over years contributes   *
*  to Alzheimer's disease.                                *
*                                                         *
***********************************************************
```

```
************************************************************
*           Many nutritional deficiencies cause vague     *
*      neurological symptoms.                              *
*           Many xenobiotic toxicities cause vague         *
*      neurological symptoms.                              *
*      ---------------------------------------------------  *
*      Add nutrient deficiencies to the xenobiotic        *
*           (chemical) overload, and it further stresses   *
*   +       an already overworked detoxication system.     *
*      ---------------------------------------------------  *
*      Results - Downward spiral of vague neurological     *
*               symptoms, difficult to diagnose.           *
*             - Progressively worse reactions as more      *
*               detox pathways are compromised.            *
*             - Finally one target organ fails and         *
*               medications are prescribed (which          *
*               further burden the detox pathways).        *
*      ---------------------------------------------------  *
*           As chemicals tear holes in membranes,          *
*      phosphatidyl choline is lost.  Acute cannibalism    *
*      occurs where the body steals choline from the brain,*
*      fostering the chemical changes of senility.  Once   *
*      senility is blamed, there's no hope of recovery.    *
*      ---------------------------------------------------  *
*           - THE SICK GET SICKER                          *
************************************************************
```

How Do You Know If Your Doctor Knows Anything About 21st Century Medicine?

One easy way is to quiz him. Ask him. You might pick any of the functional assays (Chapter 6) and say, "Dr. X did a test on me called a transketolase, but he didn't tell me what it was for. Would you please?" If he doesn't tell you it's a functional assay to measure the adequacy of vitamin B1, he doesn't know. In which case, he'll shrug it off with some glib remark to save face. Let me know what it is. I have a wonderfully funny scrap book of quotes from some very prominent medical "authorities". And after all, humor is good for the immune system.

Another surreptitious test of a doctor is to remark, "Boy, I bet you see a lot of hypochondriacs in this day and age with all the medical shows on T.V. showing people how to do everything from diagnose themselves to open heart surgery". If he agrees, or gives you some percent, that means its the percent that doesn't respond to medication. And you know what that means. One doctor in our town actually boasts that "80% of the people are hypochondriacs". Would you ever have a hope of convincing him to look at your vitamin chemistry? Not on your life. If I had 80% failure, I'd scrub floors instead.

If he is honest and just says he doesn't know when you question him, let him borrow this book. Honesty in medicine is a genuine quality worth cultivating. This guy will rarely put you down or make fun of you when you stump his diagnostic acumen. He may be very interested in knowing what's happening in the future of medicine and even want to become a part of it. He may even become the leading specialist in environmental medicine in your area in years to come. And you could be the one who kindled his fire, his burning for knowledge. Who knows, maybe he even has E.I. himself.

I am blessed with just such a friend/patient who took me under her wing. I remember the day she arrived in my office. At dinner that night, I said, "Honey! Guess what! I had one of those strange chemically sensitive people today. She's practically allergic to everything." I was so sick and so dumb in those days, that I didn't know I was also one of those "strange" chemically sensitive people.

But she never gave up on this dumb doctor. She brought me organic foods from her garden, and boxes and boxes of books on nutrition and environmental medicine at a time when I was gradually getting sicker and sicker. God has a way of looking after dumb animals and dumb physicians (see The E.I. Syndrome).

So don't give up on your doctor. We all start out as doubting Thomases. Not only that, but even after we know all of this, it takes years before puzzling events of the past start to make sense to us.

And we all know that hindsight is so much clearer than foresight. For example, I was usually at the head of my class in grade school and high school. I can't help it, I was born smart (and with a beautiful coloratura voice. A lot of other more desirable qualities I would have traded for that, but that's the package I was given). Anyway, I had wonderful grades and honor roll and honor society accomplishments through high school and won two college scholarships (good thing! I was the oldest of 7 children and no one had ever gone to college before in the history of our family, not to mention medical school. We just plain couldn't afford it).

In college, my freshman class was the first student body on a spanking brand new campus. I took one "fun" course to balance out all my biology, physics, biochemistry, embryology, comparative anatomy, botany, literature, French, and sociology. It was music appreciation. It was also the only "D" I ever got in my life. I never could figure out how I could do so poorly in anything, much less something that was a "natural" for me. But now I understand why. We listened to music in the basement classroom of this brand new building. Basements as you know have special toxic paints to make them water proof, with special fungicides to suppress mold growth. As well, the acoustical wall and floor carpeting was glued down. I would listen to music to be identified later on a test, but could never concentrate, never remember while I was in there. And I felt ill as well. But when you're a college student hell-bent on going to medical school, chemical sensitivity is the last thing you would ever think of, especially in the early 60's.

Anyway, I won a third scholarship and combined with working, I was able to go on to medical school. But to my surprise, in medical school, I actually failed the only course of my entire life. You're so smart by now that you can probably tell me what that course was. You guessed it, gross anatomy.

Every afternoon at 1:00 we would don our white lab coats (that we rarely washed because we were too tired) and slaved over our formaldehyde-soaked cadavers until dinner. Afterwards, still swaddled in the coats, we studied into the wee hours of the morning.

Our exams consisted of gathering in the dissection room where a few dozen formaldehyde-pickled cadavers were exhibited. They would have little pins stuck into them bearing numbered flags on top. We were to identify and write a copious dissertation on the structure which bore the pin.

Again, my brain was on hold in this room and I never did figure it out. Fortunately they let me take the written exam over again at the end of summer. For just a few flunkies they luckily didn't go through all the hassle of setting up the dissection room. They used pictures and toughened up the written portion instead. Naturally I passed and was on my way again.

But you can see now, how subtle the brain changes can be when one is reacting to chemicals. And how easy it is to be intimidated that it's all your own fault. A hard-working multi-scholarship winner from a poor family who has an I.Q. over 145 does not fail anything, much less a pure memory course. Yet in 20 years of school, it was my only failed course. Meanwhile I totaled five cars in six years. And even though I was surrounded by physicians, not a one had an inkling of what was happening. Nowadays we see many young medical students who have horrible brain fog from traffic and the formaldehyde in the dissection laboratories.

And to this day adhesives and formaldehyde are two of the worst chemical exposures for me, although I'm much less sensitive now than I was during the hiatus of my chemical

```
************************************************************
*                                                          *
*                                                          *
*                                                          *
*                                                          *
*                                                          *
*                                                          *
*                                                          *
*                                                          *
*                                                          *
*                                                          *
*       If you fall into a mental stupor ........          *
*                                                          *
*                                                          *
*                                                          *
*                                                          *
*                                                          *
*                                                          *
*                                                          *
*                                                          *
*                                                          *
*                                                          *
*                                                          *
*                                                          *
*                                                          *
*       ........ or have irascible mood swings by mid-     *
*       afternoon, look at what you ate or inhaled. What   *
*       else could it be?                                  *
*                                                          *
************************************************************
```

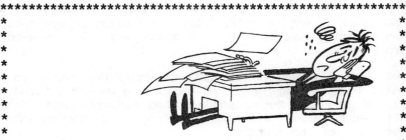

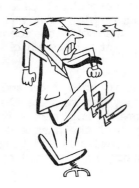

sensitivities in the seventies and eighties. There were times when my total load was at its peak, when a minuscule exposure to these left me with a headache so severe I literally could not see, or a backache so severe I had to be carried to the bathroom. At other times I was just plain brain dead, nasty and miserable.

But let that be a reminder to you. If you are not as smart, as fast, as happy, as tolerant, as creative, or as energetic as you think you should be, look for the cause. You have the information to make the diagnosis.

```
*****************************************************************
*     The Diagnosis &                                          *
*     Treatment Is As                                          *
*     Easy As 1, 2, 3           As We Described In.            *
*                                                              *
*     1.  Unload patient's                                     *
*         environment.                                         *
*         Correct nutritional    The E.I. Syndrome            *
*         biochemistry,                                        *
*            then                                              *
*     2.  Balance & initiate                                   *
*         healing & eventual     You Are What You Ate         *
*         regeneration.                                        *
*                                                              *
*     3.  How to get started.    The Macro Almanac            *
*****************************************************************
```

Meanwhile test your doctor and see if he knows 21st century medicine. If not, see if he is at least interested in learning it and working with you. It took me ten years to get where I am, so give him encouragement and admiration for having the guts to be a compassionate worker and thinker. If there is no hope for him, get rid of dead wood and sail on. Life is too precious.

The Proof Is Out There ---- Now Go For It

One physician describes a quack as someone who alleges to be ahead of his time. (Translation: anyone who is ahead of him!) Now if this isn't egocentric jealousy, I don't know what is. True, timing is of the essence. If I jogged down the street 25 years ago, someone would have thought I had a screw loose. Now it's common.

Years ago I recall coming home from ecology meetings saying to my husband, "If I start telling people there are toxic chemicals in their homes, they'll think I'm nuts. Then the formaldehyde insulation catastrophe hit and it became common knowledge.

The same thing occurred with regard to all the carcin-ogenic hydrocarbons in drinking water from industrial wastes seeping into the underground water tables. "Honey, I can't tell people there are chemicals in their tap water that can make them sick. They'll think I'm nuts!" Now it is common knowledge that it causes many to react with symptoms and the only way they'll know is to get "unmasked" and have a trial of glass-bottled spring water for 2 weeks. But by the time

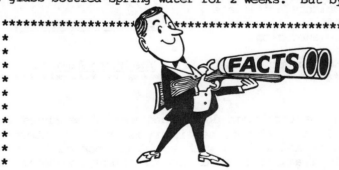

There is no longer any excuse for asserting that that there is not enough evidence for biochemical, nutritional and environmental medicine.

this information was available, it was too late for the children of Woburn Massachusetts, who died of leukemia from trichloroethylene in their tap water, or the residents of Times Beach, Missouri who developed a host of undiagnosable complaints from pesticides in theirs. If only this knowledge could have hit a little sooner.

Later I found myself saying the same with regard to radon, "If I tell people there's a radioactive gas in their basements that causes cancer, they'll know I'm nuts!"

It appears that it's pretty easy to be ahead of one's time. All it takes is a tremendous amount of sacrifice to work and read constantly. Because all the data is referenced in the scientific literature. It's all there.

The biochemistry and environmental medicine scientific literature is jammed with proof that pesticides cause brain fog and permanent, irreversible nervous system damage, like Parkinsonism; that many "normal" home and office/factory chemicals do as well; that hidden food allergies and undiscovered nutritional deficiencies also can cause any symptoms imaginable, while the brain is usually the first target organ to suffer; that presenile dementia or Alzheimer's disease can be arrested and even sometimes reversed with proper supplementation if studied and diagnosed early by a physician with adequate biochemical and environmental knowledge.

In summary, there is voluminous evidence on pesticides, chemicals, food allergy, nutritional deficiencies and abnormal bowel flora as being capable of producing chronic tiredness and the toxic brain. So why is it ignored? Because it changes all the rules of medicine. And when you usher in a new era, much of the old becomes obsolete, including those who do not have the time nor the interest to join in this exciting evolution. Remember many research grants in medical schools come from drug companies. So you're not going to get many takers for research that doesn't sell drugs.

Instead, medicine clings to antiquated, useless diagnoses like chronic fatigue syndrome, Yuppie Fatigue Syndrome, chronic Epstein-Barr Virus or chronic EBV, chronic mono, etc., etc., because these diagnoses get the physician off the hook. (Because people are so smart, use of the term hypochondriac is avoided, but psychosomatic illness or somabiform disorder are substituted). Anyway, these diagnoses (for which there are no unequivical blood tests or x-rays), provide the physician with a name so he can save face and not be stumped. At the same time it gives the unspoken message that there's nothing that can be done. You just have to learn to live with it.

And because many desperate people are eager to get relief, these diagnoses provide fresh ground for researchers in money-making high-tech substances like interferon. This is a substance the body makes to fight off viruses. But to make enough to give to someone by injection is very expensive. It reminds me of a young gal from Michigan that came to the office with a 3 year history of "chronic fatigue syndrome". She had had interferon injections ("after all else had failed") to the tune of $50 a day. It still didn't help. But on the program of environmental medicine, she described herself as 80% better than she had been in years in just the first months.

With so much evidence, there are only 3 logical things to do: find yourself a doctor, get yourself detoxed and well, then defend your right to modern molecular medicine with your insurance company. For they will actually try to push you back into antiquated drug-oriented medicine. They get much of their data indirectly through pharmaceutical firms for starters (via the academician who sits on their advisory boards but depends on drug company research grants to survive). But first, you must keep reading and getting smarter all the time. It's your only defense against those who would like to cram antiquated medicine down your throat for another 50 years.

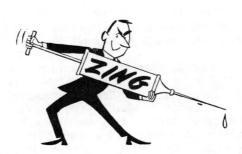

****
* Hi-tech medicine is in. But why take $50 a day of
* interferon injections that leave you only half
* well, when you can identify the causes of your
* chronic fatigue syndrome and get completely well?
****

Welcome To The Era Of Molecular Medicine

Parenthetically, you might ask, "If you knew all these things years before they hit Time and Newsweek covers, what is next? Could we have a preview?"

Sure. Beyond chemical pollution is electromagnetic pollution. You know electricity is the next level of function beyond biochemistry. For biochemistry is merely the movement of electrons. What's the difference between you dead or you alive? You're the same basket of chemicals, but the electricity is gone. How can Chinese acupuncturists anesthetize a New York City reporter enough to surgically remove his appendix while he is conversing and drinking a soda? Because they understand some of the electrical circuitry (meridians) of the body far better than western physicians. The rate of anesthetic complications could be reduced by using acupuncture in this country, but for the same reason of ego, power, politics, money, and time, we will still be gas-passers for a long time.

Anyway, your body has electricity in it, and anything that has electricity also has a field (electro magnetic field). And fields from different objects can be complementary or opposing, like the poles of a magnet. Some people react strongly to electromagnetic pollution. Remember you're always swaddled in a field when you're in a building, due to the wiring that is in the walls. It's like being inside an electrical cage. And much has been written and proven about harmful and helpful effects of electromagnetic fields on human bodies and especially minds and emotions (Becker, R.O. The Body Electric, see appendix). As an aside I would recommend you never use an electric blanket.

Suspicion of electrical sensitivity is justified if you feel worse around certain electrical devices (like a television, electric razor, computer) when they are on, versus off. Or if you feel better out of doors than indoors. You can differentiate this from chemical sensitivity, for example, by observing whether you feel improvement indoors when the circuit breaker to your room has been shut off, or when you have grounded yourself to a water pipe or by walking barefoot out doors for fifteen minutes.

With appropriate electromagnetic fields and knowledge of a person's individual frequency of response, you can make someone happy, mean, exhausted, promote healing of a non-union fracture, or cause an abortion or cancer, while others around him can remain unaffected (Electromagnetism and Life, Becker RO, Marino AA, State University of New York Press, State University Plaza, Albany, NY 12246, 1982). For since you know that all people are biochemically unique, it follows that they are electrically unique. In fact, we all have our own unique frequencies. For example, it's possible to put someone to sleep, or cause cancer or personality changes by beaming the correct frequency toward him.

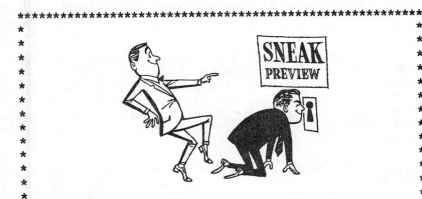

Once medicine enters the era of molecular biology, it will be ready to move on to other levels like electromagnetic fields.

But before that knowledge and research comes to fruition (it's in the making now, I just hope I live long enough to see how it turns out), medicine will discover that basic

health lies in one's diet and lifestyle. As the health care
system becomes bankrupt, you'll see the chaos that only Ayn
Rand could describe (<u>Atlas Shrugged</u>), and then educated
people will begin to take control of their health. They'll
demand whole grains in restaurants and organic foods in
groceries. They just won't buy smelly products that outgas
chemicals. They'll reduce pesticide use and find alternatives.

You've learned that by unloading your environment of
unnecessary chemicals, discovering your hidden food allergies, correcting your nutrient deficiencies and normalizing
your bowel flora that you have all the control over your
health. Furthermore, no biochemist is smarter than mother
nature, so once the deficiencies have been corrected, it's
up to you to eat as though every mouthful really counts.
Every mouthful must be of the highest nutritional quality
possible, for anything less hinders rather than helps your
body's function.

You know the scientific literature is full of papers
documenting psychiatric problems like depression, learning
disorders, senile dementia, and panic disorders that respond
to therapies with vitamins, minerals, amino acids, and
essential fatty acids. Why isn't this the thrust of medicine? Because it's just plain too much effort and not prof-
itable.

That's why the principles of environmental medicine
first have to be learned. If a man walks in my office with
9 nails in his shoe and I remove one, he'll be no better.
The next time I remove another, and still he'll be no better
and beginning to doubt if I can help him at all. It's not
until they are all gone (if he persists and reads and understands the process) that he'll get marked relief.

Fortunately the majority of folks are much easier than
the man with 9 nails. As we whittle through the total load,
we are able to progressively unload rather dramatically.
Take the average person we see with brain fog, asthma and
sinusitis, headache, irritable bowel, extreme fatigue, and
body aches. The environmental controls and mold injections

simmer down the asthma, sinusitis, and headache usually within the first month. Then, the diet clears the aches, the Candida program clears the bowel, correcting nutrient deficiencies buoys up the detox system to lift the brain fog, etc., etc.

This is what we mean when we say whittle through the total load. In most people we first look at nutrient levels. Simultaneously we'll culture the home for mold, and institute environmental control instructions. Then we might test molds since they cause so much symptomatology. Then we may evaluate the Candida program, then hidden food sensitivities, look for levels of xenobiotics in the blood, test chemicals, neurotransmitters, or assess the psychological makeup and needs.

We may possibly need much more sophisticated nutritional, biochemical, hormonal, chemical, pesticide or neurotransmitter assays. And it's exciting because the field is constantly expanding. Some need checking for electromagnetic field sensitivity, others may need detox programs, etc., etc. But in short, we will plow through that total load until we find and correct what is keeping you from feeling 100% healthy.

It sounds cumbersome, but the bottom line is it works. I had 20 years of insufferable back pain, crushed disks, osteoarthritis, spasms, and sciatica after jumping horses (or more precisely, them jumping over me). I had casts, braces, consultants, medications, physical therapy, and chiropractic, all of which helped. The bottom line was 20 years later it was better but not wonderful. Rather than accepting a fusion, I found the causes; now it's wonderful. The causes were natural gas (yes we had to throw out a perfectly good furnace, water heater, dryer, and stove .... and I'd do it again, even if I had to go to the poor house), formaldehyde (yes, we took all carpeting out of the house and office, foiled beds, etc.), meat ingestion, a marked magnesium deficiency and more. As a result of this, I ride and jump without any braces, have a huge organic garden, water ski backwards on trick skiis, windsurf in the ocean and enjoy a pain-free back. But, I can also be laid out in lavender if I throw my diet and environmental controls to the wind.

This is how we discovered many causes I never would have dreamed of, with the help of the wonderful folks who have blessed me with their friendship and refused to give up on themselves until they found the wellness they were looking for. With the help of one woman who had severe incapacitating cystitis that ruined her daily happiness, we found that the bladder was merely another target organ for multiple food and chemical sensitivities. Since then scores have recovered from this "incurable" (according to a national support group for cystitis victims) devastating malady.

And it made so much sense once she proved to me it was the cause of her symptoms. After all the brain can go into vascular spasm and have severe migraine from chocolate or MSG (or severe withdrawal from lack of coffee in a coffee addict). The lungs can go into severe spasm and you can die with ingestion of one peanut (in a peanut sensitive asthmatic). The bowel can go into ferocious spasm in the milk allergic. So why then cannot the smooth muscle of the bladder go into the same spasm? It does. And with all this spasm, you guessed it, many were also magnesium deficient as well as deficient in several other nutrients. And what a difference when a whole new life of pain-free days opened up. These women were back to college, and were into careers they had dreamed of all the years they had been house bound with this plague. There's no way any of us could ever consider drugs as our lifeline, when we can find environmental and biochemical causes and be drug-free.

Or take Jeffrey, a seven year old who made life a horror for his parents. He was vicious, malicious, hateful, nasty and immune to discipline. He had had many evaluations for this, and it was approached from many angles. What turned him into an adorable, teachable little guy and a pleasure to be around? Correcting his renal magnesium wasting syndrome that no one had found.

So as medicine continues ignoring all this, the results will continue to compound. Will we have a nation of

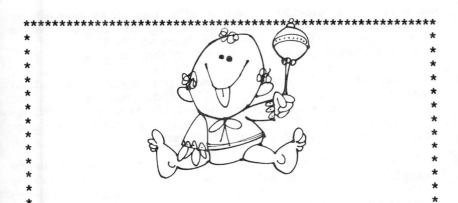

```
******************************************************************
*                                                                *
*                                                                *
*                                                                *
*                                                                *
*                                                                *
*                                                                *
*                                                                *
*                                                                *
*                                                                *
*                                                                *
*                                                                *
*                                                                *
*   If your baby isn't as smart as his parents, better           *
*   look at his toxic load.                                       *
*                                                                *
******************************************************************
```

mentally incompetent people secondary to nutritional deficiency and environmental toxicities in 25 years? Will we have schools crammed with slow learners and delinquents and nursing homes brimming with Alzheimer's?

We know that pesticides produce brain fog or toxic brain symptoms. Furthermore, we know that heavy metals (as are often found in auto and industrial exhausts, pesticide carriers, aluminum anti-caking agents in baked goods, etc.) cause permanent neurological damage. We know that inhaling formaldehyde from plastics can produce brain fog. We know that babies have immature detoxication systems.

Yet how does the intelligent middle class family care for their precious new arrival? By putting it in brand new permanent press (formaldehyde), fire-retardant and colored (carcinogenic dyes) clothes. This bundle of joy swaddled in chemicals is placed in a newly painted nursery, on a new foam mattress with more fire-retardant and pesticided, plastic sheets and crib bumpers, and then they wonder why he cries all night and seems irritable. And if mother complains, the pediatrician intimidates her into hypochondria.

Meanwhile they make his formula with tap water containing trichloroethylene from industrial run-off and added aluminum as an anti-flocculent, give apple juice which is a great way of concentrating the pesticides in apples, etc., etc.

As the kid grows, he requires special education classes because he is learning disabled. Meanwhile no one has done a biochemical assessment of his worn-out detoxication system. And I'll spare you the analysis of his diet beginning with sugared breakfast cereals.

It becomes readily apparent now the trouble we're headed for. And the solution will have to come from the individual. It's easy to keep everyone ignorant because to understand it is all encompassing. You need to understand medicine, biochemistry, psychology, toxicology, nutrition, microbiology, neurology, politics, medicine, manufacturing, and much more in order to synthesize and collate this material in order to formulate your personal plan of attack.

By now you see the light. You don't have to be a biochemist or ecologist to comprehend that <u>any symptom that a medicine can help must (by the very reason that the medicine helped) have an underlying (usually correctable) biochemical abnormality. You just need to find a physician motivated enough to find it.</u> For example, many tranquilizers, like Xanax (R) (the valium of the 80's), work as the GABA receptor in the brain, yet their effect can often be mimicked by supplying the correct amino acid precursor or correcting hypomagnesemia. Other mood elevators, like Prozac (R) and Desyrel (R), affect the serotonin chemistry, but this can also be manipulated by the correct amino acid precursors, and it's cheaper. Obviously, we don't have all the answers yet. We're the first generation of this evolution. But the accomplishments we have seen fuel us to work night and day to conquer further vistas.

We've been lulled into assuming because pollutants exist in such "low" levels that their harm is also low level. We've even set new standards now of "normal levels" (remember the New Jersey residents' blood levels?) of chemicals in the blood, because it is so rare to find someone

without any, anymore. And because the detox system has met
its match with some of these chemicals, they are not gotten
rid of. They just get stored and accumulate. Then when the
final straw comes, like moving into a new house or painting
the office, and the system breaks down, it appears to the
uninitiated that you have gotten paranoid about chemicals.

And make no mistake about it, these chemicals are so
widespread that it's impossible for you to go through a day
without exposure to them. And they do not belong in the
body. In fact they are so toxic to the body that it doesn't
know how to get rid of some of them. Furthermore, very
small levels measurable in the parts per billion can, and
have done, considerable damage to the immune system, the
hemotologic, the detox, the cardiovascular, the nervous
system and more.

When children die of leukemia because of trace "harmless" amounts of trichloroethylene in the drinking water and
adults die from leukemia from gasoline fumes, and farmers
lose their short term memory or sensation in their limbs
from a spill of pesticide on their hands, these are potent.

The reason it's so easy to lull people into this
deception is that there are so few physicians (less than
1000 out of 500,000 in the U.S.) who can diagnose these
toxicities:
1. First you must know what type of questions to ask
   to find out what might be the likely culprits.
2. Then you need to know what metabolites to look for
   in testing, because don't forget many of these
   chemicals have been altered or metabolized into
   different substances by the time we see these
   people.
3. Then you need to know what specialty labs can
   measure these chemicals at the levels you have
   remaining to the blood or fat {ppb}.
4. Next you need to know what to do with the
   information after you get it.
5. How to follow-up and what to do if your first line
   of treatment was unsuccessful. None of this is
   completely taught in any medical school in the

world as yet. {But it is taught in courses for the physician and his staff through the American Academy of Environmental Medicine}.

You can be certain of this: When you start getting tired or headachey, depressed, muscle aches, or can't think straight in the middle of the day, it has a cause. You should be smart enough by now to be sure of that. It could be the air conditioning "fresh air" intake from the roof where the heat of the sun on the tarred roof volatilizes the hydrocarbons in the tar; it could be an unsuspected wheat or sugar sensitivity or natural gas or pesticide in the restaurant where you had lunch, or withdrawal phase from your morning coffee. But it <u>has</u> a cause.

A big diagnostic problem is that some people's symptoms are not on and off, they're just always on. Without a concentrated effort, you're perennially surrounded. I was reminded of this when I knew I was having a pollutant reaction while windsurfing 2 miles out in the middle of the Caribbean.

But when I looked up in the sky I was shocked that I was sailing under the long tail of a pollutant haze that emanated from the tiny island. An island where a half dozen cruise and cargo ships dock daily, where a dozen planes land and takeoff (each one equivalent to a few hundred idling car engines), where burning is unrestricted, engine pollution is not fined, and there are too many cars, especially old ones.

On a flight into Miami one sunny day I was particularly struck by the pollutant haze. It was a beautiful sunny day and as we descended, it looked as though some artist had smeared an angry muddy hand across a beautiful painting. What really amazed me was this smudge extended about twenty miles into the ocean. That's a long ways to go just to get a breath of fresh air.

You know now that none of the poisonings are "insignificant", and that you can't depend on the government to protect you.

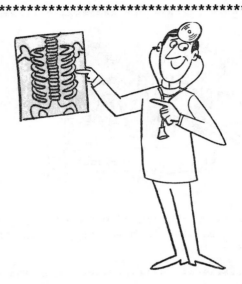

There's no question current hi-tech acute care
medicine and physicians are fantastic.

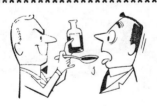

But it's also irrefutable that a headache is not
a darvon deficiency. Medicine has evolved to the
molecular biology/environmental level.

```
*********************************************************
*                                                       *
*                                                       *
```

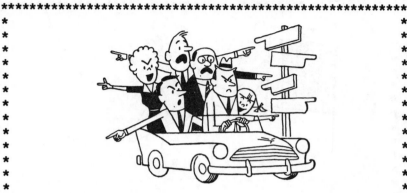

```
*                                                       *
*    And you will never run out of people arguing about *
*    which type of medicine is best for you (depending  *
*    on their vested interests).                        *
*                                                       *
*********************************************************
```

```
*********************************************************
*                                                       *
```

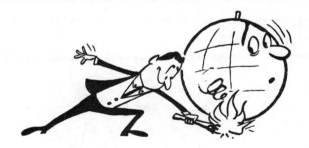

```
*                                                       *
*    But you don't have to set the world on fire in try-*
*    ing to convert everyone to your viewpoint.         *
*                                                       *
*********************************************************
```

```
**********************************************************
*                                                        *
*                                                        *
```

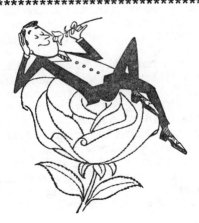

Just follow the direction to a less toxic life
style.

```
**********************************************************
```

```
**********************************************************
*                                                        *
```

And you'll come out smelling like a rose.

```
**********************************************************
```

You now know that you can not smell most pesticides and chemicals (especially when you're adapted to them), but their effects are cumulative. The symptoms can be delayed, and subtle or vague: short term memory loss, fatigue, numbness and tingling, muscle aches, inability to think straight. They can start imperceptibly, slowly.

You also know that high cholesterol is not the sole cause of heart attacks and senility any more than calcium deficiency is the sole cause of osteoporosis. There is a symphony of biochemical dysfunctions that must be identified and corrected. And by incorrectly treating these, calcium, for example, is deposited wherever the body can lay it down......in vessel walls, kidney stones, gall stones, cartilage.

In the meantime are we to ease on into any era where the majority of kids are in special education and the median age for Alzheimer's slips lower and lower?

Just because it appears that Alzheimer's or heart attacks or strokes occur overnight couldn't be further from the truth. These have been building for a long while, just as diabetes, hypertension, cancer and aging have.

Dyslexia is a terribly incapacitating specialized form of learning disability for which medicine does not have a great track record. How many doctors who treat it know that the zinc (in sweat) of children with dyslexia was only 66% of that of normal kids? (Zinc deficiency in children with dyslexia, Grant and Howard, British Medical Journal, 296, 607-609, 1988). And you know better than most many of the ways zinc affects much of the chemistry of the brain. And there are many other biochemical abnormalities published as well. But they're still waiting to discover the same abnormality in all dyslexia cases.

As I write this, there is a glimmer of hope on the horizon. The Syracuse Herald-Journal (Sept. 28, 1989) ran an article (New York Times News Service) entitled "Diuretics use raises the risk of heart attack, study finds".

Apparently Swedish doctors reported in the New England Journal of Medicine (vol. 321, issue 13, Sept. 28, 1989, p. 868) that of 60 million hypertensive Americans, 15-25 million take diuretics (fluid pills) that act "directly on body tissues to cause a sort of chemically induced diabetes and also increase blood cholesterol levels." But that is all they said! I wonder how many years it will be before researchers will collate the results of that study with the glut of evidence I've presented here so that they can teach physicians and the public how exactly diuretics cause these diseases and what they can do about it. As you now know, diuretics cause the loss of many nutrients, like magnesium. And since undiscovered magnesium deficiency is one of many common causes of hypertension (spasm or increased tone of blood vessels) and hypercholesterolemia (the body lacks the nutrients to properly metabolize the cholesterol), the use of medications, like diuretics, only serves to hasten the loss of more magnesium. This leads to conditions that become resistant to medications, so stronger, more costly, and more dangerous drugs are used. Meanwhile, with the emphasis on lowering the cholesterol with drugs and diet ("plastic foods" with trans fatty acids), the brain membranes become deficient in cholesterol and malfunction. This malfunction can be a stroke in one or senility in another. This is providing he does not die from a magnesium deficiency - induced cardiac arrhythmia first.

Meanwhile we have all this wonderful information and 25 million people are not able to reap the benefits of it. Some will die this year because of it. And some will read it and question; but as with so much in medicine, they may be told "There's not enough information yet". What we actually have is an information glut. Our creative medical minds have become constipated by an overwhelming amount of material. Who can read the over 2,000 periodic journals? We need to start a field that collates the information and puts it into practical use in our lifetimes, before we destroy our health and our planet.

Dr. John Maltzberger, a psychiatrist at Harvard Medical School agrees that if a doctor's self-esteem relies too much on his self-image, that he is vulnerable to compromising his diagnostic accuracy and treatment decisions. Dr. Robert Smith goes on to note in his study that challenging or questioning the physician's decisions is one of the most upsetting things a patient can do and may even jeopardize his care (What physicians most dislike about their patient's behavior, New York Times, 10/27/88).

Once we physicians realize that, like everyone else, we are not perfect, nor are we ever going to be, we can then get on with the fun of helping people heal through 20th century nutritional biochemistry and environmental medicine. There's no way any of us can know everything. But by being open and honest, and not saddled to our egos, we can enthusiastically embrace the medicine of the 20th century as it evolves. For those who choose not to, there are plenty of patients who still only want a pill. All we ask is honesty that is not hidden under the overworked statement, "There's no evidence for that".

It is ironic that physicians who cry for evidence can, on the same hand, choose to ignore so much evidence: it doesn't seem to alter their course when the difference in mortality among groups of patients having coronary bypass surgery versus those refusing it was statistically insignificant (Hueb, et al, Am. J. Cardiol., 63, 155, Jan. 15, 1989). Nor does a study by two doctors from the Harvard School of Public Health who called for a shift in cancer research to prevention rather than treatment, since we are losing the war against cancer (Progress against cancer?, N. Engl. J. Med., May 8, 1986).

Nor do these physicians seem to be aware that the U.S. Office of Technology Assessment offers a publication "Assessing the Efficacy and Safety of Medical Technologies" (#PB 286-929). On page 7 it says, "it has been estimated that only 10-20% of all procedures currently used in medical practice have been shown to be efficacious by controlled trial".

Additionally, for those who wish to continue to ignore all this data, "the liability of a physician should be cause for concern if a correctable occupational hazard is ignored or if a potentially compensible disability is inadequately evaluated and falsely denied" (Zaslow, J, Medical malpractice. In: Ladon, J, ed., Occupational Health Law: A Guide For Industry, NY Marcel Decker, Inc., 146-149, 1981).

There Is No Time Like The Present

Chronic glomerulonephritis is a life-threatening kidney disease that can lead to years of very expensive renal dialysis ("kidney machine" treatments). Yet hydrocarbon exposure is one of the causes in some (Zimmerman, SW, et al, Hydrocarbon exposure and chronic glomerulonephritis, The Lancet, 199-201, Aug 2, 1975; Raunskov, G, et al, Glomerulonephritis in exposure to organic solvents, Acta. Medi. Scand., 205: 575-579, 1979).

Choreic movements or tardive dyskinesia is an embarrassing problem for the elderly. You've seen it often.. ....those involuntary (uncontrollable) twitches an jerky movements of the hands or face with peculiar grimacing. Yet choline (related to the B vitamins) can stop it in many (Grawdon, JH, et al, Oral choline administration to patients with tardive dyskinesia, N. Engl. J. Med., 297: 524-527, Sept 8, 1977).

Exposures to auto and industrial exhaust can cause hidden mineral deficiencies that affect every organ, for example, causing kidney disease, as an example (Brenner, I, Cadmium toxicity, World Rev. Nutr. Diet., 32, 165-197, 1978).

Magnesium status has an important role in determining who will survive a cardiac arrest, yet it is rarely checked (Cannon, LA, et al, Magnesium levels in cardiac arrest victims: Relationship between magnesium levels and successful resuscitation, Ann. of Emergency Med., 16:11, 1195-1199, Nov. 1987).

Fatigue, dizziness, inability to concentrate, poor memory, and depression can be caused by solvents in most people's blood streams because they outgas from everyday products and work exposures, yet they are rarely looked for (Feldman, RG, et al, Neuropsychological effects of industrial toxins: A review, Am. J. Industr. Med., 1: 211-227, 1980).

Life-threatening cardiac arrhythmias can be caused by wearing a freshly dry cleaned suit, a cleaning solvent at work or typewriter correction fluid (Abedin, Z, et al, Cardiac toxicity of perchloroethylene, S. Med. J., 73: 1081-1083, 1980; Mago, L, The effects of industrial chemicals on the heart, 206-207, Balazo, T, ed, Cardiac Toxicology, CRC Press, Boca Raton, 1981; King, GS, Sudden death in adolescents resulting from the inhalation of typewriter correction fluid, J. Amer. Med. Assoc., 253: 1604-1606, 1985).

I can and want to continue until you get the message (but I also want you to be able to carry this book to the beach without a wheel barrow). AN EVOLUTION IN MEDICINE IS HERE.

If I weren't so worried about making this a twenty-five pound book, I would go on until I was sure you had the message: An evolution in medicine is upon us. But we're dragging our feet while its victims continue to suffer and prematurely die.

As The World Catches Up

It's 5:30 a.m. as I write my last pages of this book before office hours at 8. As I glance at yesterdays local paper, two articles catch my eye.

One details the over 6 million pounds of toxic gases that manufacturing firms in our small city of a third of a million spewed into just the air (not counting the water, etc.) last year (a 13% rise over the preceding year!).

The article gives in detail (The Post-Standard, Oct. 10, 1989, Factories report rising pollution, Bob Sanders, 1, A-6, A-7) the tens of thousands to even millions of pounds of pollutants that each of the top ten factories emit. These of course include, for example, over 1/3 million pounds of trichloroethane by one air conditioning manufacturer, over 1/3 of a million pounds of toluene by one plating company, and 1/3 of a million pounds of xylene by a car manufacturer.

Yes, they very chemicals that cause so much disease and that you and I have such a devil of a time ridding our homes and offices of are spewed into the air daily. This explains why many people never are able to clear their chemically induced symptoms and begin to heal in their own city.

And on another page (News Service Reports, ibid, A-2) they announced that Varmus and Bishop received the Nobel Prize for the discovery of the mechanism of cancer. Our genetic material or genes can be converted into oncogenes by exposures to chemicals. These oncogenes then go on to give the messages to our cells to grow (like a) cancer. One of the professors of Sweden's Nobel awarding committee was quoted as naively saying, "Imagine: The likely cause of cancer comes from us, and all that the outside factors have to do is to push the right button".

But how long will it be before enough people recognize the connection between the two articles and do something about it?

The cry of the procrastinator has been, "There is not enough evidence". When in truth, the exact opposite has occurred. We have so much evidence that it's overwhelming and few have attempted to tackle the enormous job of putting it together in a useful way. And when we do, we are thwarted at every cross roads while our patients are financially penalized by current insurance reimbursement programs and the politics of governing boards directed by physicians, unversed in the subject.

As our current medical reimbursement structure continues progressively into a scheme of socialized medicine, managed by cookbook computers, we can only become further removed from the reality of biochemical individuality. A headache will remain a Darvon deficiency and the nutritional biochemical and environmental causes will continue to be denigrated and ignored.

What happens in the future will be determined mostly by how much interest in his health care the consumer possesses, and how vociferous he chooses to be. And if your excuse is you don't have time, remember I wrote this book in less than a year, while teaching and lecturing all over the world and carrying a full-time private practice. I'm not a researcher, not a biochemist, and obviously not a writer. I'm more like a country doctor by nature. But having been so sick myself and having the good fortune of not only getting well, but being able to help many others like myself, I felt obliged to make this information known. What you do with it in your life is up to you.

Are you going to wait 50 years for the world to catch up? Or are you going to turn evolution into revolution? Your health is totally in your hands. Fundamental to your health is to change your diet, lifestyle, and attitude. It's a package deal. It doesn't work if you just try to fix your nutrition. Likewise just changing the diet rarely brings total well-being. Where are you going if you awaken each morning from a toxic night's sleep?

Clearly the only ones who will be able to accomplish this are those who are sick enough, or those who are smart enough. I was the former, I hope you are the latter.

You now know the answer to whether you are TIRED OR TOXIC. Now the real question is WHAT ARE YOU GOING TO DO ABOUT IT?

Environmental Health Perspectives
Vol. 76, pp. 195-198, 1987

Brief Report

Diagnosing the Tight Building Syndrome
by Sherry A. Rogers*

Formaldehyde is but one of many chemicals capable of causing the tight building syndrome or environmentally induced illness (EI). The spectrum of symptoms it may induce includes attacks of headache, flushing, laryngitis, dizziness, nausea, extreme weakness, arthralgia, unwarranted depression, dysphonia, exhaustion, inability to think clearly, arrhythmia or muscle spasms. The nonspecificity of such symptoms can baffle physicians from many specialties. Presented herein is a simple office method for demonstrating that formaldehyde is among the etiologic agents triggering these symptoms. The very symptoms that patients complain of can be provoked within minutes, and subsequently abolished, with an intradermal injection of the appropriate strength of formaldehyde. This injection aids in convincing the patient of the cause of the symptoms so he can initiate measures to bring his disease under control.

Introduction

A survey of the literature indicates homes with indoor chemical problems have higher concentrations of volatile organic compounds than houses without problems (1). The tight building syndrome is defined as a building in which worker complaints of ill health are more common than might be reasonably expected (2). Furthermore, it is assumed that nonoccupational explanations of symptoms have been ruled out. Some have called this illness in victims of the tight building the sick building syndrome (3), but medical specialists relate better to the treatment of people.

Over 25 years ago, Randolph (4) recognized that chemicals in the indoor air environment could provoke symptoms, but acceptance was delayed by lack of measurements and testing techniques which today abound. Because many of these indoor chemicals exist in outdoor air as well, a more accurate designation might be environmental illness, or EI.

Volatile organic hydrocarbons are but a part of the triggers of the tight building syndrome (TBS) or environmentally induced illness (EI). With the installation of urea foam formaldehyde insulation (UFFI), a concordant dramatic increase in symptomatology provided a vast number of victims for study. This provided us with a prototype from which we could observe the evolution and diversity of symptoms associated with an acute increase in one quantifiable indoor chemical, formaldehyde.

*Northeast Center for Environmental Medicine, 2800 West Genesee Street, Syracuse, NY 13219.

Over the last 6 years, increasing numbers of patients have presented with symptoms reminiscent of these UFFI victims (5), but they had no history of UFFI exposure (6,7). Measurements of ambient levels of formaldehyde have shown that new mobile homes, newly constructed homes with particleboard subflooring, offices recently renovated with paneling or prefabricated walls, new clothing, or even new carpeting or new furnishings, and homes with new beds and cabinetry can accumulate as much formaldehyde, as a result of offgassing, as a UFFI home (8–11). A variety of other commonly encountered volatile substances are capable of inducing the same symptoms (12–15). For example, the mean reported levels for formaldehyde in indoor air in residences was 0.03 ppm for houses without UFFI and 0.12 ppm for houses with UFFI (with and without complaints) (11). Some mobile homes had levels of 0.4 ppm, and the mean level for several hospitals was 0.55 ppm.

Guidelines are needed to facilitate diagnosis and identification of the triggering agents. Attacks of headache, nausea, inability to concentrate, mental obtundation, dizziness, lethargy, arrhythmia, flushing, laryngitis, dopiness, irritability, dysphonia, unwarranted depression, arthralgia, and extreme weakness, although nonspecific, are some of the most common symptoms of EI and frequently lead to a sequence of diagnostic evaluations which are ineffective; psychiatric evaluation is often suggested.

With proper questioning, the victim will often be able to associate the onset of disease with the purchase of new carpeting, furniture, beds, cabinets, renovation of the home or office, moving into a new dwelling, or insulating with UFFI. We now need a test that would substantiate that formaldehyde (or other chemicals) was among the triggers.

Materials and Methods

In this study, U.S.P. 37% reagent grade formaldehyde was diluted 50% with Hollister-Stier diluent and was used as a concentrate. One milliliter of this concentrate was added to 4 mL of sterile water; this made dilution 1, a 3.7% formaldehyde solution. One milliliter of dilution 1 and 4 mL of diluent made dilution 2, which thus was a 0.7% solution. Fivefold serial dilutions as described by Miller and Morris (16,17) were thus prepared out to dilution 9, a solution containing just under 10^{-6} of 1% formaldehyde (0.0000094%).

Testing of patients, who in all cases had failed to obtain relief with medical treatments elsewhere, was initiated with an intradermal injection of 0.01 cc of the dilution 3 (0.15% formaldehyde); this injection resulted in a 4 mm × 4 mm wheal. After 10 min the symptoms and wheal size were determined. If no symptoms and no growth in wheal size were observed, 0.05 cc of dilution 3 was injected, resulting in a 7 mm × 7 mm wheal. If after another 10 min both parameters were again negative, then the test was considered negative. If either parameter was positive, then 0.05 cc of dilution 4 (0.03% formaldehyde) was tested. If positive, then 0.05 cc of dilution 5 (0.006% formaldehyde) was used. Negative wheal growth and negative symptoms determined the point at which testing was terminated. If symptoms were produced with positive wheal growth and were subsequently eliminated by the dose that gave no wheal growth, the test was considered positive.

All tests were done in a single-blind fashion, and were preceded by at least one placebo injection of normal saline for baseline and placebo control. Patients were never aware of what they were being tested with until all tests had been completed.

In some cases, the blood serum level of formic acid, a metabolite of inhaled formaldehyde, was measured (SmithKline Laboratories, King of Prussia, PA). In others, a 24 hr level of formaldehyde in the ambient air of a suspect room was measured with a passive (badge) monitor.

Selected Case Examples

For brevity, only 2 of 24 cases are presented.

C.P. was a 39-year-old consulting engineer who traveled extensively. Two years ago he moved into a new home in the Syracuse, NY, area. There were new carpeting and particleboard subflooring throughout the house. Six months after moving he experienced an insidious onset of joint pain. He consulted an internist, a rheumatologist, and in spite of their treatments, he reported a year-and-a-half later that he had the same symptoms. He also indicated that he ached more after

he had been at home for the weekend, but felt well whenever he was out to town for a few days.

His blood serum level of formic acid (a metabolite of formaldehyde) was 10 µg/mL after a weekend at home, and 6 µg/mL after a day at work. A passive (badge) monitor showed an ambient 24-hr formaldehyde level of 0.06 ppm in his home. Note that current recommendations for maximum ambient air formaldehyde exposure levels range from 0.25 ppm (National Academy of Sciences) to 0.12 ppm (American Society of Heating, Refrigeration, and Air Conditioning Engineers), while concentrations below 0.06 ppm are considered of limited or no concern (18).

Single-blind testing with normal saline produced no symptoms. An injection of 0.01 cc of dilution 3 (0.15% formaldehyde) produced wheal growth and "a warm feeling"; 0.05 cc of dilution 4 (0.03%) produced "ringing in the ears and achy joints." With a 0.05 cc of dilution 5 (0.006% formaldehyde), after 10 min all of his symptoms were clear, and there was no wheal growth. Another normal saline produced no wheal growth or symptoms.

M.B. was a 41-year-old teacher who had worked in the same school for 8 years. Over summer vacation, renovations were done in the school. When she re-entered the building in the fall, she started having symptoms that with each subsequent entry came on more quickly and more severely. She would eventually lose her voice as it gradually became more hoarse over the first few hours of work. She also experienced a sore throat and tender submandibular lymphadenopathy. She would have a feeling of achiness as though a flu were starting, and became exhausted. These symptoms persisted for a day or two after leaving the building and were proportional in duration and severity to the amount of time she spent there. At home she was without symptoms. Her serum level of formic acid was 10 µg/mL after a day at school and 6 µg/mL after a weekend at home. This measurement was repeated with the same results on subsequent days. The 24-hr level of formaldehyde in the school air, measured with a passive (badge) monitor, was 0.06 ppm. Single-blind testing to formaldehyde duplicated her symptoms in the office, with administration of 0.05 mL of dilution 5 (0.006% formaldehyde) producing visible facial flushing and weakening the patient's voice. The next dose, 0.05 mL of dilution 6, cleared the symptoms.

All patients described were universally and unquestionably freer of symptoms after they had been through an intensive educational program to teach them how to lower their ambient levels of formaldehyde exposures.

Discussion

The last half decade has provided us with over 1000 patients with undiagnosed chronic symptoms, refractory to a wide variety of treatments. Single-blind testing to various chemicals generally identified a suspect chemical and provided convincing enough duplication of symptoms in patients to enable them to make inconvenient and costly environmental changes that appear to be a necessary part of a comprehensive program to bring about symptom relief for the first time. Obviously, we have extended these techniques to include other difficult-to-avoid chemicals such as toluene, benzene, xylene, ethanol, trichloroethylene, natural gas, and more, and in many instances have paired the intradermal skin tests with serum measurements before and after exposure to the suspected environmental xenobiotics (tests performed by Enviro-Health Laboratories, Richardson, TX).

In patients requiring legal proof of chemical exposure, serum levels of these chemicals are obtained after a day at work and another set after a day at home. When the levels at home are comparatively lower, we have been able to provoke and duplicate symptoms with the particular chemical, single blind or double blind, and then neutralize or terminate symptoms with the nonreacting intradermal dose in our office, which is exceptionally free of potential chemical pollutants.

To accomplish a pollutant-free environment in our office, carpets have been removed and replaced with hardwood or quarry tile floors. Wooden cabinets and synthetic chairs have been replaced with metal. As many extraneous materials as possible are kept out of the testing room. Metal lockers are provided in another area for purses, coats, and packages. No people are allowed into the office who do not pass the sniff test by nurses who are sensitive to chemicals. Nurses and all patients must be free of fragrances, fabric softeners, polyester clothes, dry-cleaning fluid, cosmetics, toiletries, tobacco smoke, home cooking odors, work odors, and, in fact, any detectable odors. Air depollution devices with charcoal and potassium permanganate filters to absorb chemicals are used extensively, and outdoor air is continually filtered and pumped inside.

It is evident that a supersensitive individual cannot be tested, for example, by a nurse wearing perfume. He can react to this trigger shortly after coming into contact with her, confusing the test results. The major problem is that the treatment dose for the chemical being tested will not stop his symptoms, because it is not the chemical that initiated them. This has been repeatedly demonstrated and has helped us attain a progressively less contaminated office and, in particular, testing area. Many people happily note the relative paucity of symptoms that they experience after they have been in our office for a period of time.

It seems that multiple changes in the immune system are triggered in part by the increasing environmental overload (19,20). The mechanism of this technique may involve in part the prostaglandin system (21). Many have pondered why only one specific dose of the same agent that causes the symptom can also abolish it, while all other doses trigger the actual symptom or are without effect. Many biological systems have dose-dependent diverse actions. Certainly, we know various biological responses have a dose that enhances and a dose of the same substance that suppresses (22). Likewise, many biological systems have a bell-shaped response curve where there is an optimum dose for response, and doses too high or too low will be ineffective. As well, nonimmunologic mediator release can even be triggered by a change in substrate concentration (23).

Two characteristics of environmentally induced illness are perhaps most worrisome; the phenomena of spreading and of heightened sensitivity. Illness in these patients was usually triggered by an over exposure to one chemical, such as formaldehyde; prolonged exposure to the initial stimulus will frequently result in the development of hypersensitivities to other chemicals, spreading to foods, or inhalants such as dusts and molds. Furthermore, once sensitized, the patient gradually reacts with heightened sensitivity to increasingly lower levels of the insulting agent.

The practitioner dealing with this select patient population is thus presented with a set of diagnostically baffling symptoms, which, despite accepted medical treatments, may become worse as weaker and less intense exposures to the initial chemical triggers symptoms. All the while, other chemicals and antigens may become triggers as well.

Formaldehyde exposure can be related to the level of formic acid measured in the blood. Formic acid is also a metabolite of endogenously produced formaldehyde. Formaldehyde oxidase normally rapidly converts aldehydes into acids, since aldehydes are harmful to the body in promoting cross-linking. But formaldehyde oxidase is limited in its production, and with ambient overload, production is unable to keep up with the increased demand. Once production is exceeded, the biochemistry switches from an oxidation reaction to a reduction reaction with alcohol dehydrogenase. This may explain the preponderance of cerebral or toxic brain symptoms as the aldehydes are reduced to alcohols (24–26).

Since these reactions require folic acid (27), often folic acid deficiency was observed, as well. Certainly, as deficiencies progressed with continual exposures, other biochemical systems would be adversely affected by a domino effect. This may explain the spreading phenomenon whereby other sensitivities develop and other target organs became involved. It is an interesting observation that rats cannot get formaldehyde toxicity because formate does not accumulate in this species. Hence, the rat would appear to be an invalid animal in which to do formaldehyde toxicity studies (27).

The diversity of symptoms of EI victims is more easily appreciated with the understanding of the extent of the damage that is rendered by inhaled xenobiotics or toxic chemicals. Toxic chemicals interfere with cellular energy metabolism by inhibiting glycolysis and mitochondrial respiration. They inhibit ATP synthesis and other enzymes, decrease the efficiency of the sodium pump, disrupt cell membranes, produce free radicals, overload the cytochrome P-450 detoxication system, and damage DNA (28). Each person's biochemical uniqueness serves to amplify the possibilities.

This paper presents a simple method for determining if a patient is sensitive to formaldehyde. We do not know the percentage of sensitivity or accuracy, nor do we understand the mechanisms, but in testing over 1000 patients with these baffling symptoms, those reacting positively have all improved after being shown how to reduce their environmental chemical overload. Treatments were based on avoidance of chemicals that were shown to duplicate symptoms.

One important caution: The testing method will not work if the physician's office has an ambient level of formaldehyde or any other triggering agent that provokes the patient's symptoms. This may explain the major cause of failure of clinical investigators who have tried these techniques and been unable to reproduce these results. The need to lower the total load or total burden of chemicals presented to the patient (in his system and in the test area) is fundamental to the success of this technique and cannot be overstressed. The same subjects, tested double blind to the same chemicals in a normal office or hospital, do not respond in a predictable manner; whereas in an office such as ours, where special measures have been taken to omit many commonly occurring chemicals, the technique appears able to turn symptoms on and off like a switch.

Basic principles used to create a safe testing environment are decreasing the amount of synthetic materials used, markedly increasing the ventilation, and filtering the air. It is important to reiterate the variability in sensitivity and target organ of man and the need to focus attention on the importance of indoor air quality on health.

REFERENCES

1. Molhave, L., Bach, B., and Pedersen, O. F. Dose-response relation of volatile organic compounds in the sick building syndrome. Clin. Ecol. 4(2): 52–56 (1985).
2. Finnegan, M. J., Pickering, C. A. C., and Burge, P. S. The sick building syndrome: Prevalence studies. Br. Med. J. 289: 1573–1575 (1984).
3. Lindvall, M. D. The sick building syndrome. Clin. Ecol. 3: 140–164 (1985).
4. Randolph, T. G. Domiciliary chemical air pollution in the etiology of ecologic mental illness. Intern. J. Soc. Psych. 16: 223–65 (1970).
5. Bardana, E. J., and Montanaro, A. Tight building syndrome. Immunol. Allergy Pract. 3: 17–31 (1986).
6. Rea, W. J. Environmentally triggered cardiac disease. Ann. Allergy 40: 243–251 (1978).
7. Godish, T. Formaldehyde and building-related illness. J. Environ. Health 44: 116–121 (1981).
8. Dally, K. A., Hanrahan, M. A., Wordbury, M. A., and Kanarek, M. A. Formaldehyde exposure in nonoccupational environments. Arch. Environ. Health 36: 277–284 (1981).
9. Gupta, K. C., Ulsamer, A. G., and Preuss, P. W. Formaldehyde in indoor air: Sources and toxicity. In : International Symposium on Indoor Air Pollution, Health and Energy Conservation. Harvard University Press, Boston MA, 1981.
10. Hollowel, C. D., and Miksch, R. R. Sources and concentrations of organic compounds in indoor environments. Bull. N. Y. Acad. Med. 57: 962–977 (1981).
11. Hart, R. W., Turturro, A., and Neimet, L. Eds. Report on the consensus workshop on formaldehyde. Environ. Health Perspect. 58: 323–381 (1984).
12. Andelman, J. Human exposures to volatile halogenated organic chemicals in indoor and outdoor air. Environ. Health Perspect. 62: 313–318 (1985).
13. Feldman, R. G., Ricks , N. C., and Baker, E. L. Neuropsychological effects of industrial toxins: A review. Am. J. Ind. Med. 1: 211–227 (1980).
14. Randolph, T. G. Human Ecology and Susceptibility to the Chemical Environment. Charles C. Thomas, Springfield, IL, 1962.
15. Rea, W. J., and Mitchel, M. J. Chemical sensitivity and the environment. Immunol. Allergy Pract. 4: 21–31 (1982).
16. Miller, J. B. Food Allergy. Provocation Testing and Injection Therapy. Charles C. Thomas, Springfield, IL, 1972.
17. Morris, D. L, Recognition and treatment of formaldehyde sensitivity. Arch. Soc. Clin. Ecol. 1: 27–30 (1982).
18. World Health Organization Report 78. WHO, 1983, p.24.
19. McGrath, K. G., Zeiss, C. R., and Patterson, R. Allergic reactions to industrial chemicals. Clin. Immunol. Rev. 2: 1–58 (1983).
20. Street, J. C., and Sharma, R. P. Alteration of induced cellular and humoral immune responses by pesticides and chemicals of environmental concern. Toxicol. Appl. Pharmacol. 32: 587–602 (1975).
21. Boris, M., Shiff, M., Weindorf, S., and Inselman, L. Bronchoprovocation blocked by neutralization therapy. (abst.) J. Allergy Clin. Immunol. 71: 92 (1983).
22. Vogt, C., Schmidt, G., Lynen, R., and Dieminger, L. Cleavage of the third complement component (C#) and generation of the spasmogenic peptide C3$_a$, in human serum via the properdin pathway: Demonstration of inhibitory as well as enhancing effects of epsilon amino-caproic acid. J. Immunol. 114: 671-677 (1975).
23. Findley, S. R., Dvorak, A. M., Kagey-Sobotka, A., and Lichtenstein, L. M. Hyperosmolar triggering of histamine release from basophils. J. Clin. Invest. 67: 1604-1613 (1981).
24. Rea, W. J. Chemical Sensitivity. Creative Informatics, Durant, OK, in press.
25. Reeves, R.A. Toxicology, Principles and Practice. Wiley and Sons, NY, 1981.
26. Jacoby, W. B. Enzymatic Basis of Detoxication, Vol. 1. Academic Press, New York, 1980.
27. Billings, R. E., and Tephly, T. R. Studies on methanol toxicity and formate metabolism in isolated hepatocytes. Biochem. Pharmacol. 28: 2985–2991 (1979).
28. Parke, D. V. Mechanisms of chemical toxicity—a unifying hypothesis. Regul. Toxicol. Pharmacol. 2: 267–286 (1982).

Environment International, Vol. 15, pp. 75–79, 1989
Printed in the U.S.A. All rights reserved.

DIAGNOSING THE TIGHT BUILDING SYNDROME OR DIAGNOSING CHEMICAL HYPERSENSITIVITY

Sherry A. Rogers
Northeast Center for Environmental Medicine, Syracuse, NY 13219, USA

EI 87-106 *(Received 18 August 1987; Accepted 18 January 1989)*

The abrupt exposure to urea foam formaldehyde insulation served as an alert to its spectrum of symptoms, including attacks of headache, flushing, laryngitis, dizziness, nausea, extreme weakness or exhaustion, arthralgia, an inability to concentrate, unwarranted depression, arrhythmia, or muscle spasms, and baffled physicians from many specialties. Later it was learned that toluene, xylene, benzene, natural gas, trichloroethylene, and many other chemicals were also capable of triggering chemical hypersensitivity. Other names for this condition include Environmentally Induced Illness (EI), the Tight Building Syndrome (TBS), the Sick Building Syndrome, and Building-Related Illness. The very symptoms patients complain of can be provoked within minutes and then subsequently alleviated with an intradermal injection of the appropriate strength of the triggering chemical. This technique aids in convincing the patient of the EI or TBS triggers so that the patient can begin to relate symptoms to environmental exposures and initiate measures to bring the disease under control. The key to safer buildings is increased ventilation, increased filtration of air, and decreased use of off-gassing synthetic materials.

INTRODUCTION

A survey of the literature indicates that homes with indoor chemical problems have higher concentrations of volatile organic compounds than houses without such problems (Mølhave et al. 1985). The Tight Building Syndrome (TBS) is characterized by a building in which worker complaints are more common than might be reasonably expected (Finnegan et al. 1984). Furthermore, it is assumed that nonoccupational explanations of symptoms have been ruled out. Some have called this illness the Sick Building syndrome (Lindvall 1985), but clearly there are those individuals who are more chemically sensitive than the rest of the population: Hence the term, "chemical hypersensitivity."

Over 25 years ago, Randolph (1963) recognized that chemicals in the indoor air environment could provoke symptoms, but acceptance of his findings was delayed by the lack of measurements and testing techniques that abound today. Because many of these indoor chemicals exist in outdoor air as well, a more accurate designation might be Environmentally Induced Illness (EI).

Volatile organic hydrocarbons are but a few of the triggers of TBS or EI. With the installation of urea foam formaldehyde insulation (UFFI), a corresponding dramatic increase in symptomatology provided a vast number of subjects for study. This provided us with a prototype from which to observe the spectrum and diversity of symptoms associated with an acute increase in one quantifiable indoor chemical, formaldehyde. It also clearly demonstrated a tremendous individual susceptibility, since some members of a household could be devastatingly ill, while others were only mildly or totally unaffected.

Over the last 6 years, increasing numbers of patients have evidenced symptoms reminiscent of these UFFI victims (Bardana and Montanaro 1986), despite having had no history of UFFI exposure (Rea 1978; Godish 1981). Measurements of ambient levels of formaldehyde have shown that new mobile homes, newly constructed homes with particle-board subflooring, offices recently renovated with paneling or prefabricated walls, new clothing, new carpeting or furnishings, and homes with new beds and cabinetry can accumulate as much formaldehyde as a result of off-gassing as a UFFI home (Dally et al. 1981; Gupta et al. 1982; Hollowell and Miksch 1981; Hart et al. 1984).

A variety of other commonly encountered volatile substances are capable of inducing the same symptoms (Andelman 1985; Feldman et al. 1980; Randolph 1963; Rea and Mitchel 1982). For example, the mean reported levels for formaldehyde in indoor air in residences was 0.03 µL/L for houses without UFFI and 0.12 µL/L for houses with UFFI (with and without complaints) (Hart et al. 1984). Some mobile homes had levels of 0.4 µL/L, and the mean level for several hospitals was 0.55 µL/L.

Guidelines are needed to facilitate diagnosis and identification of the triggering agents. Attacks of headache, nausea, an inability to concentrate, mental obtundation (the dulling of the ability to think and function when performing normal tasks), dizziness, lethargy, arrhythmia (irregular heart beat), flushing, laryngitis, irritability, unwarranted depression, arthralgia (joint pain), and extreme weakness, although nonspecific, are some of the most common symptoms of EI and frequently lead to a sequence of diagnostic evaluations that are ineffective, for instance, when psychiatric evaluation is suggested.

With proper questioning, a sufferer can often associate the onset of symptoms with the purchase of new carpeting, furniture, beds, or cabinets; the renovation of a home or office; moving into a new dwelling; or insulating with UFFI. The development of a test that substantiates that formaldehyde or other chemicals are among the trigger is thus critical.

METHODS AND MATERIALS

The skin-testing protocol for chemical hypersensitivity is described in an issue of the journal published by the National Institute of Health (Rogers 1987). Basically, as with many biological systems, there is a dose of chemical that will provoke symptoms if the individual is sensitive to that substance, and there is a dose that will terminate or neutralize the symptoms.

All testing was done single-blind, meaning that the patients were unaware of what they were being tested with, and there were many placebo controls (e.g., normal saline or salt water) used liberally throughout the testing sessions so that malingering could be ruled out. As a further measure, patients were tested again on another day, however, the chemicals were presented in a different order and many placebos were still used as well.

RESULTS: CASE EXAMPLES

C.P. is a 39-year-old consulting engineer who travels extensively. Two years ago he moved into a new house that had new carpeting and particle-board subflooring throughout. Six months later, he experienced an insidious onset of joint pain. He consulted an internist but reported that a year and a half later he had the same symptoms. He also indicated that he ached more after he had been at home for the weekend but felt better whenever he was out of town for a few days.

His blood serum level of formic acid (a metabolite of formaldehyde) was 10 µg/mL after a weekend at home and 6 µg/mL after a day at work. A passive (badge) monitor showed an ambient 24-hour formaldehyde level of 0.06 µL/L in his home.

Single-blind testing with normal saline produced no symptoms. A test dose of formaldehyde produced erythema and wheal (a redness and swelling) of 2mm, and the patient reported a "warm feeling, ringing in the ears, and achy joints." The subsequent dilution cleared or neutralized all of his symptoms, and there was no reaction on the skin.

Moving out of the house with particle-board subflooring and wall-to-wall carpeting cleared his symptoms. However, being in certain shopping malls and other places with elevated formaldehyde levels again triggered his symptoms.

M.B. is a 41-year-old teacher who had worked in the same school for 8 years. Over one summer vacation, renovations were undertaken in the school. When she returned to the building in the fall, she started having symptoms that came on more quickly and more severely with each subsequent entry. Her voice would gradually become more hoarse over the first few hours of work, and she would eventually lose it. She also experienced a sore throat and tender submandibular lymph nodes. She would have a feeling of achiness, as though a flu were starting, and would become exhausted. These symptoms persisted for a day or two after leaving the building and were proportional in duration and severity to the amount of time she had spent there. At home, she was without symptoms. Her serum level of formic acid was 10 µg/L after a day at school and 6 µg/L after a weekend at home. This measurement was repeated with the same results on subsequent days. The 24-hour level of formaldehyde in the school air, measured with a passive (badge) monitor, was 0.06 µL/L. Single-blind testing to formaldehyde duplicated her symptoms, producing visible facial flushing and weakening her voice. The next dose cleared the symptoms.

A.R. is a 56-year-old female who had 11 years of progressively worsening headaches. She could get them anywhere, but they were worse at work, where she had been employed in the same factory for 15 years. A blood test for her level of tetrachloroethylene (Accu-Chem Laboratories, Richardson, TX) after a day at work was 26.1 nL/L (N.B., the population average for this laboratory is 1.1 nL/L). After two weeks at home, it was 18.1 nL/L. Single-blind testing to the chemical reproduced or provoked her symptoms of headache, while the neutralizing dose terminated them. She was not free of headaches, even after being at home for several months, until her blood level had dropped to 1.3 nL/L.

D.B. is a 10-year-old "A" student. Over the last few months, his teacher has sent home reports indicating that he had failing grades, he was becoming disruptive in the class, and he was unteachable. Single-blind testing to common indoor chemicals was begun. Normal saline, formaldehyde, toluene, and xylene were negative. He continued to sit quietly and draw rocket ships. When phenol was tested, he suddenly began scribbling viciously and became so aggravated that he lay on the floor and kicked the wall. The neutralizing dose terminated the symptoms.

This prompted a search for the source of phenol at the school. The source turned out to be a popular phenol-based cleaning solution the teacher used to wipe down the desks. After she stopped doing this, he returned to normal.

P.S. is a 23-year-old female who was well until a few months after she started a job in a shopping mall. She began experiencing serious episodes of bizarre behavior that resulted in several hospitalizations in two different mental institutions, where she was diagnosed as being schizophrenic. She also complained of severe muscle spasms, especially in her neck, and noted that they were worse when she was in the shopping mall.

On testing, she had no symptoms when given normal saline. A test dose of formaldehyde caused muscle spasms so severe that she could not straighten her neck and lift her chin from her chest. She began laughing and rocking in the chair and thought she was Jesus' wife. The dose that produced no symptoms also had no skin growth. It restored her to normal and terminated the neck spasms and delusions within 10 minutes.

B.A. is a 53-year-old nurse who experienced swollen glands, a feeling of impending throat closure, irregular heart beat, numbness in her tongue and face,

dizziness, and an inability to concentrate when floors in the hospital were being waxed or when she was near patients smoking or wearing perfumes. The constant renovations being done at the hospital necessitated the use of many glues and strong-smelling chemicals, which she also thought caused some of her symptoms.

Single-blind testing to normal saline produced no symptoms, while testing with formaldehyde duplicated her symptoms of numbness of the tongue and the feelings that her throat was closing and her glands were swelling. The next dose, which also produced no skin growth, cleared her symptoms.

E.F. is a 63-year-old woman whose house was insulated with UFFI in 1977. Each year since, her residence has been continually upgraded with new tile floors, carpeting, couches, and construction. In 1981, she began to have severe episodes of arrhythmia, chest pain, light-headedness, arthralgias, and muscle weakness. She consulted numerous family practitioners, internists, cardiologists, ENT specialists, and rheumatologists, and yet had no confirmed diagnosis or successful therapy. After two years, she could not enter a shopping mall without using a cane or her husband's arm to lean on because she would become much weaker when in the stores. At age 23, she had had polio involving her right arm and leg. During symptomatic episodes these areas in particular were affected, making it impossible to carry her purse on her right arm or to walk without dragging her right foot. After being outdoors for a while, her symptoms would clear and her gait and strength again became normal.

Single-blind testing duplicated her symptoms of chest pain. Sleeping in the bedroom, which had two foam-insulated walls, on a new foam-filled mattress and bed with a particle-board headboard gave her a serum formic acid level of 10 μg/mL and symptoms. Sleeping on an old cot in the living room, where the furnishings were much older and which had only one foam-insulated wall, most of which was dominated by a large glass window, she had a level of 5 μg/mL and reduced symptoms. Removing the new carpeting and replacing the new furnishings reduced her symptoms.

J.K. is a 30-year-old female lab technician who began experiencing episodes of facial flushing, a feeling of strained breathing, and heavy eyes. She also complained of pronounced dizziness and a feeling of faintness. After these episodes, she felt extremely tired for hours and had to sleep.

Single-blind testing to normal saline produced no reaction, while her symptoms wee reproduced with formaldehyde. The next dose of formaldehyde eliminated the symptoms.

I.C. is a 43-year-old woman who, within six months of having her house insulated with UFFI, developed a severe hoarseness that reduced her voice to a nearly inaudible whisper. Over the next year and a half, she consulted at least ten physicians in an attempt to have her voice restored. The only thing that would restore her voice would be staying out of her house for two weeks.

The study was repeated over the next few months, several times in a double-blind fashion (with neither the tester nor the patient knowing the content of the syringes), and the same results were observed; loss of voice occurred within four minutes of administration of the test dose of formaldehyde, but the voice returned within several minutes of administering the neutralizing dose.

All patients described were universally and unquestionably freer of symptoms after they had been through an intensive educational program to teach them how to lower their ambient levels of formaldehyde exposures (Rogers 1986).

DISCUSSION

The last half-decade has provided us with well over 1,000 patients with undiagnosed chronic symptoms refractory to a wide variety of treatments. Single-blind testing to various chemicals generally identified a suspect chemical and provided convincing enough duplication of symptoms in patients to enable them to make sometimes inconvenient and costly environmental changes that appear to be a necessary part of a comprehensive program to bring about symptom relief for the first time.

This technique of provocation-neutralization of symptoms to diagnose chemical hypersensitivity has been used by hundreds of physicians over the last 20 years. Some of the chemicals tested have included the more frequently identified indoor chemicals that are difficult to avoid, including chemicals such as toluene, benzene, xylene, ethanol, trichloroethylene, and natural gas.

One important caution: The testing method will not work if the physician's office has an ambient level of formaldehyde or any other triggering agent that provokes a patient's symptoms. This may be a major cause of the failure of clinical investigators who have tried these techniques to reproduce the results. The need to lower the total load or total burden of chemicals presented to the patient (in the system and in the treatment area) is fundamental to the success of this technique and cannot be overstressed. The same subjects tested double-blind to the same chemicals in a normal office or hospital do not respond in a predictable manner; however, in an office where special measures have been taken to omit many commonly occurring chemicals, the technique appears able to turn symptoms on and off like a switch.

To accomplish a relatively pollutant-free environment in our office, carpets have been removed and replaced with hardwood or quarry tile floors. Wooden cabinets and synthetic and plastic chairs have been replaced with metal. As many extraneous materials as possible are kept out of the testing room. Metal lockers for purses, coats, and packages are provided in a separate area. No one is allowed into the office unless they pass a sniff test administered by nurses who are hypersensitive to chemicals. Nurses and all patients must be free of fragrances, fabric softeners, polyester clothes, dry-cleaning fluid, cosmetics, toiletries, tobacco smoke, home cooking odors, work odors, and, in fact, any detectable odors. Air depollution devices with charcoal and potassium permanganate filters are used extensively to absorb chemicals, and outdoor air is filtered continuously before being pumped inside.

It is evident, for example, that a supersensitive individual cannot be tested by a nurse wearing perfume, since the individual can react to this trigger shortly after coming into contact with the nurse, thus confusing the test results. Many people happily note the relative paucity of symptoms they experience after they have been in our office for a period of time.

Basic methods used to create a safe testing environment include decreasing the amount of synthetic materials used, markedly increasing the ventilation, and filtering the air. In testing over 1,000 patients with these baffling symptoms, those reacting positively have all improved after being shown how to reduce their environmental chemical overload. Treatments were based on the avoidance of chemicals shown to duplicate symptoms.

Once a chemical has been identified as one that is elevated in the blood and which provokes the very symptoms the person is complaining of, the patient must then know where the sources of this chemical are in his environment and how to avoid them. This has been described elsewhere (Rogers 1986).

Since we are the first generation exposed to such "tight buildings" containing an unprecedented number of out-gassing materials, many of the rules of medicine may become obsolete when it comes to understanding chemical hypersensitivity. Clearly, the patients presented have demonstrated some of the principles of chemical hypersensitivity:

1. The symptoms are unpredictably variable and break many of the rules of medicine. This, unavoidably, will usher in a new era of medicine, and never again can we be content to tell someone that baffling symptoms "are all in your head," or "there is no known cause," or "nothing can be done about it."

2. From the very beginning of our identification of people with UFFI in their homes, we began to discern a tremendously varied individual susceptibility in symptoms, even among members of the same family (who have far more similar genetics than the average office population).

3. In spite of years of exposure to chemicals, an individual can develop a hypersensitivity to them at any point in time.

4. Places of old injury or previous disease (like polio) are often the target for chemical hypersensitivity. This inevitably will be a source of confusion, since one is more likely to blame back pain, for example, on an old injury than to consider a possible chemical hypersensitivity.

We also have observed (but not included case examples to demonstrate) that once symptoms are triggered many people will suddenly begin manifesting hypersensitivities to many other chemicals that previously did not bother them, and that the total body burden or load of these chemicals at any one point in time is directly proportional to the ease with which symptoms can be provoked.

Much work remains to be done: for example, we have no idea of the amount of false negatives. But clearly, we have a technique that has been useful in pointing patients in the right direction in identifying and eliminating exposure to chemicals that were provoking baffling symptoms.

REFERENCES

Andelman, J. Human exposures to volatile halogenated organic chemicals in indoor and outdoor air, Environ. Health Perspect. 62, 313-318; 1985.

Bardana, E.J. and Montanaro, A. Tight building syndrome, Immunol. Allergy Pract. 3, 17-31; 1986.

Dally, K.A., Hanrahan, M.A., Wordbury, M.A. and Kanarek, M.A. Formaldehyde exposure in nonoccupational environments, Arch. Environ. Health 36, 277-284; 1981.

Feldman, R.G., Ricks, N.C. and Baker, E.L. Neuropsychological effects of industrial toxins: review, Amer. J. Ind. Med. 1, 211-227; 1980.

Finnegan, M.J., Pickering, C.A.C. and Burge, P.S. The sick building syndrome: prevalence studies, Br. Med. J. 289, 1573-1575; 1984.

Godish, T. Formaldehyde and building-related illness, J. Environ. Health 44, 116-121; 1981.

Gupta, K.C., Ulsamer, A.G. and Preuss, P.W. Formaldehyde in indoor air: sources and toxicity; Harvard University Environ. Inter. 8, 349-358; 1982.

Hart, R.W., turturro, A and Meimet, L., editors. Report on the consensus workshop on formaldehyde, Environ. Health Perspect. 58, 323-381; 1984.

Hollowell, C.D. and Miksch, R.R. Sources and concentrations of organic compounds in indoor environments, Bull. N.Y. Acad. Med. 57, 962-977; 1981.

Lindvall, M.D. The sick building syndrome, Clin. Ecol. 3, 140-164; 1985.

Mølhave, L., Bach, B. and Pederson, O.F. Dose-response relation of volatile organic compounds in the sick building syndrome, Clin. Ecol. 4(2), 52-56; 1985.

Randolph, T.G. Human Ecology and Susceptibility to the Chemical Environment, Charles C. Thomas, Springfield, IL; 1963.

Randolph, T.G. Domiciliary chemical air pollution in the etiology of ecologic mental illness, Intern. J. Soc. Psych. 16, 223-265; 1970.

Rea, W.J. Environmentally triggered cardiac disease, Ann. Allergy 40, 243-251; 1978.

Rea, W.J. and Mitchel, M.J. Chemical sensitivity and the environment, Immunol. Allergy Pract. 4, 21-31; 1982.

Rogers, S.A. The E.I. Syndrome, Prestige Publishing, Syracuse, NY; 1986.

Rogers, S.A. Diagnosing the tight building syndrome, Environ. Health Perspect. 76, 195-198; 1987.

A CASE HISTORY

PROVOCATION-NEUTRALIZATION OF COUGH AND WHEEZING IN A HORSE

Sherry A. Rogers, MD

Sherry A. Rogers, M.D., F.A.A.E.M., F.A.A.F.P., F.A.C.A.*

KEY WORDS:

Provocation
Neutralization
Asthma
Heaves
Double-blind

ABSTRACT:

Heaves in horses includes coughing and wheezing, and can be thought of as the equine equivalent of human asthma. In a double-blind trial, the symptoms were provoked with intradermal injections of antigens. Using a serial dilution of these antigens, a dose was found that terminated the symptoms. Therapy with these doses successfully controlled the symptoms on a daily basis. Two weeks after testing and the initiation of therapy, dramatic improvement was reported in the severely afflicted animal, as he was able to be ridden for the first time in six years without provoking disabling cough and wheezing.

E quine asthma, or heaves, has been recognized as a disease of possible immune origin and has often been treated with such immune suppressive agents as azathioprine, corticosteroids, and cyclophosphamide (1). Successful long-term therapy is difficult, and the prognosis for young animals diagnosed with heaves is poor (2). Miller and many others (3-10), have described the use of minute amounts of extracts of offending foods to neutralize the symptoms of food sensitivities in humans; and other authors have likewise reported the successful use of homologous allergens to control sensitivities to inhalants (11-13) and chemicals (14).

In 1982, McMichael (15) reported the adaptation of Miller's techniques to test and treat over fifty horses with heaves. The significance of this work was two-fold in that it both permitted the control of a disease in horses that was previously considered sufficiently incapacitating as to warrant euthanasia, and it also provided an animal model free of placebo influences for evaluating the efficacy of various therapeutic modes for treating hypersensitivity in humans.

ACKNOWLEDGEMENT
The author wishes to thank Dr. John McMichael, Ph.D., formerly of Milkhaus Laboratory, Cambridge Springs, PA, for preparing the antigens for the study, Donald W. Hostettler, D.V.M. of Cambridge Springs, PA for examining the horse during the study, Mrs. Shirley Gallinger, allergy technician from Syracuse, NY, for administering the antigens, and Mrs. Judy Acker of Saegertown, PA for the use of her horse.

*Northeast Center for Environmental Medicine
2800 West Genesee Street
Syracuse, NY 13219

The following is a case report of a nine year old gelding Apaloosa horse with heaves of six years duration which responded to immunotherapy with histamine, mold and grass pollen extracts. In the past five years the horse was not able to be ridden because incapacitating cough and wheezing would start within the first few hundred feet.

METHODS AND MATERIALS

The subject of this study had heaves diagnosed by his veterinarian. He had not been studied previously, nor had he been treated in any manner similar to the one employed during the study, nor had he been seen by any participant in the study other than the veterinarian (who also examined him during the study).

From the horse's case history it was decided to test two allergens, grass pollens and mold mix A (Holister-Stier), as well as histamine (Table 1). Serial five-fold dilutions in phenolated saline were prepared; the diluent alone served as the placebo. An area approximately nine centimeters square was clipped on the lateral surface of the neck. The initial evaluation was performed by the veterinarian.

The horse was tested by intradermal inoculation of 0.05cc of test material or placebo into the clipped area, with dimensions of the resulting wheals measured and recorded immediately after injections and again five minutes later. The same protocol was used as it is used on humans.(16) The attending veterinarian reported the condition of the horse with respect to lung sounds, degree of definition of the subcostal heave lines, snorting, nostril flaring, and/or agitation before and two to three minutes after each injection and again five minutes later.

Neither the technician administering the injections, the veterinarian, the horse owner, nor the physician videotaping the trial was privy to the contents in any syringe or the frequency with which placebos would be employed.

Following completion of the study, injections were prepared for the horse using neutralizing endpoints of

Table 1
Allergenic Materials Employed in Testing and Therapy

Allergen	Source	Rationale for Inclusion
Timothy Extract	Hollister-Stier	Primary grass in hay
Mold Mix A	Hollister-Stier	Exposure to dusty(moldy) hay, mold growth in barn
Histamine Phosphate	E. Lilly Co.	Heaves when drinking, with temperature changes, and when humid

each allergen. The injections were formulated such that each 0.5cc injection contained 0.05cc of the neutralizing dose of antigen, with that dose being defined as the highest concentration of antigen that resulted in a negative wheal and produced no symptoms. A negative wheal was one that, after five minutes, gave less than a two millimeter growth in two dimensions (Table 2).

The neutralizing dose found for histamine was #4 (1:625), for Timothy #3 (1:125) and for mold mix A #3 (1:125). The horse owner was instructed to administer these prepared doses subcutaneously on alternate days for one week beginning on the day following testing. After the first week, injections were given weekly.

RESULTS

Table 2 records the results of sensitivity testing with the extracts and the placebo with respect to both linear measurements of wheals and veterinary assessment. It can be seen that placebo injections given three times consistently provoked neither wheal growth nor symptoms. In contrast, relatively higher concentrations of some antigens, e.g. mold mix A #2, induced symptoms which were subsequently neutralized by injection of the same antigen in a lower concentration (#4) but not by the placebo.

Two weeks after initiation of therapy the owner reported that the horse could be ridden harder and longer than at any time in the previous six years, that he could run at full speed in the pasture for extended periods and that his symptoms at rest were greatly diminished. The owner was contacted after one year and again after two years. It was reported that the effect of treatment was persisting.

DISCUSSION

Successful neutralization or de-sensitization of a hypersensitive individual is known to be a concentration-dependent phenomenon with respect to the allergen used in the neutralization process (17). Miller and others (3-14) have reported that with varying concentrations of allergen, symptoms can be provoked with a high dose and neutralized with a lower dose.

From the double-blind trial reported herein, it appears that the horse with heaves serves as a satisfactory animal model for the evaluation of neutralization. Not only did the horse exhibit positive wheal growth and symptoms when tested intradermally with relatively high doses of antigen, but his symptoms cleared within minutes when a lower, neutralizing dose of the same antigen was given. Furthermore, placebo injections failed to either induce or relieve symptoms.

Test #5 (using the third mold dilution) provoked symptoms without the anticipated corresponding wheal growth. The five minute time period for development of wheal growth and symptoms was half that used by Miller (4), and wheal growth might have occurred had

Table 2
Response of Horse to Intradermal Injections of Three Extracts and Placebo

Test #	Allergen	Dilution Number*	Initial Wheal(mm)	5 Minute Wheal(mm)	Veterinarian's Assessment
0	No injection				Baseline breathing
1	Histamine	2	6x6	11x11	Increased dyspnea and wheeze
2	Histamine	3	7x7	9x9	Dyspnea persists
3	Histamine	4	5x5	5x5	Same as baseline status
4	Placebo	-	7x7	7x7	Same as baseline status
5	Mold Mix A	3	7x7	7x7	Increased dyspnea and wheeze
6	Mold Mix A	2	7x7	9x9	Dyspnea persists, nostrils flared, heave line accentuated
7	Mold Mix A	4	7x7	7x7	Same as baseline status
8	Placebo	-	7x7	7x7	Same as baseline status
9	Histamine	2	7x7	11x11	Coughing, increased wheeze and heave line
10	Histamine	4	7x7	7x7	Same as baseline status
11	Timothy	2	7x7	7x11	Increased wheeze and heave line
12	Timothy	3	7x7	7x7	Same as baseline status
13	Placebo	-	7x7	7x7	Same as baseline status

* Refers to the number of five-fold dilutions made to arrive at that dose. Eg, #3 refers to the third five-fold dilution (1:125) of the allergen in question.

the reaction time been increased. While this is merely a single horse study, studies with a larger number of horses need to be carried out to confirm the validity of neutralization.

It has been noted (McMichael et al, in preparation), that the volumes and concentrations used to neutralize a two thousand pound horse are the same as those for a two pound rat. Such might occur if the target cell possesses not only specific membrane receptors for the regulating molecule in question, but also specific intercalation with sites on the DNA or RNA into which the molecule in question can "lock into place" and consequently repress, or de-repress, various metabolic functions of the cell. Clearly this study on an asthmatic horse has confirmed what has been reported in humans, namely that stronger doses can provoke symptoms and weaker ones can neutralize or terminate them. Further studies are required to confirm this finding.

REFERENCES

1. MaCaffey LW. Respiratory Conditions in Horses, *Vet Res.*, 74, 1295-1314, 1962.
2. *The Merck Veterinary Manual*, Rahway, Merck & Co.,
3. Miller JB. *Food Allergy: Provocation Testing and Injection Therapy*, Springfield, Thomas, 1972.
4. Miller JB. A Double-Blind Study of Dood Extract Injection Therapy: A Preliminary Report, *Ann Allergy* 38:185-191, 1977.
5. O'Shea J, Porter S. Double-blind study of children with hyperkinetic syndrome treated by multi-allergen extract sublingually, *J Learning Disability* 14:189-190, 1981.
6. Rapp D. Double-blind confirmation and treatment of milk sensitivity, *Med J Aust* 1:571-572, 1978.
7. Rapp D. Food allergy treatment for hyperkinesis, *J Learning Disability* 14:189-190, 1981.
8. Rapp D. Weeping eyes in wheat allergy. *Trans Am Soc Ophthalmol Otol Allergy* 18:149-150, 1978.
9. Rea WJ, Podel RN, Williams ML, et al. Elimination of oral food challenge reaction by injection of food extracts. *Arch Otolaryngol* 110:248-252, 1984.
10. Morris DL. Use of sublingual antigen in diagnosis and treatment of food allergy. *Ann Allergy* 27:289-94, 1969.
11. Boris M, Schiff M, Weidorfs, et al. Broncho-provocation blocked by neutralizing therapy. *J Allergy Clin Immunol* 71:92, 1983.
12. Morris DL. Treatment of respiratory disease with ultra-small doses of antigens. *Ann Allergy* 28:494-500, 1970.
13. Morris DL. Recognition and treatment of formaldehyde sensitivity. *Clinical Ecology*,1: 27-30, 1982.
14. Rogers SA. Diagnosing the Tight Building Syndrome. *Environmental Health Perspectives* 76: 195-198, 1987.
15. McMichael J. The Control of Heaves in Horses as a Model for Human Allergy Therapy, presented at symposium, Man and His Environment in Health and Disease, Dallas, 1982.
16. Rogers, SA, Resistant Cases: Results of Mold Immunotherapy and Environmental and Dietary Controls. *Clinical Ecology* V:3: 115-120; 1987-88.
17. Macher E, Chase MW, Studies on the Sensitization of Animals with Simple Chemical Compounds. *J Exp Med*: 129: 81, 103, 1969.

Case Studies

RESISTANT CASES: RESPONSE TO MOLD IMMUNOTHERAPY AND ENVIRONMENTAL AND DIETARY CONTROLS

Sherry A. Rogers, MD, FACA, FAAEM*

KEY WORDS

Mold spores
Allergy
Immunotherapy
Fungi

ABSTRACT

Diverse recalcitrant allergic symptoms may be caused by sensitivity to fungi. In this study patients with symptoms resistant to current therapy, including eczema, hyperactivity, depression, asthma, edema, cystic acne, vasculitis, urticaria, dizziness, migraine, weakness, exhaustion and atopic dermatitis underwent five-fold serial dilution end point titration with 21 different fungal extracts. All fungi were tested individually and some also as components of mixes. If testing with the mix and all of its components produced the same end point for wheal growth, the mix was used therapeutically. If none of the fungal components had the same end point as the entire mix, the positive fungi were given individually. If most of the component fungi had the same end points as the mix, the mix was given. Patients concurrently followed an elimination diet, avoiding common allergenic foods such as milk, wheat, corn and especially foods containing fermentation products, such as bread, cheese, alcohol, vinegar, salad dressing, mayonnaise, ketchup, mustard, chocolate and processed foods. Ten cases are cited, describing significant improvements in symptoms. Symptoms returned with double-blind substitution of saline placebos for treatment injections, and were cleared on reinstitution of treatments. Removal of carpet, washing of surfaces with borax, permeating the home with vinegar and chlorine bleach fumes, and installation of electrostatic precipitators and ultraviolet lights are discussed as ways to reduce indoor fungi.

* Northeast Center for Environmental Medicine, 2800 W. Genesee St., Syracuse, NY 13219

Fungi produce some of the most potent toxins, hallucinogens, and antibiotics known to man and are indispensable to the food industry (1). They can thrive in conditions inimicable to many other living organisms and under certain climatic conditions can produce billions of spores. During the height of the pollen season it is not unusual for the ratio of *Cladosporium (Hormodendrum)* spores to pollen to be 1,000:1 (2).

Fungi have been shown to produce symptoms in the allergic individual (3-5). Allergists usually test a patient's degree of sensitivity to the major molds, *Hormodendrum, Aspergillus, Alternaria* and *Penicillium*, and test a dozen or fewer other fungi on an individual basis.

In a previous study (6) we showed that by substituting a medium of malt agar extract for Sabouraud's medium, by increasing plate exposure time from 10 minutes to 1 hour, and by saving plates for up to three weeks to allow the slow growers to appear, we produced a 32% yield increase for cultured fungi. We then showed that the fungal flora was in a state of constant change, and that for best results gravity plates should be placed during periods of human activity, between knee and shoulder height (7). A third paper gave an updated view of our region's fungal flora (8).

The purpose of the present study was to determine the practical and clinical significance of incorporating fungi we had previously isolated into a scheme for treating a variety of recalcitrant allergic symptoms.

Materials and methods

Twenty-one fungi were selected for this trial and divided into mixes as shown in Table 1.

Table 1.
Components of mold mixes used

Mix A	*Aspergillus, Alternaria, Hormodendrum (Cladosporium), Penicillium*
Mix B	*Epicoccum, Fusarium, Pullularia (Aureobasidium)*
Mix D	*Fomes, Mucor, Phoma, Rhodotorula*
Mix E	*Cephalosporium, Botrytis, Geotrichum, Helminthosporium, Stemphyllium*

Trichophyton, Candida, Epidermophyton, Rhizopus and *Sporobolomyces* were tested individually.

We tested with several different strengths of each fungus to assess the relative degree of sensitivity to each. Five-fold serial dilutions (9) were prepared for each fungus, as described previously for chemical testing (10). Dilution #1 was four parts Hollister-Stier diluent and one part of the concentrate. Dilution #2 was four parts diluent and one part #1, and so on. Intradermal testing began

with an injection of 0.05 ml of #5. Only that amount was injected to produce a 7x7mm wheal. If no wheal growth occurred, 0.05 ml of #4 was applied, and so on until a 2mm wheal growth was obtained. Again, each time only the amount necessary to produce a 7x7mm wheal was injected. The last negative dilution (no wheal growth) which preceded the first positive wheal growth was the treatment dose. If #2 dilution produced no growth, the test was considered negative. If #5 showed 2mm wheal growth, it was considered positive and weaker dilutions were tested until the first negative dilution was found. This first negative was used as the treatment dose.

All fungi were tested individually and as components of the respective mixes. If testing the mix and all of its components produced the same end point for wheal growth, the mix was used therapeutically. If none of the fungal components had the same end point as the entire mix, the positive fungi were given individually. If most of the component fungi had the same end points as the mix, the mix was given.

The mixes were prepared with equal parts of their constituent fungi and serially diluted five-fold just as the individual fungi were, as described above. The dose administered for all antigens was held constant at 0.05cc twice weekly for one month and weekly thereafter. The doses were not raised.

All patients were tested in the winter to avoid pollen exposure. Those sensitive to pollens had them included in their immunotherapy schedules. Likewise, patients shown to be sensitive to housedust and housedust mite *Dermatophagoides pteronyssinus* had those antigens included in their medication.

At the beginning of the test period, patients were placed on a major elimination diet which prohibited such commonly consumed foods as milk, wheat, corn, and ferments (bread, cheese, alchohol, vinegar, salad dressing, mayonnaise, ketchup, mustard, chocolate and processed foods). They were allowed to eat foods they knew to be safe and that they did not normally eat more frequently than once a week.

Results

The following cases represent the results observed in many of over a thousand patients treated in this manner. For brevity, the original cases selected have been reduced.

Case 1—K.W., a 33-year-old male, had facial, arm, torso and leg eczema since childhood. For the previous 11 years he had severe eczema with marked exfoliation of his lichenified skin. He also suffered from chronic diarrhea. He had been thoroughly examined at several major hospitals in the northwest and treated without improvement by four allergists and three dermatologists. He lived in a trailer in the woods and suspected that molds were part of his problem.

Laboratory findings revealed increased T-4 cells of 60.2% (normal 38-53%) and B cells of 18.9% (normal 7-11%), decreased T-8 cells of 10.3% (normal 18-30) and NK cells of 2.1% (normal 6-13%) and IgE of 33,088 I.U. Unlike the typical patient with hyper-IgE syndrome, he had not had so much as a cold in five years. He knew that milk caused severe exfoliation within a day and his milk RAST was moderately positive.

Within 13 days after initiation of therapy his skin was totally cleared by maintaining the elimination diet and receiving his dust, dust mite and mold injections. This was the first time in 11 years that he had been free of eczema, in spite of many medications, including oral steroids, and immunotherapy trials. His IgE went from 33,088 I.U. to 8,809 I.U. after four months and to 6,456 after six months. After one year it was 2,305 I.U., and after 2 years it was 1,321. He has remained clear for over four years. His severe total body eczematous dermatitis recurs with dietary indiscretion or with double-blind substitution of normal saline for his mold-mite-dust injections. (See before and after photos , Figure 1)

Figure 1
Case 1 K.W.

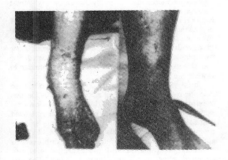

Before immunotherapy   **After one month's**
                              immunotherapy

Case 2—C.V., a 37-year-old female, had severe facial atopic dermatitis for six years with large erythematous, tender, pruritic papules. Her IgE was unremarkable at 17 I.U. She thought that molds were a problem since her face would burn and tingle when she went outdoors in the

fall. Many foods were avoided and the remaining foods rotated on a four day cycle to control symptoms. After receiving injections her facial dermatitis cleared, except when normal saline placebos were substituted double-blind. (Figure 2)

Figure 2
Case 2 C.V.

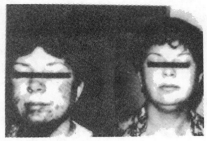

Before immunotherapy   **After three month's**
                              immunotherapy

Case 3—C.H., an 8-year-old boy, was on 10mg Dexedrine t.i.d. for hyperactivity. He was tested with the fungal extracts and placed on appropriate immunotherapy. Within one month he was able to discontinue the Dexedrine, his attention span improved to the point where he was teachable, his behavior was markedly improved, he grew in height and teeth had erupted after a 2 year arrest.

Before sensitivity testing for molds, he could draw a flower and write his name at a level compatible with his age. Testing with molds reproduced his hyperactivity and his best effort at repeating what he had drawn just five minutes earlier was more compatible with that of a 3-year-old. When the treatment dose was used, his hyperactivity ceased and his writing and drawing returned to normal. (Figure 3)

After four months this boy, who was previously unable to be taught, was earning A's in school. One year later a placebo was substituted for his active medication unbeknown to the allergy nurses administering the injections, to the patient, and to the boy's parents. Within two weeks the mother presented with a black eye the boy had given her for no apparent reason. At that time she stated that his behavior suggested that he was no longer receiving his injections. Also within that two week period two school teachers had gone to the principal and requested that he not be allowed to return the next year. Furthermore, he had been taken by the police to their station twice for discipline after he had come home from school and made calls to the police advising them of non-existent emergencies at his home. When his injections were reinstated, his life returned to normal.

Figure 3
Case 3 C.H.

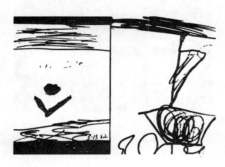

While being tested with pollen extracts	While being tested with mold extracts*

* When he was given the neutralizing dose, his drawing returned to normal

Case 4—F.N., a 48-year-old barber, for 6 years had had up to 25 severe headaches a month. They began with the right eye becoming glassy. The right side of his face would swell, the eye would tear, and incapacitating pain would leave him bedridden for two days, contemplating suicide. No amount of analgesics, beta blockers, antihistamines or vasoconstrictors had alleviated the problem. With appropriate injections the headaches ceased. One year later they recurred for the first time, after the injections had been stopped for 10 days.

Case 5—W.B., 41, was a college professor and chairman of his department. Eighteen months prior to his first office visit he developed what he thought was the flu, but it never resolved. He had constant non-vertiginous dizziness, headache, and incapacitating

weakness that would fluctuate in intensity without ever completely abating. His prior workups included hospitalization with CAT scans of the brain and a lumbar puncture.

He reported a distinct improvement after being tested with the mold extracts and receiving his first therapeutic injection. The second injection a few days later cleared all symptoms for the first time since the onset 2 years previously. His symptoms now recur every fourth day and disappear within 30 minutes after an injection. He remains clear as long as he obtains his injection twice a week. Double-blind placebo substitution for his injections causes symptoms to recur.

Case 6—M.E. was a 68-year-old orthopedic surgeon. He had experienced cardiac arrhythmia accompanied by diarrhea and weakness over the previous months. The weakness had become incapacitating to the point where he feared walking across a room. After one week of mold injections he described himself as 80% better than he had felt in the preceding 10 years, and has continued that way on immunotherapy. He also had a history of anosmia for 30 years, thought to be secondary to chronic atopic sinusitis and recurrent polypectomies. His sense of smell returned after injections began.

Case 7—R.S. was a 36-year-old severely asthmatic woman who worked in a family-owned bakery. Wheat RAST was strongly positive. IgE was 70 I.U. Cultures from her bedroom yielded 16 colonies of *Sporobolomyces*, 1 of *Fusarium*, 48 of bacteria, 2 of yeasts, and 1 of sterile fungus. The bakery yielded 1 of *Penicillium*, 1 of *Rhodotorula*, 5 of *Sporobolomyces*, and 3 of bacteria. After two months on immunotherapy her asthma cleared. She was able to stop all medication and she has continued to work in the bakery.

Case 8—S.K. was a 57-year-old carpenter who became cyanotic merely from walking across the room. He was maximally medicated for asthma and was on oral steroids as well. Pulmonary specialists had hospitalized him for a bronchoscopy and bronchograms and his prognosis was guarded. His IgE was 5,666 I.U. With appropriate immunotherapy he began to improve. His cyanosis disappeared and his exercise tolerance increased. After one year on immunotherapy his IgE was 2,146, he no longer needed steroids and had dropped many of his medications. After two years his IgE had fallen to 1,370 I.U. and he only needed albuterol occasionally.

Case 9—M.D. was a 30-year-old housewife with five years of chronic total body pruritis, headache, and rhinitis. All her symptoms cleared within two months of injections and diet.

Case 10—K.L. was a 41-year-old housewife with a seven month history of giant urticaria. She incidentally had had headaches for 20 years and a perennial rhinitis. On appropriate immunotherapy, all symptoms cleared in less than two months and recurred if injections were late.

Discussion

The above case histories are representative of many successfully treated patients. The findings suggest a treatment method for a variety of allergic disorders which have failed to respond to other forms of treatment. The indications of the specificity and appropriateness of immunotherapy with fungal antigens was reinforced by the use of double-blind placebos and the serendipitous failures of patients who were unable to maintain what proved to be critical restrictive diets.

These cases of resistant asthma, eczema, acne, pruritic dermatoses, weakness, migraine, dizziness, and hyperactivity also represent the basic target organs we observed to be affected. Most patients also complained of perennial allergic rhinitis or sinusitis, but that was secondary to their major complaint. This symptom also cleared when the major complaint cleared.

In these as well as hundreds of other similarly treated cases, the brain was a target organ. Hyperactivity, severe headaches, and non-vertiginous dizziness were the major symptoms in many, and were usually accompanied by profound weakness and/or exhaustion. This program brought dramatic relief to many of these patients. These patients reverted to pre-treatment status with double-blind substitution of placebo injections or dietary indiscretions.

Ambient fungi and commonly ingested foods may cause symptoms in a variety of target organs not customarily thought to be affected in atopic diseases. When the top tolerated dose is determined by intradermal testing and frequently ingested foods are eliminated, dramatic responses occurred. Eventually patients added back foods one a day to identify those that triggered symptoms. The offending foods were unique for each case, although the commonest offenders were the ferment foods, meaning those derived from yeasts (breads, cheeses, alcohols, vinegars, processed foods). This is not surprising since processed foods are high in fungal antigens. Many preservatives, enzymes, vitamins, pigments, stabilizers, and flavorings are derived from the fermentation process (1). It is possible that cross-antigenic stimulation is at work.

The techniques described here provide one more tool with which the allergist can demonstrate the impact of the environment on a sensitized individual. Appropriate treatment terminates the adverse effects caused by the interplay between man and his environment.

Recommendations for environmental control

Testing and treating for sensitivity to indoor fungi can clear recalcitrant conditions. Methods for reducing the prevalence of fungi also need to be developed.

In this study over 500 mold plates were exposed in bedrooms before and after a variety of environmental controls. Although these have not yet been subjected to statistical analysis, it is evident that washing the entire room with a borax solution, removing carpet, and closing off forced air ducts reduced ambient fungi.

Because there was such wide variability in patient home location and construction as well as financial resources, a number of different modalities were evaluated in terms of effectiveness in lowering fungi levels.

Simply cleaning all surfaces thoroughly and removing carpet and unnecessary clutter reduced fungi in many bedrooms.

One inexpensive and labor-saving method was to seal the rooms and allow evaporation for 48 hours from an open bowl of one cup of vinegar and one cup of chlorine bleach. Occupants were allowed back into the area 48 hours after removing the mixture. In some cases no improvement was seen, but in over 50%, there was significant reduction in colony counts.

In one case use of the mixture for 48 hours in a bedroom reduced the *Penicillium* colony count from 26 to 2 and the *Sporobolomyces* count from 14 to 1.

Prior to the use of the mix, cultures in the bedroom of a patient with chronic sinusitis yielded 12 colonies of *Cladosporium*, 84 of bacteria, 5 of *Alternaria*, 5 of *Rhodotorula*, and 3 of sterile fungi. After using the mixture, no organisms could be grown on the gravity plates.

More beneficial was the use of a single-room electrostatic precipitator. Mold plates indicated that one week of 24-hour operation reduced ambient fungi by 50-100%.

Although most fungi fall within the size range of one micron to 400 microns, the average size of fungi identified on the plates is around 10 microns. With *Cladosporium*, the commonest mold, one species (*C. sphaerospermum*) has a 3-4.5 micron diameter, another (*C. herbarum*) measures 8-15 by 4-6 microns, while other species can be up to 60 microns long. The electrostatic precipitator we recommended had a capacity of 255 cfm and precipitated particles down to 0.1 micron size (11-13).

Most dramatic of all, however, was the use of ultraviolet fluorescent lights. Placement of these in 8-foot ceilings prevented all fungal growth after two weeks. Further studies are being done to determine optimal spacing of these lights.

One disadvantage of this procedure is that the lights must be wired so they are turned off when animals or people enter the room, since eye damage can result within minutes of exposure. They are not as unobtrusive as a single air pollution control device, but they may be useful for particularly moldy environments such as basements.

Increased ventilation is an important way to reduce

indoor chemical air pollution, but our study showed that increasing ventilation by opening windows increased levels of fungi regardless of which control method was used. Hence, heat exchangers should be used and incoming air should be filtered rather than forgo ventilation.

Most of our efforts were aimed at reducing fungi in bedrooms, since we were attempting to create a hypoallergenic oasis for the patient for at least one-third of the day. Extension of some of these methods to the rest of the home or to business environments would be difficult and/or costly and would clearly require the help of a heating, ventilation and air conditioning (HVAC) engineer.

Hopefully, collaborative efforts between the specialist in environmental medicine and the HVAC engineer would prove synergistically beneficial and prevent others from becoming sensitized to ambient fungi.

References

1. Beuchat LR. *Food and Beverage Mycology.* Westport, CT:AVI Publ., 1978.

2 Lehrer SB, Aukrust L, Salvaggio JE. Respiratory allergy induced by fungi, in Symposium on Immune Factors in Pulmonary Disease. *Clinics in Chest Medicine* 4:23-41, 1983.

3. Holst PE et al. Asthma and fungi in the home. *New Zealand Med J* 96:718-20, 1983.

4. Mazar A, Baum GC, Segal E et al. Antibodies to inhalant fungal antigens in patients with asthma in Israel. *Ann Allergy* 47 (5 Part I):361-364, 1981

5. Salvaggio JE, Aukrust L. Mold-induced asthma. *Allergy Clin Immunol* 68:327-46, 1981.

6. Terracina F, Rogers SA. In-home fungal studies. *Ann Allergy* 49:1;35-37,1982.

7. Rogers SA. A comparison of commercially available mold survey services. *Ann Allergy* 50:37-43, 1983.

8. Rogers SA. A thirteen-month assessment of local work-leisure-sleep fungal environments. *Ann Allergy* 52:338-41, 1984.

9. Willoughby JW. Diagnosis of allergy by serial dilution end-point titration. *Continuing education for the family physician* 11:3, 1979.

10. Rogers SA. Diagnosing the tight building syndrome. *Env Health Persp* 76: 195-198, 1987.

11. Ellis MB. *Dematiaceous Hyphomycetes.* London: Commonwealth Mycological Inst., 1971.

12. Querholts LO. *The Polyporaceae of the United States, Alaska, and Canada.* Ann Arbor: University of Michigan Press, 1983.

13. Lincoff GH. *The Audubon Society Field Guide to North American Mushrooms.* New York: A.A. Knopf, 1981.

A COMPARISON OF COMMERCIALLY AVAILABLE MOLD SURVEY SERVICES

SHERRY A. ROGERS, M.D., F.A.C.A.

Plates from the County Laboratory, Hollister-Stier and our lab were simultaneously placed in the same locations. Comparisons show increased yield comes from a combination of the latter two and the greatest over-all yield came from our lab. Also multiple-placed plates in the same room show the flora is not static.

IN A PREVIOUS STUDY we found several modifications of mycologic techniques to increase the yield in our home fungal studies.[1] In the present study we were interested in with yet another commercially available service. Some of their plates were saved to assess the effects of shipment on culture results.

Because we had no known standard with which to compare the results, and because we were suspicious that even in the home the fungal flora was not a static phenomenon, we performed an additional study. In this we looked at several plates placed at different heights and locations within the same room. This arrangement was repeated several times in the same room at three different locations within a 24-hour period. This latter study was with our plates only.

Methods

This first study, completed in one day, was conducted in three suburban homes in opposite ends of the city. The resident of each house placed plates in the bedroom, family room, basement and outdoors (June). At least three plates were placed in each location. These were a malt agar plate from our laboratory, a Sabouraud dextrose from the County Laboratory and a Rose-Bengal agar from the Hollister-Stier Laboratory. (The latter plate marked "outdoors" does not contain the Rose Bengal ingredient as the four indoor plates do.) The County plates were all exposed for 10-min periods. Ours and those of Hollister Stier were exposed one-half hour outdoors and one hour indoors. They were all exposed according to each laboratory's instructions and taped shut. The County's were returned to their laboratory and Hollister-Stier's were mailed to them. We also kept some

Doctor Rogers is in Private Practice Allergy and is Attending Physician, Community General Hospital, Syracuse, New York.

County and Hollister-Stier plates to read ourselves. Our plates were processed as described in our preceding paper.[1] Great care was taken to open the lid only far enough to obtain a sample of the mold being identified under sterile conditions.

Because the County Laboratory plates and those of Hollister-Stier were transported greater distances than ours (the former by Courrier Service, the latter by the U.S. Postal Service), there was a chance that showering of spores would occur with rough handling. Therefore no attempt at quantitation was made.

Results

When all the plates were read the data were tabulated as follows. The total individual genera obtained in each house were listed individually for each house. No quantitation of each organism was attempted. The results of this experiment are shown in Table I.

Our plates of malt agar had a larger number of genera than did Hollister-Stier or County Lab plates. No new genera were found on the County Lab plates. Also, several molds which we found were not reported by them. In the previous paper we gave many reasons for this.[1] Hollister-Stier reported fewer fungi than we did but more than the County. However, they also reported some fungi which our plates did not produce.

Second, for a few randomly selected rooms we set out duplicate County and Hollister-Stier plates, keeping one set to read for ourselves while returning the other set for the official report as stated above. The comparative results are shown in Table II.

The County Laboratory did not report as many genera of fungi as the plates read by our mycologist but we retained the plates for a few weeks to give the slow growers a chance to form colonies.

Although Penicillium was not detected on our plates or on those reported by Hollister-Stier, we did detect a

Table 1. For Each of Three Houses, Five of Our Malt Agar Plates, Five Sabouraud Agar Plates From The County Lab (Co) and Five Of Rose-Bengal Agar (H.S.) Were Exposed. Fungi Reported From Each Of The Three Labs Are Tabulated. At The Asterix H.S. Actually Reported Polyporus (A Basidiomycete).

	FM's house			SG's house			CF's house		
	Ours	Co	HS	Ours	Co	HS	Ours	Co	HS
Cladosporium	+	+		+	+	+	+	+	+
Penicillium	+	+	+	+	+		+		+
Sterile		+			+	+		+	+
Basidiomycetes	+	+	+*	+	+		+	+	+
Alternaria	+			+			+		+
Aureobasidium	+			+			+		+
Epicoccum	+			+			+		
Yeast				+			+		
Paecilomyces	+					+			
Aspergillus									+
Bacteria				+					
Geotrichum								+	
Rhodotorula								+	
Mortierella	+								
Rhizopus				+					
Curvularia				+					
Sphaeriodaceae				+					
Trichoderma								+	
Botrytis								+	
Fusarium									+
Stemphylium									+

Table II. In The Bedroom of CF's House, One of Our Malt Agar Plates, Two Sabouraud Agar Plates (Co) and Two Rose-Bengal Plates (H.S.) Were Exposed. We Saved One of Each To Read Ourselves and Compare With The Commercial Reading.

	Our malt*	County-SD		HS-Rose Bengal	
		They read	We read	They read	We read
Cladosporium	+	+	+	+	+
Alternaria	+		+	+	+
Basidiomycetes	+	+			+
Penicillium			+	+	
Fusarium				+	+
Epicoccum	+		+		
Sterile	+	+			
Botrytis			+		+
Aureobasidium	+				
Yeast			+		
Bacteria			+		

Basidiomycete and Botrytis which were not detected by Hollister-Stier plates. This divergence led us to perform the last part of the experiment.

Mold surveys using malt agar only were conducted 11 months later in one room of two houses studied. Simultaneously three plates were exposed in each room at varying heights and locations within the room. In addition, additional malt agar plates were exposed in the same locations every six to 12 hours for a total of 24 hours. The results of this study are given in Tables IIIa and IIIb. As can be seen in Table IIIa, multiple plates exposed in the same room at the same time did not demonstrate the same fungi. Also, at 6:00 p.m. during the period when air turbulence is at its maximum due to human traffic, more fungi were detected on the plates. Samples at high locations (e.g., refrigerator top) revealed fewer molds than samples at low locations such as countertops and floors. Minimum levels of molds were found at midnight. In the second household, similar quantitative results were obtained with regard to numbers of mold.

Discussion

A knowledge of the ambient fungal flora is important to the management of allergic patients.[3] However, all methods of sampling have some degree of inefficiency.[2] First, there is no perfect sampling device. Although gravity plates are easily manageable and economical, only viable numbers of spore are detected. Moreover, viability does not necessarily equate with antigenicity. Many factors other than the presence of spores influence fall-out into the plate. These include room air currents as well as the physical characteristics of the spores, such as size and density, also static spore traps have a layer of dead air space over their surfaces, tending to minimize spore fall-out.[4]

Suction devices and moving impactors are often expensive, clumsy to use for patient home sampling, collect debris other than mold spores, often necessitate spore identification (which is more difficult than identification from a growing colony) and tend to by-pass the smaller spores.[5]

Moreover, there is no optimal medium on which to grow these fungi. Malt agar and Sabouraud dextrose agar plates have been reported to be superior to Rose Bengal,[6] a finding we cannot substantiate in our small study. The antibiotic in Rose Bengal inhibits the growth of some fungi entirely. None of these media support many of the Basidiomycetes such as the rusts and smuts. Some studies have attempted a variety of methods[7] and indeed at this point it is probably best to persist in individualizing the needs of each allergic patient.[8]

Not only does the amount of physical activity in the environment increase the yield, as we and others[9] have seen, but also affects the number of genera.

38

Table IIIa. Our Malt Agar Plates Were Exposed at Three Different Locations Within the Same Room of SG's House, Every Six Hours for 24 Hours. The Molds Recovered Are Shown.

	6:00 a.m.			12 noon			6:00 p.m.			12 midnight		
	C	R	F	C	R	F	C	R	F	C	R	F
Cladosporium	+		+	+		+		+	+	+		+
Sterile	+	+	+			+	+	+	+	+		
Penicillium				+	+			+	+		+	+
Aspergillus				+	+			+	+		+	+
Aureobasidium	+			+			+	+	+	+		
Yeast			+		+	+	+	+	+			
Bacteria	+			+	+		+	+	+			
Geotrichum	+	+	+							+		
Rhodotorula							+	+	+			
Actinomycetes						+		+	+			
Alternaria								+	+			
Phoma							+		+			
Basidiomycetes			+							+		
Epicoccum			+									

C—Kitchen counter
R—Top of refrigerator
F—Floor

Table IIIb. Our Malt Agar Plates Were Exposed at Three Different Locations Within the Same Room of CF's House, Three Times Within 24 Hours. The Molds Recovered Are Shown.

	6:00 a.m.			6:00 p.m.			12 midnight		
	F	T	D	F	T	D	F	T	D
Penicillium	+	+	+	+	+	+	+	+	+
Yeast		+	+	+	+	+	+	+	+
Sterile	+	+	+	+		+	+	+	+
Cladosporium	+	+	+	+	+	+			+
Aureobasidium		+	+		+	+		+	+
Geotrichum	+	+	+		+		+		+
Aspergillus	+	+		+					+
Rhodotorula	+		+	+	+	+			+
Actinomycetes		+		+	+	+			
Bacteria				+	+			+	
Black yeast				+		+	+		
Alternaria	+			+					
Phoma				+				+	
Verticillium								+	
Basidiomycetes	+								
Rhizopus					+				

F—living room, fireplace
T—top of TV
D—floor by door

In our previous study[1] we showed that Sabouraud's media used by the County, employing shorter exposure and incubation times gave a lower yield of fungi. The results of the present study shown in Table I demonstrate the effects of these variables. We next evaluated the effects of the size of the plates and length of transit times in shipping on the yield of organisms. No evidence to substantiate this was obtained. Comparative studies with Rose Bengal and malt agar would determine whether the discrepancy lies in the medium itself. Because Rose Bengal did detect fungi that we did not obtain, there seems to be additional benefit in having a Rose Bengal plate as well. There is, of course, the question of which is preferrable, a malt agar plate and a Rose Bengal plate or several randomly placed malt agar plates at peak activity time, repeated throughout the year.

Conclusion

In this study our malt agar plates detected far more genera of fungi in houses than Hollister-Stier's Rose Bengal plates, which far exceeded those employed by the County Laboratory. Each plate detected individual genera of fungi not detected by the other. No additional fungi were found using the County plates. It appears that a malt agar and Rose Bengal plate should give increased yield. Also, increased yield was observed by exposing plates during the time of peak activity in the home (6:00 p.m.) and having plates at a level of four feet or lower. Multiple plates will decrease the chance of missing some ambient spores.

Summary

Plates from the County Laboratory, Hollister-Stier and our lab were simultaneously placed in the same locations. Comparisons show increased yield comes from a combination of the latter two and the greatest over-all yield came from our lab. Also multiple placed plates in the same room showed variations in flora.

Acknowledgments

I acknowledge with gratitude the preparation and reading of all our plates by Fred Terracina, Ph.D., taxonomic mycologist, at the State University of New York, College of Environmental Science and Forestry.

Also appreciation goes to Kathleen Ascioti for typing of the manuscript.

References

1. Terracina F and Rogers S: In-home fungal studies. Ann Allerg 49: 35, 1982.
2. Solomon WR: In Allergy: Principles and Practice, Middleton E, Reed C and Ellis E (Eds.). St Louis: C. V. Mosby Company, 1978.
3. Chapman JA: The enhancement of the practice of clinical allergy with daily pollen and spore counts. Immunol & Allerg Pract IV: 1, 1982.
4. Mallock D: Molds: Their Isolation, Cultivation and Identification. University of Toronto Press, p. 37, 1981.
5. Solomon WR, Burge HA, Boise JR and Beelen M: Comparative particle recoveries by the retracting rotorod, rotoslide and Burkard Spore Trap sampling in a compact array. Int J Biometeor 24, 2: 107–116, 1980.

6. Burge HP, Solomon WR and Boise JR: Comparative merits of eight popular media in aerometric studies of fungi. JACI 60, 3: 199–203, 1977.

7. Kozak P, Gallup J, Cummins LH and Gillmon SA: Ann Allergy 45: 85, 1980.

8. ibid II. Samples of problem homes surveyed. 45: 169, 1980.

9. Burge HP, Boise JR and Solomon WR: Fungi in libraries: an aerometric survey. Myopathologia 64: 2, 67–72, 1978.

Requests for reprints should be addressed to:
Dr. Sherry A. Rogers
280 West Genesee Street
Syracuse, New York 13219

AN EXCHANGE OF NOTES

"... We cannot dedicate, we cannot consecrate, we cannot hallow, this ground. The brave men, living and dead, who struggled here, have consecrated it, far above our poor power to add or to detract ... It is for us, the living, rather, to be dedicated here, to the unfinished work that they have thus far so nobly carried on. It is rather for us to be here dedicated to the great task remaining before us; that from these honored dead we take increased devotion to that cause for which they here gave the last full measure of devotion; that we here highly resolve that these dead shall not have died in vain ..."

From President Lincoln's "remarks" at
the dedication of the National Soldiers'
Cemetery at Gettysburg, November 19, 1863.

"... I would be glad if I could flatter myself that I came as near to the central idea of the occasion in two hours as you did in two minutes ..."

Note from Edward Everett, orator at the
dedication.

"... In our respective parts yesterday, you could not have been excused to make a short address, nor I a long one. I am pleased to know that, in your judgment, the little I did say was not entirely a failure ..."

President Lincoln's reply to Mr. Everett.

IN-HOME FUNGAL STUDIES: METHODS TO INCREASE THE YIELD

FRED TERRACINA, Ph.D., and SHERRY A. ROGERS, M.D., F.A.C.A.

This paper shows that by increasing the exposure time from 10 minutes to one hour, substituting malt agar for Sabouraud's dextrose agar and observing the plates beyond one week for four to six weeks, an increase in the variety of genera was noted, above that previously reported.

Introduction

IN A RECENT STUDY of patients with inhalant allergies the incidence of mold allergy was 86%.[1] Airborne fungi are frequently associated with allergic manifestations.[2] There is a growing armamentarium of commercially available mold extracts. However, over the last decade the reports from our local county laboratory on mold surveys done in our patients' homes and offices generally fell into one of three categories: (1) no growth, (2) Basidiomycetes, (3) one or more of the "four mold" group Cladosporium (Hormodendrum), Alternaria, Penicillium and Aspergillus.

The high frequency of Basidiomycetes and the low frequency of genera other than the basic four molds raised the following questions. The first was whether this survey reflected the genera present. The second was whether the Sabouraud's dextrose agar used by our county laboratory and commonly used in medical laboratories would give different results from malt agar, which is commonly used by non-medical mycologists who generally study airborne fungi. Third, we were also interested in whether longer exposures than the 10 minutes exposure recommended by our county laboratory would yield more genera. The fourth was whether plates incubated longer than four days, which was the incubation time used for the county surveys, would yield other genera.

Therefore we decided to do a small study of 10 plates in each of seven residences within the Syracuse metropolitan area.

Materials and Methods

Sterile, disposable Petri dishes (90 × 15 mm) containing Sabouraud's dextrose Agar (Difco-B109) or 3% malt extract plus 2.0% agar were exposed for one hour in the following four rooms of seven houses: (1) master bedroom, (2) basement, (3) family room and (4) major bathroom. Another exposure for 15 minutes was done with both media in the family rooms of each home. Descriptive data of each house were taken which summarized site location (i.e., city, suburb, rural), type (ranch, cape, etc.) construction (brick, wood, block), heating method, humidification and insulation type, if any. The presence or absence of stored wood was also noted as well as electrostatic precipitators.

The plates were marked, taped shut and incubated in the dark at 24°C. Each plate was examined at the end of four days and bi-weekly thereafter for four to six weeks. Identifications were made from slides made directly from the exposed plates or from subcultures plated onto the appropriate diagnostic media, depending on the fungus being studied.

Results

The results from 70 plates are tabulated in Tables I and II. The order of listing in both tables is based on decreasing frequency. Nineteen taxa were identified. Eighteen of the taxa (95%) were collected on malt extract agar. Twelve taxa (63%) were collected on Sabouraud's dextrose agar.

Although plates from individual rooms remained sterile, no houses examined were free of fungal growth. Bacteria were present in every house sampled and constituted the second most frequently occurring taxon. Aspergillus was also present in every house sampled. Penicillium was common in five of the seven houses examined. Trichoderma did not become identifiable until well after the first week. Basidiomycetes were found in four of the seven houses. They were also more frequently found on malt agar than Sabouraud's agar.

Fred Terracina, Ph.D., is a Taxonomic Mycology Research Associate, College of Environmental Science & Forestry, S.U.N.Y., Syracuse, New York.

Doctor Rogers is in the private practice of allergy, Attending Community General Hospital, 2800 W. Genesee Street, Syracuse, New York 13219

The populations displayed on the media were rather similar, with the most frequently appearing organisms appearing on both media (11 of the 19 taxa involved). Sorenson's Quotient of Similarity[3] was used to estimate the similarity between the two media.

$$Q = \frac{2J}{A + B} \times 100$$

where J = # of taxa in common
A = # of taxa on malt extract agar
B = # of taxa on Sabouraud's dextrose agar
In this analysis identical communities would have a Q of 100. Our results yielded a Q of 80.

Table I. Comparison of Rates of Recovery of Fungi Utilizing Two Different Culture Media

Taxa	Malt agar (%)	Sabouraud dextrose agar (%)
Cladosporium spp.	57	34
Bacteria	43	46
Aspergillus spp.	29	26
Penicillium spp.	23	26
Yeasts (other than Rhodotorula)	29	17
Basidiomycetes	26	20
Rhodotorula sp.	14	9
Trichoderma viride Pers ex Fries	14	3
Epicoccum purpurascens Exrenb ex Schlect	3	6
Alternaria alternata (Fr.) Keissler	9	3
Microsphaeriopsis olivacea (Bonord) Hohn	6	6
Aureobasidium pullulans (De Bary) Arnold	6	0
Sterile moniliaceous	0	6
Sterile dematiaceous	6	0
Phialophora heteromorpha (Nannf.) Wang	3	0
Scytalidium lignicola Pesante	3	0
Stachybotrys atra Corda	3	0
Stephanosporium cerealis (Thum.) Swart	3	0
Wallemia sebi (Fr.) v. Arx	3	0

Discussion

Gregory[4] and Hirst[5] summarized many outdoor surveys of airborne fungi. Indoor surveys are not as frequently performed.[6] Lacey[7] presents a concise overview of the aerobiology of conidial fungi. Recent trends in residential energy conservation (retrofitting) include reducing air infiltration of existing homes, replacing air conditioners with large ceiling circulating fans, increasing humidity and placing insulating materials within the exterior walls that, under elevated moisture conditions, support the growth of many fungi. These considerations, then, may lead to increased numbers of kinds of fungi within the living spaces, particularly during the long winter months in the north temperate zone. Our study was not large enough to draw clear conclusions in this area.

We recognize that our listing of taxa contains elements at various classification ranks and, therefore, our frequency levels are not strictly comparable because of unequal numbers of species are represented in several taxa. Nevertheless, this practice is common with almost all other published studies in this area[8,9,10] and therefore our results may be compared with other workers'.

In our study the genus Cladosporium (Hormodendrum) was isolated more frequently than any other taxon. This is consistent with Lumpkins et al[6] as well as Hirsch & Sossman[9] and many previous studies of outdoor samples.[7] Within this taxon three different species were collected: C. cladosporoides, Fresen (deVries), C. herbarium Link ex Fr. and C. sphaerospermum Penzig.

Examples of the genus Aspergillus recovered included Aspergillus flavus group (resembling A. flavus Link var. columnaris Rapar and Fennell), Aspergillus fumigatus Fresenius, Aspergillus niger V. Tiegh and Aspergillus clavatus Desm.

The most frequent Penicillia isolated in our study were Penicillium notatum Westling and Penicillium thomii Maire. The frequency of the genus Trichoderma in this

Table II. Frequency of Isolation of Fungi from Individual Patient Residences

Patient														
A		B		C		D		E		F		G		
SD*	M**	SD	M	SD	M	SD	M	SD	M	SD	M	SD	M	
+	+	+	+	−	−	+	+	+	+	−	+	+	+	Cladosporium spp.
+	+	+	+	+	+	+	+	−	+	+	+	+	+	Bacteria
−	+	+	+	+	+	−	+	+	+	+	+	−	+	Aspergillus spp.
−	+	−	−	+	+	+	+	+	+	+	−	+	+	Yeasts (other than Rhodotorula)
−	+	−	+	+	+	−	+	+	−	−	−	+	+	Basidiomycetes
−	+	−	−	−	−	+	+	+	+	−	−	+	+	Rhodotorula msp.
−	−	−	+	−	−	−	+	−	+	+	+	−	−	Trichoderma viride
−	−	−	−	+	+	+	+	+	−	−	−	−	−	Epicoccum purpurascens
−	−	−	−	−	+	+	+	−	−	+	−	−	−	Alternaria alternata
−	−	+	−	−	−	−	−	−	−	+	−	−	−	Microsphaeriopsis olivacea
−	−	+	−	−	−	−	−	−	−	−	−	−	−	Aureobasidium pullulans
+	−	−	−	−	−	+	−	−	−	−	−	−	−	Sterile Moniliaceous
−	+	−	−	−	−	−	−	−	−	−	+	−	−	Sterile Dematiaceous
−	−	+	−	−	−	−	−	−	−	−	−	−	−	Phialophora hetoromorpha
−	−	−	−	−	−	+	−	−	−	−	−	−	−	Scytalidium lignicola
−	−	−	−	−	−	+	−	−	−	−	−	−	−	Stachybotrys altra
−	−	−	−	−	−	−	−	+	−	−	−	−	−	Stephanosporium cerealis
+	−	−	−	−	−	−	−	−	−	−	−	−	−	Wallemia sebi

* SD = Sabouraud dextrose agar.
** M = malt agar.

study is higher than one usually finds in the literature.[7] It may be reported as a sterile fungus if plates are discarded prematurely.

No attempt was made to identify the yeasts other than to confirm that the pink yeasts recovered were in the genus Rhodotorula rather than Sporobolomyces.

Several kinds of Basidiomycetes were found but we were not able to identify them using either Nobles[11] or Stalpers[12] keys. Frequent oidia and small clamps were invariably found in those cultures we designated as Basidiomycetes. We suspect that identification of Basidiomycetes to the generic level (e.g., Polyporus and Fomes) can not be accomplished except for laboratories having large collections of referenced cultures available for matings, which is often required for identification at the generic and specific levels. Four of the seven houses we examined yielded Basidiomycetes. This result may indicate that they are more frequent than commonly thought because of changing environmental conditions or that they are missed by other investigators who commonly discard plates before two weeks. They are frequently associated with decaying wood.

Neither medium collected all the taxa recovered but the malt extract agar seemed to have a broader spectrum than the Sabouraud's dextrose agar. No Actinomycetes were found and this may be due to the types of media used.

The frequency of appearance of molds on gravity plates does not allow quantitative estimates of the numbers of fungi present per unit volume. However, it is apparent that the qualitative data they provide when ranked by frequency of appearance of taxons closely mimics the rank order found when quantitative viable methods are used.[13,14] It is likely that the numbers of conidia per unit volume of air exhibits short-term periodic fluctuations depending upon biological fluxes and external environmental factors. We are not convinced that the added expense and inconveniences associated with quantitative collection devices warrants their use for routine investigations of patients' residences.

The high incidence of yeasts, Rhodotorula in particular, and Basidiomycetes bears acknowledgement and further study.

Additional findings worth noting are that the top seven isolates from our 70 plates in order of prevalence were Cladosporium (Hormodendrum), bacteria, Aspergillus, Penicillium, yeasts (other than Rhodotorula), Basidiomycetes and Rhodotorula.

In summary, the results of the present studies indicated the following. (1) There were indeed no houses with no growth. Also there were many more genera present than Basidiomycetes and the basic four molds. (2) Malt extract agar yielded 95% of the fungi, while Sabouraud's dextrose agar yielded 63%. This suggests that the malt extract agar has a better retrieval rate. (3) No plates were overgrown by bacteria to an extent where they interfered with the identification of fungi. (4) Many of the genera were not identifiable during the first week, thus plates should be observed longer.

Therefore, by increasing exposure time from 10 minutes to one hour, substituting malt agar for Sabouraud's dextrose agar and, rather than discarding plates prior to one week, by examining the plates for four to six weeks, the over-all number of genera observed was increased by 32%.

References

1. Speer F, Denison TR, and Baptist JE: Aspirin allergy. Ann Allerg 46: 123–182, 1981.
2. Hyde HA: Atmospheric pollen and spores in relation to allergy. J Clin Allergy 2: 153–159, 1972.
3. Sorensen T: A method of establishing groups of equal amplitude in plant society based on similarity of species content. K Danske Vidansk Selsk 5: 1–34, 1948.
4. Gregory PH: Microbiology of the Atmosphere, Second Edition. Leonard Hill, Aylesbury, 1973.
5. Hirst JM: A trapper's line. Trans Br Mycol Soc 61: 205–213, 1973.
6. Lumpkins E, Corbit SL and Tiedeman GM: Airborne fungi survey. I. Culture-plate survey of the home environment. Ann Allerg 31: 361–370, 1973.
7. Lacey J: The aerobiology of conidial fungi. In Biology of Conidial Fungi. Volume 1, Cole GT and Kendrick B (Eds.). New York: Academic Press, 1981, pp. 373–416.
8. Levitan E and Horowitz L: A one-year survey of the airborne molds of Tulsa, Oklahoma. II. Indoor survey. Ann Allerg 41: 25–27, 1978.
9. Hirsch SR and Sossman JA: A one-year survey of mold growth inside twelve homes. Ann Allerg 36: 30–38, 1976.
10. Richards M: Atmospheric mold spores in and out of doors. J Allerg 25: 429–439, 1954.
11. Nobles MK: Identification of cultures of wood inhabiting Hymenomycetes. Can J Bot 43: 1097–1139, 1965.
12. Stalpers JA: Identification of wood-inhabiting aphyllophorales in pure culture. Stud Mycol 1:248, 1978.
13. Burge HP, Boise JR, Rutherford JA and Solomon WA: Comparative recoveries of airborne fungus spores by viable and non-viable modes of volumetric collection. Mycopathologia 61: 27–33, 1977.
14. Kozan PP, Gallup J, Cummins LH and Gilman SA: Currently available methods for home mold surveys. II. Examples of problem homes surveyed. Ann Allerg 45: 167–176, 1980.

Requests for reprints should be addressed to:
Dr. Sherry A. Rogers
2800 W. Genesee Street
Syracuse, New York 13219

A 13-MONTH WORK-LEISURE-SLEEP ENVIRONMENT FUNGAL SURVEY

SHERRY A. ROGERS, M.D., F.A.C.A

Thirty plates per month for 13 months were exposed in patients' work-leisure-sleep environments in central New York State. Results show the months of highest mold prevalence in decreasing order were October, September, May and July. These months are also typically our high pollen months.

The categories of highest prevalence in decreasing order were yeasts, mycelia sterilia, Cladosporium, Penicillium, Rhodotorula, bacteria, Alternaria, Aureobasidium, Epicoccum, Aspergillus, Geotrichum, Basidiomycetes, Actinomycetes and Phoma. These were present in at least 14% of all 390 plates.

The present study includes a discussion of the value of these findings in an allergy practice.

Introduction

PREVIOUSLY WE PRESENTED a method to increase the yield of fungi isolated in our in-home fungal studies.[1,2] We found a different media, a longer exposure time and a longer reading time gave increased yields. In the light of these findings the purpose of the present study was to assess the fungal environment in our area over a period of 13 months. Surveys were done of work-leisure-sleep areas to obtain data that would more nearly reflect a patient's 24-hour exposure.

Materials and Methods

One-hundred and thirty allergy patients were randomly selected from an allergy practice. Each month for 13 months (June, 1981, to June, 1982), 10 different patients exposed three plates each in their environments.

For all patients culture plates were exposed in the bedroom. For the second plate most chose the family room or basement, depending upon where they spent leisure time. The third plate was exposed at the place of employment which was often an office, home kitchen, barn or outdoors. Thus we attempted to obtain a representation of the fungal exposures for a person who has three major areas of exposure: work-leisure-

sleep. All people lived within a 100-mile radius of the city of Syracuse, New York. The plates contained 3% malt extract plus 2.0% agar and were exposed for one hour. Plates were marked, taped shut and stored at room temperature. They were examined twice a week, semi-permanent slides in lactophenol were made and taxa were identified from slides until new colonies ceased to appear, usually two to three weeks.

Results

The data from 390 plates, 30 each month for 13 months, were tabulated. Table I shows the genera of fungi isolated or other taxonomic groups that were identified within the limits of practicality. They are arranged in decreasing order of prevalence based on the percentage of plates from which each was isolated. One hundred percent would mean that taxon was present on all 390 plates.

Figure 1 is a bar graph illustrating the 14 most prevalent taxa. These were also present in at least 14% of the 390 plates.

The six most divergent months from the 13-month average were February, March, May, July, September and October. February and March had far fewer fungi isolated than all the other months. May, July, September and October were the months of highest mold prevalence, well above the average for the year. For each taxon, the order from top to bottom in the bar graphs is May, July, September, October 1 to the 13-month average.

Some of the recent changes in fungal taxonomy

Presented at the 39th Annual Congress of the American College of Allergists, January 29–February 2, 1983, New Orleans, Louisianna.
Dr. Rogers is in private practice in allergy and is Attending Physician at Community General Hospital, Syracuse, N.Y.

Table I. Percentage of Plates on Which Present (Total 390 Plates).

1.	Yeasts	78%	11.	Geotrichum	16%
2.	Mycelia sterilia	65	12.	Basidiomycetes	16
3.	Cladosporium	63	13.	Actinomycetes	16
4.	Penicillium	52	14.	Phoma	14
5.	Rhodotorula	45	15.	Dematiaceous fungi	8
6.	Bacteria	44	16.	Fusarium	6
7.	Alternaria	44	17.	Rhizopus	5
8.	Aureobasidium	40	18.	Trichoderma	5
9.	Epicoccum	23	19.	Paecilomyces	3
10.	Aspergillus	23	20.	Beauveria	3

Present on 1% of plates

Monocillium	pycnidial-producing (non-Phoma)
Stachybotrys	Acremonium
Arthrinium	Botrytis
Scopulariopsis	Candida
Gilmaniella	Ulocladium
Zygomycetes	

Only one colony each

Monodictys	Graphium
Helminthosporium	Crysosporium
Sepadonium	Thysanophora
Oidiodendron	Nigrospora
sclerotial-producing	Gliomastix
Custingophora	

include *Cladosporium* (*Hormodendrum*), *Aureobasidium* (*Pullularia*) and *Acremonium* (*Cephalosporium*).

Discussion

September is not only the height of the ragweed season but also the month of second highest airborne fungal prevalence. The results of published studies suggest that in some patients we may be identifying the wrong etiologic allergen, at least underestimating the total antigenic load.

During the month of October the largest number of fungi were recovered. This may in part account for the "persistence of symptoms" after the ragweed season (i.e., the first October frost). Lopez et al and Santilli et al have suggested that the basidiomycetes may be in part responsible for fall symptoms.

The yeasts were the predominant category identified each month. How antigenic these and other categories are remains to be elucidated. Moreover, the complete identification of yeasts is beyond the expertise of most allergists. Possibly a large percentage is represented by only a few of the many genera of yeasts that exist.

The yeast *Rhodotorula* is distinguished by its glistening pink globular colonies and therefore was categorized separately. Adding *Rhodotorula*, the fifth most prevalent category, to the yeast category, which is the number one most prevalent category each month, makes this taxon even more assuming. Candida is also a yeast but can be identified to genus by its white to cream-colored yeast-like colonies at 25 C° and the presence of pseudomycelia.

The bacteria, number 6 in prevalence and present in 50% of the cultures, were also not further differentiated

since these require diagnostic media and techniques not employed in the present studies.

Aureobasidium (*Pullularia*) is number 8 in prevalence. Our area has many transient people who upon transfer here enable us to see previous allergy records from all over the country. This genera is not frequently tested.

The basidiomycetes were identified only if a clamp connection was seen. Some of the mycelia sterilia may have been basidiomycetes as well. In other laboratories many plates may be discarded before the laborious task of seeking clamp connections has been undertaken, leaving them to be added to the mycelia sterilia category. This may be an important observation since mycelia sterilia constitute the second most common classification. Basidiomycetes do not lend themselves easily to further differentiation in culture and rusts and smuts would not be expected to be detected on this medium, since they are basidiomycetes which are strict plant pathogens. Many deuteromycetes are pleomorphic, in that in spite of possessing one genotype, they can produce two or more phenotypes. This may be dependent upon availability of nutrients. This leads to the speculation among taxonomic mycologists that many deuteromycetes (and this includes yeasts) represent the asexual phase of organisms that really belong to the class basidiomycetes.[5a]

The actinomycetes, a group of organisms closely related to bacteria (pro-karyotes), were a surprising observation since our media and methods were not ideal for the isolation of these organisms.[6]

This category might be more prevalent if studies were to be done under conditions appropriate for their growth.

In addition to basidiomycetes, the mycelia sterilia may represent imperfect fungi Again, many of these fungi may have nutrient requirements not provided for in the present studies. The inclusion of petri dishes containing other media in a survey may help further identifications of unsuspected fungi.[2,5b]

The pycnidial-producing organisms included all the Sphaeropsidales except *Phoma*, which is easy to identify by its characteristic large black pycnidium.[7]

Some of the dematiaceous fungi could have been included in the mycelia sterilia, making it even more expansive, but were easily separated due to their dark mycelia. The categories were not all at the same taxonomic level but identification was taken as far as was practical.

Because *Rhodotorula*, *Aureobasidium*, *Epicoccum* and *Geotrichum* are fungi that are commonly isolated but infrequently tested for, it may be worthwhile testing patient reactions to extracts of these in addition to the four that are commonly tested for (*Cladosporium*, *Penicillium*, *Alternaria*, *Aspergillus*). Perhaps other fungi should be tested for antigenic importance if they are significant in the patient's 24-hour exposure.

339

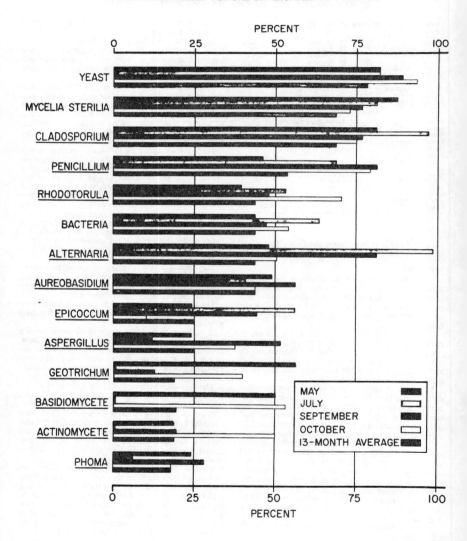

Conclusion

In view of the improvement in our techniques and lack of recent local surveys, a 13-month survey was done to assess the local work-leisure-sleep environments. The times of highest fungal prevalence occurred concurrently with the highest pollen seasons and worst seasons, symptom-wise, for many patients. Yeasts and bacteria have high prevalence but are not commonly tested for reactivity in allergic individuals. Basidiomycetes and actinomycetes were also prevalent. All four of these taxonomic groups require sophisticated studies to further identify their members. Additional studies may also be required to see if antigenicity exists for type 1 atopy.

Rhodotorula, Aureobasidium, Epicoccum, Geotrichum and *Phoma* seem to merit placement in intradermal test sets along with the four commonly tested major fungi (*Cladosporium, Penicillium, Alternaria* and *Aspergillus*). Other fungi could be tested depending upon the results of patients' individual 24-hour environmental culture results.

Acknowledgments

The author is grateful for the reading of all plates by Mr. Chin Shan Yang, word-processing by Mrs. Bonnie Worden and the generous technical advise of Dr. Fred Terracina, taxonomic mycologist, and illustrative services of Mr. Doug Whitman.

References

1. Terracina F., Rogers, SA.: In-home fungal studies: methods to increase the yield. Ann Allergy 49: 35–37, 1982.
2. Rogers, SA.: A comparison of commercially available mold survey services. Ann Allergy 50, #1: 37–40, 1983.
3. Lopez, M., Salvaggio, J. and Butcher, B.: Allergenicity and immunogenicity of basidiomycetes. JACI 57 #5: 480–488, 1976.
4. Santilli, J., March, DG., Collins, RP, Alexander, JF. and Norman, PS.: Basidiospore sensitivity and asthma. JACI 69, #1, Part 2: p. 98. 1982.
5a. Al-Doory Y. and Domson F.: *Mould Allergy.* Lea & Febiger, Philadelphia, chapter 2, 1984.
5b. Ibid, chapter 3.
6. *Fungi of Pulp & Paper in New York,* Wang, CJK. Technical Publication #87. State Univ. College of Forestry at Syracuse Univ., p. 92–95, 1965.
7. *Illustrated Genera of Imperfect Fungi,* Barnett, HL., and Hunter, DB. Burgess Publ. Co., Minneapolis, Minnesota 1972.

Requests for reprints should be addressed to:
Doctor Sherry A. Rogers
2800 West Genesee Street
Syracuse, New York 13219

Advice for the Physician

"Sometimes give your services for nothing, calling to mind a previous benefaction or present satisfaction. And if there by an opportunity of serving one who is a stranger in financial straits, give full assistance to all such. For where there is love of man, there is also love of the art. For some patient, though conscious that their condition is perilous, recover their health simply through their contentment with the goodness of the physician. And it is well to superintend the sick to make them well, to care for the healthy to keep them well, also to care for one's self, so as to observe what is seemly."

Hippocrates

A CASE OF ATOPY WITH INABILITY TO FORM IgG

SHERRY A. ROGERS, M.D., F.A.C.A.

SINCE ISHIZAKA'S DISCOVERY of the reagenic homocytotropic antibody IgE and Szentivanyi's elaboration of the partial beta-adrenergic blockade theory, allergists are more aware of the multiple defects present in the atopic patient. There appears to be a deficient recognition system whereby IgE antibodies are made to materials which are normally not recognized as pathogenic by the rest of the population. There is a defect in the T suppressor cells which apparently would normally inhibit this type of reaction.[1] There is also an apparent cholinergic imbalance with a decreased beta receptor sensitivity within the cell wall[2] and there is an increased sensitivity for histamine release (G_{50} dose) within the cell which appears to be antigen specific.[3,4]

We understand how immunotherapy works to some extent.[5] There is an increase in the serum IgG antibodies and an increase in IgG and secretory IgA antibodies in the secretion as well. IgE antibodies in the serum are generally reduced after several years of immunotherapy but are never eliminated. Several measures of lymphocyte function in the presence of specific antigen are reduced and mediator-containing cells at times show reduced reactivity or sensitivity. The IgG antibody produced appears to have a higher affinity for tissue mast cells than does the IgE. It attaches to the mast cells preferentially, thereby blocking the attachment of IgE which would in turn release the mediators of allergic reactions.[6] As allergists, there are bound to be times when we will discover a patient who is not able to make IgG or who makes extremely small amounts of it. It would intrigue us to know if we could stimulate the formation of IgG in a person who is deficient in it.

Case: M.L. is a 20-year-old Caucasian male who was referred by a chest surgeon for an allergy evaluation. He was the product of a normal pregnancy and delivery and was healthy, tolerating the routine immunizations of childhood until the age of seven. At that time he developed rubella and severe rubella pneumonia. Since that time, for the last 13 years, he has had recurrent bouts of sinusitis and pneumonia innumerable times each year. At age 15 he was operated on for bronchiectasis

of the middle and lower lobe of the right lung. Post-operatively he manifested an empyema requiring completion of a lobectomy on that side. The patient did receive transfusions of blood during his surgery at age 15 without any problem. He never has had occasion to receive gammaglobulin injections and the predominant organism in all of his chest cultures has always been Staphylococcus.

He enjoyed better health for the next four years, having about five episodes of pneumonia a year and still a great deal of sinusitis. At age 19 he presented again to the chest surgeon complaining of repetitive bouts of "flu" with cough, hemoptysis and copious sputum. Chest X-ray showed an infiltrate in the upper lobe of the right lung and bronchography was done again. This was normal, however. At this time studies for cystic fibrosis were negative and immune globulins were done in a local hospital lab which were interpreted as showing IgG decreased in amount, IgA not present, IgM not present, beta 1C normal, A2 macroglobulin normal, albumin normal. Further immunologic studies were not done at that time.

At age 20 the patient was referred to this office for an evaluation to see whether he was allergic. He stated he still had recurrent sinusitis, constant postnasal drip and frequent pneumonias. He was on antibiotics more often than he was off them and it was difficult to perceive where one infection ended and another began.

On examination, he was a normal appearing young man and did not seem chronically ill. He had the normal amount of lymphadenopathy (which, in view of his abnormal amount of infection, was abnormal for him), constant sniffling, some nasal congestion and, otherwise, an unremarkable exam. He complained of chronic sinusitis, postnasal drip and recurrent pneumonias. His father and sister had hay fever and chronic sinusitis.

The laboratory reported a normal CBC, with a differential with 5% serum eosinophilia and a slightly elevated total eosinophil count of 288 eos/mm³. A complete chemical profile was normal except the total protein was slightly reduced at 5 gm/dl and the A/G ratio was elevated to 2.9/1. HDL cholesterol was in the equivocal range (41 mg/dl), suggestive neither of high nor low risk for coronary artery disease. ASO titer was 170 Todd units. Blood type was group A negative, Duffy factor negative, rubella antibody titer was 1:64. There were no anti-A antibodies and the titer for anti-B antibodies was 1:2. Total complement was normal. IgA was nonexistent. IgG was 139 mg/% (normal for his age should be 0.7 to 1.6 gm/dl). IgM was normal at 138 mg/dl. Febrile agglutinins to Salmonella A, B, C, E, D, typhoid and Proteus OX-2, -19 and -K were all negative. Brucella antibodies negative. IgE was 38 U/ml. Urine and serum creatinine were normal. Total urine protein was elevated to 12 mg/dl (normal 2 to 8 mg/dl). A protein electrophoretic breakdown of these components revealed that 75% of this was in the albumin fraction (albumin should only be 38% of the total) and the other 25% was in the gammaglobulin fraction (this should only account for 3% of the total urinary protein). Alpha 1 and 2 globulins and beta globulins were not present at all and these should contribute to 59% of the urinary protein. Additional studies were done on the serum and there were large amounts of Lambda Bence-Jones proteins detected in the serum. These were not, however, detected in the urine.[7]

While awaiting the results of these studies, intradermal tests were done. There were large positive reactions to only Alternaria, cat, Cephalosporium, lambs quarters and tomatoe. Nasal provocations induced sneezing to Aspergillus and Hormodendrum. Nasal provocations were negative to the control talcum, Alternaria and Penicillium. RAST tests were performed to timothy, house dust by Hollister-Stier, *Alternaria tenuis*, oak tree, common ragweed and *Dermatophagoides farinae*. These were all negative.

Diagnosis: (1) dysgammaglobulinemia A and G; (2) benign monoclonal gammopathy; and (3) recurrent chest infections and sinusitis, most likely the result of the dysgammaglobulinemia.

Because allergy is only one constituent of the differential diagnosis of recurrent infection, as allergists we must be sure that patients with abnormal amounts of infection do not have chemotactic deficiencies, immune globulin deficiencies or complement deficiencies. As well, we need to be sure that their T and B cell functions are normal.

Discussion

It is intriguing to think that immunotherapy would possibly stimulate this young man to form more IgG and help with the control of his symptomatology, had he proved to be atopic. However, with the presence of a monoclonal gammopathy, the chance of this being triggered to become a full-blown case of multiple myeloma is far too great. At this point, we can call him benign merely because he is without myeloma symptoms and without macroglobulinuria but no one can tell how long he will remain unchanged or at what point in time he will evolve into a myeloma.[8]

There is also increasing evidence that this type of lambda chain is the precursor for amyloidosis.[9,10]

As for the negative RAST screen, nowhere in the literature has anyone demonstrated that all the antigenic sites of the antigen molecule are exposed as it is attached to the polymer. This may account in part for the better correlation of high degrees of allergy with positive RASTs. We have all noted low degrees of allergy with negative RASTs. The same holds true with the increased frequency of elevated IgE levels seen in severe allergy as compared with lower frequency in milder allergies.[11] However, the results in this case seem to contradict the possibility of atopy.

As with all IgA deficient patients, it is important that they not receive regular gammaglobulin prophylaxis for hepatitis exposure and that they not receive transfusions unnecessarily since, at any time, they could make IgA antibodies and have a resultant anaphylaxis.[12] IgA antibodies were not measured in this patient. It would be interesting to know whether he had them since he had had transfusions with his surgery.

Unfortunately, he became discouraged that surgery could not cure his repeated infections and that he would not be a candidate for immunotherapy. He, therefore, elected to cease any further medical treatment and would not undergo a bone marrow and further diagnostic studies.

References

1. Ishizaka K and Ishizaka T: In *Allergy, Principles and Practice,* Middleton E, Reed C and Ellis E (Eds.). St. Louis: C. V. Mosby Co., 1978.
2. Gold WM: In *Asthma, Physiology, Immunopharmacology and Treatment,* Austen KF and Lichtenstein LM (Eds.). New York: Academic Press, Inc., 1973.
3. Norman PS and Lichtenstein LM: In *Immunological Diseases,* Samter M (Ed.). Boston: Little, Brown & Co., 1971, p. 851.
4. Pruzansky, JJ and Patterson R: Histamine release from leukocytes of hypersensitive individuals. II. Reduced sensitivity of leukocytes after injection therapy. J Allerg 39: 44, 1967.
5. Norman, PS: A Review of Immunotherapy. Allerg 33: 62, 1978.
6. Patterson R, Liebeimer P, Irons JS, Pruzansky JT, Melone HL, Metzger WJ, Zeins CR: Ibid (1).
7. Courtesy of Dr. Thomas Burgess, Upjohn Laboratory Procedures, Inc., Prussia, Pennsylvania.
8. Kyle RA and Bayrd ED: The monoclonal gammopathies in *Multiple Myeloma and Related Plasma Cell Disorders.* Springfield, Ill: Charles C Thomas, 1976, p. 284.
9. Thaler MS, Klauser RD and Cohen HJ: *Medical Immunology.* Philadelphia: J. B. Lippincott Co., 1977, p. 337.
10. Terry WD, et al: Structural identity of Bence-Jones and amyloid fibril proteins in a patient with plasma cell dyscrasia and amyloidosis. J Clin Invest 52: 1276, 1973.
11. Johnson EE, Irons JJ, Patterson R and Roberts M: J Allerg & Clin Immunol 54: 94, 1974.
12. Ammann AJ and Hong R: In *Immunologic Disorders in Infants and Children,* Stiehm ER and Fulginiti VA (Eds.). Philadelphia: W. B. Saunders Co., 1973.

Requests for reprints should be addressed to:
Dr. Sherry A. Rogers
2800 West Genesee Street
Syracuse, NY 13219

APPENDIX

For everyone - physicians and lay:

For any questions, read:
The E.I. Syndrome, by Sherry A. Rogers, M.D.
Box 3161
3502 Brewerton Rd.
Syracuse, NY 13220
$15 + $3 (postage & handling in U.S., $6 elsewhere)
(This book also contains a large "Resources" section.)

and You Are What You Ate, by Sherry A. Rogers, M.D.
Box 3068
3502 Brewerton Rd.
Syracuse, NY 13220
$10 + $3 (postage & handling in U.S., $6 elswhere)

and The Macro Almanac ... from the same publisher.

For mold plates (petri dishes with culture agar) to expose
in your home so you can determine if it is too moldy and
what types of molds are present:
Northeast Center for Environmental Medicine
Mold Survey Service
2800 W. Genesee St.
Syracuse, NY 13219
$15 per plate*
*This price includes a mold plate, a mailer box and address
label in which to return the plate. In 7 weeks or less
(when new molds stop appearing), the molds will be identified and the report mailed to you.

Books of Interest to Physicians

Chemical Sensitivity, by W.J. Rea, M.D.
In press. Write to address below for release date:
8345 Walnut Hill Ln. Ste. 205

Dallas, TX 75231

Casarett and Doull's Toxicology, Basic Science of
Poisons, Third Edition, 1986, Editors: Klaasen, C.D.,
Amdur, M.O., Doull, J., MacMillan, New York

Nutritional Biochemistry and Metabolism, Editor:
Linder, M.C., 1985 Elsevier Science Publishing Company
52 Vanderbilt Ave. New York, NY 10017

Enzymatic Basis of Detoxication, Volumes I and II,
1980, William B. Jakoby, Academic Press

Biologic Basis of Detoxication, J. Caldwell and W.
Jakoby, 1983

Metabolic Basis of Detoxication, W.B. Jakoby, J.R.
Bent, J. Caldwell, Academic Press, New York 1982

Enzymology and Molecular Biology of Carbonyl
Metabolism, Aldehyde Dehydrogenase, Aldo-Keto
Reductase, and Alcohol Dehydrogenase, vol 232, H.
Weiner and T.G. Flynn, Alan R. Liss Inc New York, 1987

Anti-Oxidant Adaptation, Its Role In Free Radical
Pathology, Steven Levine, Ph.D. 1985 Allergy Research
Group, 400 Preda St., San Leandro, CA 94577-1985

Biochemistry, Third Edition, 1988, L. Stryer, W.H.
Freeman and Company, New York

Magnesium Deficiency, Editors: Halpern, M.J., Durlock,
J., 1985, S. Karger, A.G., PO Box CH-4009 Basel,
Switzerland

Nutritional Toxicology, Volume 2, Editor: J.N.
Hathcock, 1987, Academic Press Orlando, FL 32887

Fats and Oils, Udo Erasmus, 1986, Alive Books, PO Box
67333, Vancouver, British Columbia Canada V5W3T1

Harper's Review of Biochemistry, D.W. Martin, P.A.

Mayer, V.W. Rodwell, D.K. Gravner, Lange Medical Publications, Los Altos, CA 94023, 1983

Aldehyde Adducts in Alcoholism, M.A. Collins, Alan R. Liss, Inc., New York, 1985

The Healing Nutrients Within, Facts, Findings, and New Reasearch on Amino Acids, Braverman, ER, Pfeiffer, CC, Keats Publ., Inc., New Canaan, CT, 1987

Enzymology and Molecular Biology of Carbonyl Metabolism, Aldehyde Dehydrogenase and Aldo/Keto Reductase, vol 114, H. Weiner and B. Wermuth, Alan R. Liss Inc., New York, 1982

Beta-Carbolines and Tetrahydroisoquinolines, F. Bloom et al, Alan R. Liss Inc., New York, 1982

Occupational Medicine, Principles and Practical Applications, 2nd Ed. C. Zenz, Year Book Medical Publishers, Inc. Chicago, 1988

Current Topics in Nutrition and Disease, Clinical, Biochemical and Nutritional Aspects of Trace Elements, vol. 6, A. Prasad, Ed., Alan R. Liss, Inc. New York, 1982

1984-85: A Year In Nutritional Medicine, J. Bland, Ed., Keats Publ. Inc., New Canaan, CT, 1986

Metabolism of Trace Elements in Man, vol. 1, O.M. Rennert, W. Chan, CRC Press, Boca Raton, FL, 1985

Molecular Biochemistry of Human Disease, vol I, G. Feaer, F. de la Iglesia, CRC Press, Boca Raton, FL, 1985

Toxicology: Principles and Practice, vol. I, A.L. Reeves, Ed., John Wiley and Sons, NY, 1981

Current Topics in Nutrition and Disease, Volume 2, Chromium in Nutrition and Disease, Saner G, Alan R.

388

Liss Inc., NY, 1980

Zinc: Clinical and Biochemical Significance, S.C.
Cunnane, CRC Press, Boca Raton, FL, 1988

A Guide To General Toxicology, F. Hamburger, J.A.
Hayes, E.W. Pelikin, Karger, New York, 1983

Sulfation of Drugs and Related Compounds, G.J. Mulder,
CRC Press, Boca Raton, FL, 1981

The Metabolic Basics of Inherited Disease, Scriver,
CR, et al, 6th ed., Vol I and II, McGraw Hill, NY,
1989

Taurine and Neurological Disorders, Barbeau, A,
Huxtable, RJ, Raven Press, NY, 1978

Indoor Air '87, Proceedings of the 4th International
Conference on Indoor Air Quality and Climate, Vol. 1,
2, 3, 4; Institute fur wasse-, Boden-und Lufthygiene,
des Bindes gesundhertsantes, Corresplatz, D-1000
Berlin 33 (in English), 1987

Healthy Buildings '88, Swedish Council for Building
Research, Stockholm, Sweden, 1988

Acupuncture Medicine, Its Historical and Clinical
Background, Omura, Y, Japan Publ., Inc., NY, 1982

Human Ecology and Susceptibility To The Chemical
Environment, Randolph, TG, Charles C. Thomas Publ.,
Springfield, IL, 1962

Disposition of Toxic Drugs and Chemicals in Man, 3rd
ed., Baselt RC, Cravey RA, Yearbooks Medical Publ.
Inc., Chicago, 1990

Omega-3, The Fish Oil Factor, Newton WL, Omega-3
Project, Inc., 10615-6 Tierrasanta Blvd., St. 347,
San Diego, CA 92124, 1986

Essential Fatty Acids and Immunity In Mental Health,
Bates C, Life Sciences Press, PO Box 1174, Tacoma, WA
98401, 1987

Bowes and Church's Food Values of Portions Commonly
Used, Pennington JAT, Church HN, JB Lippincott Co.,
Philadelphia, PA, 1985

Books of Interest To Lay and Physicians:

A Bitter Fog, Herbicides and Human Rights, Van Strum,
C, Sierra Club Books, San Francisco, 1983

Peace, Love and Healing, Siegel, BS, Harper and Row
Publ., Inc., NY, 1989

The Body Electric, Becker, RO, Selden, G, William
Morrow and Co., NY, 1985

Nutritional Influences On Illness, Werbech, MR, Third
Line Press, Tarzana, CA, 1987

Mercury Poisoning From Dental Amalgam – A Hazard To
Human Brain, Stortebecker, P, Bio-Probe, Inc., PO Box
58010, Orlando, FL 32858-0160, 1985

How to build or renovate a non-toxic home:
Your Home, Your Health and Well Being, by
D. Rousseau, W.J. Rea, J. Enwright
Hartley & Marks, Publ.
3663 W. Broadway
Vancouver, B.C. VGR 2B8
1988

The theory of macrobiotics:
The Book of Macrobiotics, by Michio Kushi
Japan Publ. Inc.
(Harper and Rowe), New York
1986

A physician who cleared prostate cancer

with macrobiotics:
Recalled By Life, by A.J. Sattilaro, M.D.
Avon, New York
1984

A young housewife who cleared metastic cancer of the
    ovaries:
Recovery, by Elaine Nussbaum
Japan Publications, ibid.

For companion theory and practical cookbooks on macrobiotic
    management of allergies, arthritis, etc:

Macrobiotic Health And Education Series
    by Michio Kushi

Allergies - A Natural Approach
Arthritis - A Natural Approach
Diabetes and Hypoglycemia - A Natural Approach
Infertility and Reproductive Disorders - A Natural
    Approach
Obesity, Weight Loss and Eating Disorders - A Natural
    Approach

Macrobiotic Food And Cooking Series
    by Aveline Kushi

Allergies - Cooking for Health
Arthritis - Cooking for Health
Diabetes and Hypoglycemia - Cooking for Health
Infertility and Reproductive Disorders - Cooking for
    Health
Obesity, Weight Loss and Eating Disorders - Cooking
    for Health

Japan Publ. Inc.
(Harper & Row), New York
Or order above books from:
Natural Lifestyles Supplies
16 Lookout Drive
Ashville, NC 28804
704-254-9606

Or from:
N.E.E.D.S.
602 Nottingham Rd.
Syracuse, NY 13224
1-800-643-1380 (continental U.S., including NY)

For general, non-technical information on vitamins:
Super-Nutrition, Megavitamin Revolution,
by R. Passwater
Pocket Books
(Simon & Schuster, Inc.), New York
1975

Nutrition and Vitamin Therapy,
by M. Lesser
Grove Press, Inc.
196 W. Houston St.
New York, NY 10014
1980

The Nutrition Desk Reference,
by R.H. Garrison
Keats Publ. Inc.
New Canaan, CT 06840
1985

For more general information on clinical allergies:
An Alternative Approach to Allergies,
by T.G. Randolph, R.W. Moss
Bantam Books
1987

For more information on Candida:
The Yeast Connection, by W.G. Crook
Professional Books
PO Box 3494
Jackson, TN 38301
1986

and   The Yeast Syndrome by J. Trowbridge and M. Walker
Bantam Books, NY

<u>Hypoallergenic Nutrients Formulated for the Ecologist</u>
(send for catalogues)

Allergy Research Group
400 Preda St.
PO Box 489
San Leandro, CA   94577
1-800-545-9960
415-639-4572

Klaire Laboratories Inc.
1573 W. Seminole St.
San Marcos, CA   92069
1-800-533-7255
619-744-9680

Cardiovascular Research
1061-B Shary Circle
Concord, CA   94518
415-827-2636

Probiologic (T.E. Neesby Inc.)
1803-132nd Ave. NE
Bellevue, WA   98005
1-800-426-1047
1-306-581-8218 (WA)

N.E.E.D.S.
602 Nottingham Rd.
Syracuse, NY   13224
1-800-634-1380
Catalogue of most of the items needed for a less toxic
lifestyle (supplements, air cleaners, foods, books,
etc.). Will ship any where.

HEAL (Human Ecology Action League)
PO Box 49126
Atlanta, GA   30359-1126
A national organization with chapters throughout the
world, formed as a resource and support group for

people with E.I.

<u>Primary Seminars and Courses</u>, for physicians and their staff
    (emphasis on all aspects of total load)

For annual scientific seminars and basic, intermediate, and
    advanced training courses:

    American Academy of Environmental Medicine*
    Box 16106
    Denver, CO 80216

*   If you send $3 and a self-addressed, stamped envelope
    they will send you a list of physician members in your
    region of the country. Bear in mind, there is a wide
    variation in level of practice expertise, for we are
    all at different levels of learning.

    Annual World Conference
    Man and His Environment in Health and Disease
    c/o Dr. William J. Rea
    8345 Walnut Hill Ln., Suite 205
    Dallas, TX 75231
    (214) 368-4132

<u>Secondary Seminars and Courses</u>

Emphasis on nutrition:
    North American Nutrition and Preventive Medicine Assc.
    in conjunction with the University of Georgia
    c/o Ms. Bonnie Jarrett, Director
    9895 Buice Rd.
    Alpharetta, GA 30201

Emphasis on Candida:
    International Health Foundation
    PO Box 3494
    Jackson, TN 38303

Emphasis on beginner level:
    Pan American Allergy Society

PO Box 947
Fredericksburg, TX 78624

Emphasis on beginner level and RAST testing:
American Academy of Otolaryngic Allergy
1101 Vermont Ave. NW
Washington, D.C. 20005

Audio Recordings of Seminars
    (If you have a hobby where you can wear a cassette
    player, you'll get a fantastic education from these
    tapes of all the courses and seminars you've missed.)

Instatape
PO Box 1729
Monrovia, CA 91016
1-800-322-TAPE

For Specialized Blood Tests

    Pesticides and Other Xenobiotics
    Dr. John Laseter
    Accu-Chem Laboratories
    E.H.S. Inc.
    990 Bowser Suite 800
    Richardson, TX 75081

Testing of Nutrient Levels
    Doctor's Data Inc.
    PO Box 111
    West Chicago, IL 60185
    1-800-323-2784
    312-231-3649

    Monroe Medical Laboratories
    Rt 17 PO Box 1
    Southfields, NY 10975
    914-351-5134

For Other Difficult to Find Specialized Tests
        in Nutritional Biochemistry
    Meridian Valley Chemical Labs

24030-132nd SE
Kent, WA 98038
1-800-234-6825

Interpretation of Biochemical Data
   Bionostics
   John Pangborn, Ph.D.
   PO Drawer 400
   Lisle, IL 60532

For highly chemically sensitive people in need of hospitalization, surgery, nutritionally monitored sauna programs, or chemically less-contaminated transient living quarters to reduce chemical load:

   American Environmental Health Center
   c/o Dr. William J. Rea
   8345 Walnut Hill Lane, Suite 205
   Dallas, TX 75231

Literature search sources include:

Special thanks to Dr. Wagdy Tadros, Dr. Abdel Amin, Dr. Mohan Mysore, and Dr. Arnold Yeadon of Respiratory Search, a professional service of Rorer Pharmaceuticals, Engelwood, New Jersey, for computer searches and providing abstracts:
   1-800-426-8440 or 1-800-338-0176

   Ms. Diana Reinstein
   Medical Librarian
   Community General Hospital
   Syracuse, NY

   Family Health Foundation of America
   (A philanthropic arm of the American
   Academy of Family Physicians)
   8880 Ward Parkway
   Kansas City, MO 64114-0418
   1-800-274-2237

For Doctors Only:

You can copy the following protocol for the oral magnesium loading test on your letterhead and use as a patient handout to explain the rationale and instructions for doing the oral magnesium loading test. Being an oral challenge, it, of course, has the drawback of relying on normal renal function and absorption. But you'll find more magnesium deficiency this way than trying to convince people to have magnesium given I.M. or I.V. You can, of course, when the suspicion arises of malabsorption, switch to 0.2 mEq/kg body weight of either magnesium chloride or magnesium sulfate (Clinical Ecology, vol 4, #1, pg 17-20, Rea, WJ, 1986).

For parenteral loading challenge, the percent of excretion is calculated by dividing the baseline excretion plus the challenge dose into the challenge excretion and multiplying by 100. Magnesium deficiency is defined as less than 80% excretion.

For the oral challenge, omit adding the challenge dose in the calculation and call it positive if there is over 40% retention. In other words, divide the "after" magnesium into the "before"; certainly anything over 50% retention deserves a trial. In most cases, a therapeutic trial cleared resistant symptoms, affirming that this isn't a bad estimate. Further refinement is under way.

In devising this protocol, I used Slow-Mag because it is made by a pharmaceutical firm. This makes it universally available for standardization and many patients have insurance prescription coverage. Also absorption characteristics have been studied. It has drawbacks, in that the many additives are not always tolerated by the chemically sensitive patient. In this case, you will need to substitute a magnesium formulation that is tolerated by your patient.

In the case of patients who have an above normal excretion, these are termed renal magnesium wasters. A trial of injectable magnesium sulfate (one 50 mg ampule I.M. two times at least, an hour apart, being sure there are good patellar reflexes before each injection) will give a better idea of magnesium pools. Collect a 24 hour urine magnesium the day of the injections and calculate the percent retention from that. Also the injection will often correct the renal magnesium wasting, making a return to oral supplementation possible.

Note: After evaluating the first 300 people with this test, we found that there was a percentage who actually put out less magnesium on the single urine magnesium follow-up than they had on the "before" urine of the magnesium loading test. Because these people had dramatic improvement in symptoms with the follow-up test, we did a complete "before" and after loading test after they had followed the follow-up protocol. What we found was they had now saturated, but had much lower baseline retentions. They had markedly improved their daily conservation of magnesium, or reset their renal conservation threshold.

Protocol For Oral Magnesium Loading Test

MAGNESIUM DEFICIENCY.......The Silent Epidemic

An unsuspected magnesium deficiency is almost epidemic and potentially life threatening. U.S. Government studies (Science News, vol 133 June 1988) show that the average American diet supplies about 40% of the recommended daily amount (RDA) of magnesium. Taking medications (like diuretics for blood pressure or fluid retention), having chronic symptoms, sweating, alcohol, eating fast foods, poor absorption because of inflamed bowel (as from Candida), being on IV's in a hospital and many other things serve to lower magnesium at a faster rate. Many magnesium authorities (Dr. Mildred Seelig, Dr. William Rea) suggest that at least 80% of the population has a hidden magnesium deficiency.

Since magnesium is important in over 300 enzymes, the symptoms of deficiency can be anything from just plain feeling tired, depressed, irritable or weak to having muscular spasm problems. Remember, calcium makes a muscle contract, while magnesium (or death) makes it relax. So a magnesium deficiency will result in unopposed calcium induced contraction or spasm. Diseases of spasm include migraines (brain blood vessel smooth muscle spasm), asthma (bronchial smooth muscle spasm), colitis (intestinal smooth muscle spasm), coronary artery disease, cystitis, strokes, uterine hemorrhage, chronic back pain, infertility and hypertension. Other symptoms of magnesium deficiency may include osteoporosis, uncorrectable potassium deficiency, chronic back pain, phlebitis, irritability, chronic muscle or joint pain, mental confusion, dizziness, balance problems, diabetes, depression, exhaustion, kidney stones, heart attack, cardiac arrhythmias or palpitations, arteriosclerosis, insomnia, seizures or twitchy lung; for really any symptom is possible especially those that defy categorizing or are "undiagnosable".

Because nutrition has taken a back seat ever since patent medicines became so powerful, magnesium deficiency is rarely thought of in a differential diagnosis process. Because it is readily depleted by sweating, for example, and because it causes muscle spasm, it is responsible for many cases of sudden death in seemingly healthy athletes. When the smooth muscles around delicate coronary (heart) blood vessels go into spasm, the heart muscle is deprived of oxygen. When this happens, it can respond by becoming very irritable or excited and go into fibrillation, an arrhythmia that may cause instant death. There's much likelihood that physically fit joggers who had sudden death were magnesium depleted from excessive sweating.

In spite of all this, a magnesium deficiency is rarely diagnosed. This is partly because a magnesium serum test is nearly useless. Because of a protective balancing mechanism of the body's called homeostasis, by the time that the serum magnesium becomes abnormal, you are in dire straights in an emergency room with convulsions or arrhythmia (if you live that long). An RBC (red blood cell) or erythrocyte magnesium is great if it's abnormal, but studies have shown (Rea, Clinical Ecology, vol 4, #1, 17-20, 1986) that if it's normal, the individual can still be devastatingly low in magnesium. This was proven when an intravenous test dose of magnesium quickly turned off symptoms. The best test at present is the magnesium loading test (M.L.T.)

The Magnesium Loading Test

To do the magnesium loading test, first start with a 24 hour urine test for magnesium. This will measure how much magnesium you excrete in 24 hours under normal circumstances. When you awake in the morning, discard the very first urine and then collect every drop of urine for the next 24 hours. This means you must put your jug on top of the toilet seat so you won't forget, especially in the middle of the night. Be sure to collect the first morning urine of the following morning (since you did not collect it the preceding day), as this marks the end of your 24 hour collection period).

You must carry your jug wherever you go. (You can put it in a shopping bag so that it won't be noticed.) Refrigerate the jug after collection of the "before" urine is complete. Refrigeration during collection is not necessary.

For the next stage of the magnesium test, begin your Slow Mag prescription, 2 tablets three times a day. They are best taken with breakfast, lunch and dinner. It can be started right after you collect the last urine (first morning) for the "before" urine test. On day two of the magnesium prescription, begin the second urine test. Again discard the first morning urine and collect all the urine all day long, all night long, and the first morning urine of the next day. Remember, the second urine collection will be on the second day of magnesium ingestion, taken as two tablets three times a day. If you forget a dose, make it up as soon as you remember, even if it means you have to take 4 at a meal. You could then take two before the meal and two after the meal to avoid gastric upset. At the end of the urine collection, refrigerate the second container as well, until you take both urine bottles back to the laboratory or office you obtained them from.

The laboratory will measure the amount of magnesium excreted in both containers (the "before" and "after"). These values are used by the doctor to make a calculation to see if your body soaked up all this magnesium like a sponge (because it was deficient), or if it put it out in the urine because there was sufficient magnesium already in the system. The percentage of magnesium that was retained shows whether you seem deficient or sufficient in magnesium. (However, even this is not fool proof, since you may be a poor absorber of magnesium. Injections can be used if there is suspicion of this.)

In the meantime, continue the magnesium for the 2 week trial that is on your prescription and finish up all the pills, 2 three times a day to see what effect this magnesium load may also have on your symptoms. If it produces a beneficial effect, be sure to let the doctor know in writing what exact symptoms were better so that more can be prescribed. Do not phone the office to tell your symptoms or ask for a prescription or lab test results. The personnel are not equipped with this information and it is an interpretation that requires interaction between the doctor and patient. It is not a cut and dried absolute test of pass or fail. Remember, medicine is constantly learning so never discount the feedback that your body provides, since the bottom line is how you feel and not how any laboratory test looks on a piece of paper.

For example, one gal had a perfectly normal magnesium loading test on paper. But when she came to the office, I learned that she felt fantastic on the magnesium and it stopped six different symptoms she had been plagued with for years. On closer questioning, the day she did the second magnesium, she had been suffering from "a wicked sunburn". Her urine volume was extremely small, since most of the water had gone to the skin to help healing. Repeating the test showed she was extremely deficient and gave us a good idea on how much correction she needed.

You might question, "Why don't we just forget the two 24 hour urine tests and just take a trial of magnesium?" The reason is clear: Normally if the second test shows that say 80% of the dose of magnesium was excreted (and 20% was retained), then you do not store the extra magnesium because your body already has sufficient storage of it. But if you found that after your two week trial of magnesium, that some of your symptoms were markedly improved, it would suggest a different story. It would suggest that you are magnesium deficient, and the reason you are is that your kidneys waste or get rid of too much magnesium. They don't know enough to conserve it when you are deficient. Only the urine test would tell us that your kidneys are unable to conserve magnesium appropriately. This is a very important fact, because it tells us additionally that you'll need much higher doses of magnesium than normal and careful monitoring over time.

Interestingly, man has discovered the usefulness of magnesium in the past without being directly aware of it's relaxant properties: epsom salts for sprains, milk of magnesia for cramps, magnesium injections for eclampsia of pregnancy (a life threatening condition with extremely high blood pressure and convulsions and coma in the pregnant mother), and all the new calcium channel blockers for heart problems, (if magnesium is low, it makes it appear to the body that calcium is disproportionately high, so expensive drugs are used to block the calcium).

Remember, there are two ways to treat a symptom. Cover it up with drugs or find the cause and correct it. With the magnesium loading test we have one more important tool to help us identify and correct the cause.

Note: If your magnesium prescription from the doctor has a dose different from the above, follow your prescription directions in place of the above 2 tablets 3 times a day.

Note: The urine containers contain a small but necessary amount of dangerous hydrochloric acid. Do not touch it nor discard it.

	M.L.T. ------ REVIEW
FRIDAY	*Throw away first urine. *Save all the rest of urine all day and night.
SATURDAY	*Save 1st morning urine. Now refrigerate the bottle and print name, date, and "before" magnesium on it. *Now start magnesium tablets (Slow Mag) 2 three times a day: {2 at breakfast {2 at lunch {2 at dinner *Continue these 2 tablets 3 times a day until the Rx of 100 is finished.
SUNDAY	*On day 2 of the magnesium test, do another 24 hour urine for magnesium (only this time you are taking your magnesium 2 three times a day). Again discard the first urine and collect all of it (every drop) all day and night.
MONDAY	*Collect first morning urine to go into the container. Label the container

"after" and add your name and date.
Failure to follow these directions
exactly will waste your time and
money and give no helpful information
about your body. Return both containers to the office or laboratory where you
got them.

TUESDAY *Be sure to continue the magnesium prescription until it is finished and report in
writing to the doctor if the magnesium
helped in any way or made you feel better.
(This is an important part of the test that
doesn't get reported by the lab!)

*Schedule an appointment to go over the
results with the doctor in 3-4 weeks.
Do not call the office to merely report your results or to find out the
results of your test. This is not a
cut and dried normal or abnormal
test. It must be interpreted in
light of many factors which the staff
are not prepared to evaluate. As
always, however, you should call the
office if you have any problem.

It's exciting to be at the entry of the era of molecular biochemistry into medicine. As part of environmental
medicine, it continues to change the rules of medicine by
making the patient an intergral part of the medical team.

Case example: LR was a chemically sensitive young woman
when she was exposed to traffic exhaust, perfumes, and certain other chemicals. She would get frightening throat
spasms. The magnesium loading test showed 75% retention of
the initial dose. Magnesium cleared her symptoms and she no
longer has throat spasms when exposed to chemicals.

Doctor: Once you have found your patient to be suspicious for magnesium deficiency, you'll want to not only saturate his stores of magnesium, but verify that this has been done. Also you'll want a follow-up 24 hour urine magnesium to determine just how useful this test is and whether it might need modification. Furthermore, you'll want to re-assess the magnesium status within a year to determine if this deficiency is a recurrent problem. Hopefully your patient will be eating better by then (organic whole foods) so that it won't be a recurrent problem.

The following magnesium follow-up protocol can then be given when you see them to go over the results of the loading test.

If they always have 50% or more retention (or 50% or less excretion), then you'll want to consider a parenteral trial to bypass absorption problems.

Obviously an oral test has drawbacks of relying on normal digestion and assimilation, bowel transit time and renal function. Magnesium sulfate injections can be given during the "after urine" if poor absorption is suspected. Once confirmed, gastric analysis for sufficient hydrochloric acid is in order. The Heidelberg test or Levine tube method can be used. Hypochlorhydria appears to be second in importance as a factor in hypomagnesemia; first being a diet low in nutrient density.

If the Slow Mag (6 tablets) were not tolerated, Magnesium Complex (Bronson) (2 tabs) or Magnesium solution 18% (Cardiovascular Research, Ltd.) (3tsp), magnesium taurate (Cardiovascular Research) (3 tabs), Magnesorb (Neesby) (3 tabs), or magnesium sulfate injections (2 a day) may be used.

MAGNESIUM FOLLOW UP PROTOCOL

If your retention was 50% or higher or you felt demonstrably
better on the magnesium, this suggests that you were very
magnesium deficient. Now you want to take 2 Slow Mag twice
a day for 2 months. At the end of that time, pick up one
more jug for a 24 hour urine for magnesium, then switch back
to 2 Slow Mag three times a day. On the second day of the
Slow Mag get the 24 hour urine, as you did before.

How Long	Dose	Comments
2 months	two twice a day (or a more tolerable substitute if necessary)	
2 days	two 3 times a day (or whatever other special dose you had before; this dose should be exactly the same as the first time you did the test)	on second day you will be collecting 24 hr. urine for magnesium again.

Finish the magnesium one twice a day.

After that is done, then finish your magnesium as one twice
a day and do not get more after it is done. When we receive
the magnesium we will be able to calculate whether you have
finally saturated your magnesium stores and now have less
than 40% retention, which is normal. You should definitely
be under 50%. We will contact you if your results are abnormal. If you don't hear anything, it is normal.

By then you should be stable enough to have changed your
diet to more whole grains and vegetables and gotten off
processed foods, cokes, coffee and junk foods so that you
will never get magnesium deficient again. Also, organic
foods possess far more magnesium than commercially grown

foods. If at any time you suspect you are low, please come in so that we can help you balance it early to avoid unnecessary symptoms. For if your stores get periodically depleted, you may need a maintenance dose. Remember magnesium is crucial in over 300 enzymes and a deficiency of it can cause any symptom you can think of. So it's very crucial to your overall mental and physical health and future well-being. But when it is treated without optimal knowledge, the balance of over a dozen other minerals can be upset; so it must be done judiciously.

You might say, "Well, if I feel better why do I need to repeat this urine test?" The reason is that it's the only way to know that the stores and all 300 enzyme sites are filled or saturated. Because if they are not, you'll continue to have "vague" symptoms and problems that will be chalked up to "aging", like loss of teeth requiring expensive bridge work, osteoporosis that tests won't show for 20 years when it is not longer correctable, easy sprains, muscle problems, etc., etc. ------- any symptom is possible. Symptoms will bounce around from one target organ to another as the body "robs Peter to pay Paul" in an attempt to put the magnesium where it is needed the most at the moment.

It's exciting that we have the biochemical tools for wellness. Now it is up to us to use them to our maximum benefit.

Please fill out and mail to the office so we can learn more about you and magnesium:

Name: _____
Date: _____

When I finished the 2 day magnesium loading test and took 2 weeks of magnesium, it helped these symptoms:

_____ _____

_____ _____

It caused these adverse reactions:

_____

When I did the two months of magnesium it helped these symptoms:

_____

_____

It caused these adverse reactions:

_____

Overall, the magnesium helped make me feel (circle one)

25% better   50% better   75% better   100% better

no change

Comments:

****

Note: If you had to switch horses in mid-stream and change to another form of magnesium, you'll need a before and after urine for the follow-up (just as you did for the initial loading test). Also if you were a renal magnesium waster initially, you'll need 2 urines for follow-up, since often the wasting corrects, so the baseline is reset.

GLOSSARY and INDEX

acetaldehyde - an intermediary metabolite in the breakdown
of some chemicals and brain hormones, also made by
Candida; highly toxic to the body if it stays in this
stage and doesn't get metabolized further into an excretable and less toxic acid. 65, 99, 105, 161, 162
233, 249, 252, 313.

acetylcholine - a neurotransmitter, a chemical that is responsible for memory and transmission of information
between nerves and muscles. 111, 148, 161, 175, 184,
319, 354.

adaptation - the process whereby the body "gets used to" or
begins to tolerate something that could be harmful for
it; the process requires energy and uses up enzymes
and nutrients. 79, 85-87, 91, 92, 261, 290, 302, 305,
310, 353, 378.

adducts - dangerous metabolites that attach to DNA, for
example, and change it forever; often causing cancer
or target organ destruction. 84, 163, 310.

adrenal gland test - cortrosyn stimulation test. 329.

adrenalin - epinephrine, the "fight or flight" or stress
hormone of the body. 111, 148, 161, 163, 325.

alcohol dehydrogenase - an enzyme that changes the alcohol
stage to an aldehyde; a Phase I detox enzyme. 48, 56,
101, 153, 167, 170, 173, 186, 191.

aldehyde - a general category of intermediate metabolites
that are toxic to the body if a bottleneck or block
occurs here. 24, 31, 47, 48, 51, 55, 56, 65, 99, 101-
105, 111, 115, 142-144, 153, 161-163, 165-168, 170,
175, 186, 187, 196, 226, 233, 235, 245, 249, 318, 319,
324.

aldehyde dehydrogenase - the enzyme that metabolizes toxic aldehydes to safer acids that can be excreted. 65, 81, 115, 153, 168, 233, 319, 321.

aldehyde oxidase - another enzyme that metabolizes aldehydes, requires molybdenum and iron. 48, 153, 167, 170, 173, 319.

aldehyde reductase - another enzyme that metabolizes aldehydes back to alcohols. 116.

aliphatic - simply means the carbon atoms in the molecule form a chain (see aromatic). 34.

aluminum - an element found in the brains of Alzheimer's patients; it can get there from inhaling aluminum in city industrial smog, using aluminum beer and soda cans, cookware, it's an anti-caking agent in salt, baking powder, etc. 60, 270, 272, 275, 281, 371, 372.

Alzheimer's - a disease where one becomes prematurely senile. A surgeon in his 50's, for example, in one year's time can become so incapacitated that he has only the skills of a 3 year old and not a quarter of the memory retention; could not even appropriately dress self or cross the road, no recent memory, cannot recall what he ate one hour ago. 93, 148, 161, 212, 213, 269, 270, 353-355, 363, 371, 378.

amino acid - building blocks of proteins, essential for life. 9, 25, 40, 41, 45, 52, 54, 55, 60, 94, 96, 140, 148, 153, 157, 170, 172, 175, 180, 181, 184-187, 190-192, 230, 231, 251, 257, 266, 294, 306, 318, 319, 324, 329, 352, 354, 368, 372.

aneurysm - a weakening and ballooning of a section of vessel wall that can lead to rupture and death. 169, 243.

angina - chest pain due to spasm or cholesterol blockage of coronary (heart) blood vessels, so not enough oxygen gets to the heart. You know how painful a muscle can be if you use it constantly and don't rest it? The heart never gets to rest. 159, 226, 240, 241.

antioxidants – the vitamins and minerals that control dangerous free radicals and keep them from damaging the body (examples, vitamins A, C, E). 140, 269, 296, 354.

anti-parietal antibody – a protein made in the body that attacks cells in the stomach making it impossible for oral vitamin B12 to be absorbed. 181.

aorta – the main large artery of the heart. 169, 229.

arachidonic acid – one of the end metabolites of Omega-6 fatty acids that are responsible for producing undesirable symptoms (like asthma). 207.

aromatic – merely describes the structure of hydrocarbon chemicals and means the carbons in a chemical structure form a ring (see aliphatic). 24, 34, 53, 166, 321.

arrhythmia – irregular heartbeat, palpitations; since the heart (a pump) is not beating properly it can lead to poor delivery of oxygen to heart or brain and be fatal. 51, 74, 153, 154, 157, 159, 216, 231, 241, 242, 325, 379, 382.

arteriosclerosis – hardening of the arteries where the walls become rigid and plugged with cholesterol, thereby raising the pressure as well as restricting the flow to end organs, causing disease in many organs. 24, 63, 153, 176, 187, 206, 209, 211, 212, 214-218, 228-232, 235, 237, 240, 241, 252, 254, 255, 257, 329.

arthritis – inflammation of joints with pain and stiffness and often swelling; can be caused by a reaction to an everyday food and/or chemical, or other factors. 12, 14, 28-30, 33, 62, 63, 70-73, 83, 98, 99, 108, 109,

142, 150, 157, 163, 190, 209, 220-222, 251, 252, 257, 316, 333, 336, 339, 340, 369.

ataxia - poor balance.   126, 135.

ATP - adenosine triphosphate - the tiny molecular storage and transport form for energy in the body.   44, 146, 329, 330.

auto-cannibalism - where the body literally eats itself; for example; if the body is deficient in some substance in one area, it will "rob Peter to pay Paul" and steal it from one place to put it elsewhere; if the substance is phosphatidyl choline and is stolen from the brain membranes to be used, for example in the detox membranes, the brain membranes become deficient and Alzheimer's can result.   270, 354, 355.

auto-immune - allergenic to itself, for example, rheumatoid arthritis is an auto-immune disease, because the body makes antibodies against the joint tissues and attacks them as though they were a foreign invader, hence inflammation and pain.   33, 63, 147, 332.

Benveniste, Dr. Jacque - the French researcher who proved homeopathy.   25, 346, 347.

benzene - a common chemical in indoor air from carpets, gasoline, rubber, etc.; it is known to initiate leukemia.   16-19, 23, 24, 36, 67, 83, 88, 89, 125, 129, 141, 142, 279, 295, 296.

BHT - a toluene derivative that is in food to stop it from going bad {toluene is methyl-benzene, or benzene with a methyl (CH3) group attached}.   24.

bile - substance secreted by the gall bladder; is the exit route for many chemicals to go from the liver to the gut and be excreted.   40, 41, 42, 54, 56, 60, 96, 131, 165, 184, 217, 232.

bioaccumulation - the dangerous result of the input of chemicals exceeding the ability of the body to get rid of them, hence they get stored in body tissues, usually lipids. 79, 88, 105, 124, 128, 132, 176, 201, 304, 310.

biochemistry - the study of chemistry of living things. 8, 9, 34, 35, 43, 47, 50, 57, 68, 70, 72, 80, 83, 89, 94, 97-99, 102, 105, 143, 150, 155, 163, 166, 168, 174, 176, 181, 187, 196, 203, 205, 217, 218, 237, 241, 244, 257, 294, 302, 303, 306, 309, 310, 318, 320, 332-335, 345, 346, 351-354, 358, 361-363, 366,367, 369, 370, 372, 378, 380, 383, 384.

biotransformation - using the body to change a substance to a different chemical, usually to make it less toxic and excretable, synonymous with detoxication. 36, 43, 44, 91, 115.

bipolarity - the existence of opposite phases for the same trigger resulting in a stimulatory phase initially and a depressant phase with withdrawal eventually as adaptive enzyme systems become depleted. 90, 105, 304, 305.

bottleneck - a stricture (figure of speech); like a traffic jam; a common pathway for many metabolites, where a blockage or slowing of function will cause serious backlog and eventual shift of metabolites to alternative routes. 24, 47, 55, 65, 99, 104, 105, 111, 115, 116, 125, 153, 161, 162, 165, 170, 186, 226, 229, 233, 235, 249, 319, 323.

Brassaciae - the family of cabbages, broccoli, cauliflower, Brussel sprouts, turnips, etc., also known as Cruciferae. 55.

calcification - getting hard and brittle and degenerating faster than normal, due to deposition of the unmetabolized mineral, calcium. 237, 240, 243, 244.

calcium - a necessary mineral in bone, nerve and muscle function, etc. 95, 156, 159, 171, 192, 193, 219, 226,

227, 231, 232, 234, 236-244, 254, 255, 269, 270, 311, 322, 329, 378.

calcium channel blockers – expensive drugs to regulate heart and blood pressure that usually mean someone forgot to do a magnesium loading test. 9, 241, 242.

Candida – a fungus or mold or yeast that is normal in the intestine if it grows in normal amounts; its growth is accelerated by antibiotics and sugars. 30, 62, 90, 95, 103-105, 108, 161, 166, 167, 233, 247-253, 257, 262, 263, 293, 313, 331, 369.

carbon monoxide – a gas in the exhausts of industry, autos, furnaces; in the bloodstream it is a poison. 17, 21, 37, 84.

carbon tetrachloride – a common chemical solvent and also a highly potent liver toxin, CCl_4. 19, 20, 125.

carcinogen – an agent that can help lead to cancer growth by poisoning the growth regulatory system of a cell, usually occurs slowly and silently over many years. 13, 162.

carcinogenic – able to cause cancer. 18, 55, 67, 114, 225, 275, 321, 326, 362, 371.

catalyze – augment, help along.

catecholamine – a category of hormones, includes adrenalin (epinephrine, the flight or fight hormone). 162, 163.

cerebral – having to do with the brain. 63, 143, 167.

chemical sensitivity – can be any symptom that results from the body's inability to detoxify the everyday chemicals that are in everyone's bloodstream. 13, 21, 24, 25, 28-31, 37, 46, 47, 52, 57, 65-67, 82, 84, 87, 98, 102, 105, 106, 108, 112, 115, 116, 129, 137, 146, 162-166, 180, 185, 333, 336, 339, 359.

chloral hydrate - "Mickey Finn" or knock-out drops, also made in the brain if detox path is overloaded. 24, 32, 46, 48, 56, 61, 102, 111, 137, 143, 167, 170, 313.

chloroform - an anesthetic that can form in your shower from the aerosolization (spray) of the contaminating chemicals that are in most city water supplies. 19, 20, 125, 296.

chlorpyrifos - Dursban, a commonly used toxic organophosphate pesticide in schools, homes and offices. 117, 135.

cholesterol - a necessary fat in the body, but becomes dangerous if sufficient nutrients are not available for its proper metabolism; then it just lays down on damaged blood vessel walls in attempt to patch them up, creating arteriosclerotic plaques. 24, 77, 95, 154, 169, 211-219, 227-235, 252-254, 327, 329, 378, 379.

choline acetyl transferase - an enzyme necessary for the metabolism of the brain and nerve hormone acetyl choline. 161.

chromium - a necessary mineral for sugar and lipid metabolism, also in the digestive enzyme trypsin; lack of it can cause diabetes or arteriosclerosis, it is in whole grains but removed when they are processed to flours. 63, 191, 192, 194, 211, 213-215, 226-232, 235, 239, 254, 257, 311, 336, 349.

chronic fatigue syndrome (CFS) - the name given for a constellation of symptoms, which include fatigue, by doctors untrained in environmental medicine; provides a presumed rationale for stopping the search for a further cause. 6, 11, 59, 151, 181, 190, 338, 363-365.

chronic mono - same as CFS, only there are positive blood tests for the Epstein-Barr virus; (there possibly are actually people who have this and cannot get better.

I just haven't seen any who cannot get better). 6, 59, 70, 190, 364.

claudication - blockage of a vessel (through spasm or cholesterol deposits) causing pain in the muscle that should be fed by this vessel. 226.

CoA - short for acetyl coenzyme A, an important metabolite in many reactions in the body. 54, 140, 175, 184.

complement - one of the proteins in the pathway leading to inflammation. 248.

complement sequence - the cascade or multiple reaction stages that the proteins that cause inflammation go through in order to damage the body. 163.

confusion - inability to concentrate, poor thought process. 21, 22, 124, 126.

conjugation - coupling of a chemical with a protein so it can be flushed out of the body easier. 41, 44, 52, 54, 56, 116, 140, 153, 160, 165, 166, 173, 175, 184–186, 232, 306, 318, 324, 333, 354.

copper - a mineral important in over a dozen enzymes; low levels can cause high cholesterol and aneurysms. 156, 168–173, 191–193, 232, 237–239, 307.

coronary - having to do with the heart blood vessels. 24, 153, 219, 223, 224, 230, 234, 239, 241, 336, 380.

corrective - a temporary and intentionally unbalanced nutrient program, designed to dove-tail with and correct an existing deficiency. 145, 173, 174, 195.

cortrosyn stimulation test - 190, 329.

cross linking - the making of abnormal chemical bonds that can accelerate aging and lead to cancer; usually caused by a chemical or free radicals. 162.

cruciferous - see Brassaciae. 55, 324.

cyanide - a poison found in some pesticides that has particular propensity for the white matter of the brain. 19, 36, 125.

cysteine - an amino acid crucial to Phase II detox. 41, 52, 56, 96, 116, 140, 153, 165, 166, 171, 172, 184-186, 193, 195, 252, 269, 354.

cystitis - inflammation and spasm of the urinary bladder, common causes are magnesium deficiency and hidden food allergy. 70, 98, 159, 240, 274, 370.

cytochrome C oxidase - an enzyme involved in electron transfer and energy synthesis in the body. 168-169.

cytochrome P-450 - the enzymes in the endoplasmic reticulum which initiate the Phase I detox process. 51-52, 64, 65, 142, 173.

cytosol - the substance inside the cell, outside of the nucleus. 39, 40, 52.

D-6-D - delta-6-desaturase, the enzyme that helps metabolize essential fatty acids. 206, 207, 217, 219.

degenerative disease - all disease processes (degenerate or deteriorate the body). 75, 79, 91, 98, 160, 210, 213, 220, 225, 226, 240, 302, 351.

dehydrogenation - adding an electron. 37.

depollution - detoxifying. 141, 143, 144, 192, 282.

depression - abnormal lack of interest in anything (often due to being "stoned" on some chemical or a bad diet). 5, 12, 14, 23, 29, 70-75, 82, 85, 90, 92, 94, 102, 111, 124, 126, 129, 137, 139, 148, 149, 158, 159, 165-168, 179, 190, 237, 240, 245, 251, 261, 314, 317, 338, 368, 381.

detoxication – making less toxic. 9, 11, 34–39, 41, 43–68, 79–89, 91–106, 111, 114–116, 119–123, 128, 131, 135–153, 160–176, 184–186, 191–197, 201–205, 231, 235, 246, 249, 253, 257, 259, 261, 271, 274–281, 289, 290, 296, 302–309, 321, 330, 334, 352–356, 371.

detoxification – see detoxication.

D-glucaric acid – one of the de-pollution enzymes, an indicator of stress to the detox path. 140–143.

diabetes – abnormal glucose or sugar metabolism, often secondary to chromium and other mineral deficiencies. 63, 85, 159, 187, 190, 220, 226, 228–231, 257, 323, 332, 336, 337, 378, 379.

DNA – deoxyribose nucleic acid, the genetic material that resides inside the cell nucleus. 15, 46, 67, 84, 173, 185.

domino effect – the spreading phenomenon, where each defect leads to several other defects, generating a massive breakdown or cascade of malfunctions in the system. 63, 165.

dopamine – a brain hormone (neurotransmitter). 111, 148.

dopa oxidase – a copper-containing enzyme for metabolizing dopamine. 168, 169.

double blind – testing performed while neither the patient nor the nurse tester knows what is being tested. 6, 29, 30, 347, 354.

downward spiral – getting worse by leaps and bounds; cascade of malfunctions where the sick get sicker. 50, 105, 165, 166, 170, 185, 356.

Dursban – see chlorpyrifos. 122, 135.

dysfunctional detoxication – malfunctioning system that is supposed to clean chemicals from the body before they create damage and disease. 24, 30, 32, 62, 128, 139, 151, 310, 311.

EBV – Epstein-Barr Virus, the presumed cause of infectious mononucleosis. 6, 59, 364.

eclampsia – a potentially fatal attack of severe magnesium deficiency in the last weeks of a pregnancy. If the patient lives, it can result in a stroke, coma, and loss of the fetus or death of the mother. 159.

EFA – essential fatty acids; there are 2 types, Omega 3 and Omega 6. 9, 25, 45, 192, 207-209, 217, 221, 254.

E.I. – environmentally-induced illness, or environmental illness, for short. 42, 47, 55, 56, 72, 115, 116, 121, 123-128, 142, 150, 151, 174, 185, 189, 253, 291, 299, 302, 303, 314, 335, 348, 357.

eicosapentaenoic acid – or EPA for short, the Omega 3 essential fatty acid. 210, 223.

electron – a charged particle, all substances are made of molecules which have electrons in them, it can be thought of as the electro-chemical base of all matter. 39, 160, 165, 175, 226, 366.

endocrine – having to do with glands and hormones. 33, 61, 85, 86, 91, 98, 201, 301, 306, 310, 332.

endoplasmic reticulum – the set of membranes in the cell where detox occurs. 39, 40, 51, 59, 61, 63, 64, 205, 232, 270, 310, 319, 330, 354.

environmental medicine – the first and only medical specialty that deals with detox and finding the causes of symptoms whether they be from sensitivities to the environment (pollens, dusts, molds, chemicals, Candida) or foods, or from nutritional deficiencies. 2, 10, 18, 25, 59, 72, 78, 90, 99, 109-111, 124, 131, 141, 145, 156, 202-205, 244, 302, 304, 336, 352, 353, 357, 358, 362-364, 368, 380.

enzyme - a protein that makes a reaction proceed. 9, 41,
   44-65, 84-101, 114, 116, 120, 136, 140-144, 152-154,
   160-163, 167-173, 179, 184-186, 191, 193, 195, 206,
   209, 211, 217, 219, 231, 240, 244, 248, 250-253, 265,
   299, 302-306, 310, 312, 317-332, 353.

epinephrine - adrenalin, the stress hormone. 148, 161, 163,
   166, 184.

epoxides - dangerous intermediates that cause cancer, E.I.;
   they poison the immune system, damage genetics. 53,
   55.

essential fatty acids (EFA) - the Omega-3 and Omega-6 lipids
   which we can't live without. 9, 25, 45, 94, 175, 186,
   192, 206-215, 219, 229, 231, 237, 254, 257, 294, 306,
   311, 336, 352, 368.

excrete - get rid of through excretions like urine or stool.
   36, 39-41, 47, 56, 60, 125, 128, 131, 153, 200, 237,
   322.

fatty acids - only two forms are essential to the function
   of body membranes, omega 3 and 6. 60, 91, 211, 213-
   215, 329.

flora - the types of living things contained therein
   (usually refers to the normal bacteria and yeasts and
   molds that inhabit the gut to break down our food).
   91, 144, 192, 248, 251, 252, 302, 310, 320, 322, 363,
   368.

food processing - the removal of many vitamins and minerals
   and the addition of many chemicals (preservatives,
   colorings, additives, chemical flavorings) to make
   food tasty, quick to prepare and slow to deteriorate.
   92, 185, 238.

formaldehyde - a ubiquitous chemical in exhaust fumes as
   well as outgassing from "foam" products and many
   others. 12-20, 23, 24, 29, 36, 64, 82, 83, 89, 99,

103, 144, 161, 162, 186, 191, 276, 295, 303, 307, 310, 311, 314, 359, 360, 362, 369, 371.

formic acid – a metabolite of formaldehyde in the body, hence an indicator of whether the body can detox formaldehyde appropriately. 28, 140, 143, 144, 191, 307.

free radical – crazy naked electrons that result from chemical reactions; their danger is that they eat holes in membranes and cause cell damage (and hence diseases like arthritis if, for example, the damage is in the joint lining tissues) and death; they can also damage or derange the regulatory enzymes and the genetic material (this is how they can initiate cancer). 61, 67, 140–143, 160, 162, 165, 169, 175, 186, 193, 226–228, 254, 305, 322, 354.

gamma amino butyric acid – a neurotransmitter or brain hormone; many tranquilizers work at this level. 111, 161, 251.

gastroenterologist – a specialist in bowel problems; oddly enough, they have no training in complicated food allergies. 29, 76, 290.

gene repair – the constant upkeep and renewal of our genetic material (that governs all of the body functions). 84, 173, 185, 191, 309.

genetic – having to do with heredity (genes); also these nucleic acids regulate our future health (and can be damaged or changed by environmental chemicals). 15, 40, 41, 45, 46, 55, 59, 60, 66, 67, 83, 84, 91, 115, 121, 139, 142, 162, 179, 180, 186, 250, 290, 299, 306, 309, 332, 346, 350, 353, 383.

glutathione – GSH, a tripeptide that conjugates chemicals so the body can excrete them. 41, 46, 52, 62, 95, 116, 131, 136, 140, 153, 160, 165, 166, 175, 185, 193, 306, 318, 322, 326, 327.

glutathione peroxidase - GSH PX a selenium dependent enzyme that helps protect the membranes from lipid peroxidation, and as it "neutralizes" the peroxides, it triggers glutathione to conjugate with and carry away the remaining part of the xenobiotic. 52, 62, 140, 143, 173, 179, 186, 192.

glutathione reductase - the vitamin B2 requiring enzyme that restores unused glutathione (GSSG) to the usable form (GSH). 52, 179, 192.

glutathione S-transferase - an enzyme used in metabolizing glutathione. 89.

glutathione synthestase - an enzyme that helps form glutathione (requires magnesium). 160, 173.

glycine - an amino acid; when it conjugates with chemicals it puts hippuric acid into the urine which can be measured as proof of chemical overload. 41, 52, 54, 184.

GSH - glutathione. 41, 46, 52, 62, 95, 140, 165, 173, 175, 184, 185.

GSH PX - glutathione peroxidase. 52, 62.

health - not the absence of disease, but optimum vitality and function. 1-10, 28, 34, 72, 79, 103, 106, 108, 119, 123, 129, 150, 187, 195, 203, 211, 218, 220, 229, 235, 241, 259, 266, 267, 297, 299, 300, 304, 309, 316, 317, 336, 347, 349, 351, 367, 368, 384.

hexane - a hydrocarbon in exhaust fumes. 16, 17.

hexanol - the alcohol of hexane. 17, 18.

histamine - a substance the body makes excess of in allergic reactions and in the presence of magnesium deficiency. 102, 111, 159, 248, 321.

homeostasis - the balancing out that the body constantly strives for in attempting to compensate for deficiencies and environmental overload. 160, 192.

hydrocarbon - a chemical compound of hydrogen and carbon (most are derived from coal products). 17-24, 31, 34, 62, 80, 103, 126, 166, 299, 306, 321, 362, 374, 381.

hydrogen - an element. 19, 39.

hyperactivity - a name for a childhood condition of excessive motion and usually accompanied by poor learning; current treatment prescribes dangerous drugs related to street "speed" (amphetamines), but most children have treatable causes once environmental triggers and nutrient deficiencies are found. 74, 75, 90, 109, 225, 336.

hyperacusis - normal noises seen uncomfortably louder. 126.

hypercholesterolemia - high cholesterol in the blood. 95, 311, 354, 379.

hypertension - high blood pressure, often due to magnesium and other nutrient deficiencies, also overload of xenobiotics and wrong foods. 33, 64, 95, 148, 154, 159, 187, 190, 220, 222, 231, 240-243, 257, 325, 378, 379.

hypochondriac - a non-entity; commonly thought of as a patient who complains but has nothing wrong. (Why would he be complaining then if he were healthy and happy?) 5, 9, 32, 34, 50, 69, 71, 77, 83, 357, 364, 371.

hypoglycemia - low blood sugar; can cause mood swings, sweats, fainting, and headaches, often caused by undiscovered chromium deficiency. 90, 190, 228.

IgE - immunoglobulin E, or one of the allergic antibodies. 106, 252, 302, 352.

immune system - includes the parts of the body that make antibodies (that cause allergies and that also fight off disease). 30, 33, 56, 61, 84, 86, 98, 105-107, 119-121, 163, 196, 201, 209, 284, 303, 321, 352, 357, 373.

immunosuppression – turning off of the good protective parts of the immune system; usually caused by a chemical and can lead to severe and even fatal vulnerability to infection. 55.

impotency – inability to have an erection (can be caused by nutrient deficiencies; diabetes, arteriosclerosis, etc. are blamed as the cause often, while the underlying deficiency is not looked for). 49, 226.

individuality – one of the underlying principles of environmental medicine which recognizes we are all biochemically different or unique. 8, 9, 45, 66, 68, 70, 72, 83, 89, 92, 105, 107, 122, 124, 150, 191, 192-194, 237, 245, 250, 267, 302, 304, 309-313, 329, 340, 353, 367, 383.

inert ingredients – refers to the hydrocarbon solvent carrier or vehicle for pesticide sprays; is far from harmless and can be more toxic than the actual pesticide. 114, 125, 126, 326.

intermediary metabolite – one of the chemicals formed on the way to forming the end result of a pathway. 233.

intravenous – injected into the vein. 129, 157, 242, 255.

Kroker, Dr. George – 340, 342.

laryngitis – inflammation of the larynx or throat. 12, 14, 245.

lipid – fat; crucial in cell membranes, but damaging in blood vessel walls if deposited here because of lack of nutrients to properly metabolize it. 23, 24, 40, 44, 61-63, 80, 141, 142, 205, 210, 219, 229-232, 243-244, 326.

lipid peroxidation - the free radical attack on cell membranes leading to their damage and dysfunction, can lead to a chain reaction of destruction if antioxidants are lacking. 67, 146, 147.

lipid peroxides - free radicals (that result from chemical detoxications) that cause the membrane damage that leads to disease and aging. 140-143, 147.

lupus - system lupus erythematosis is a disease of the connective tissues of the body; can cause disease in any organ and even death; like most other disease names, usually biochemical deficiencies and environmental triggers can be identified so that health is restored without the use of drugs. 33, 70, 73, 98, 150.

macrobiotics - a way of eating and living in harmony with nature; many people have cured "incurable" end stage cancers with this. It translates into "large life" and emphasizes whole grains, vegetables, beans, seaweeds, and seeds to maximize balance and nutrition. 273, 298, 306, 307, 314, 317, 318, 322-336.

magnesium - a very essential mineral in the body; helps muscles relax; nature's tranquilizer and calcium channel blocker. 9, 55, 57, 63, 65, 94, 95, 99, 102, 103, 129, 138, 153-163, 168-170, 179-181, 188, 192-194, 208, 211, 213-216, 223, 232, 234, 235, 239-244, 253-255, 265, 270, 303, 307, 311, 314, 323, 336, 349, 369, 370, 379, 381.

magnesium loading test - a 2-part urine test that is a more reliable way of diagnosing magnesium deficiency than any blood test. 154, 157, 159, 172, 191, 223, 228, 240, 323, 398-407.

maintenance - a prescribed program of supplements which is made after deficiencies are corrected; takes into account individual's needs and still requires monitoring periodically for appropriateness. 229.

manganese - an essential mineral. 160, 161, 169, 170, 173,

189, 192, 193, 208, 231, 234, 237-239, 254.

manic depression - a form of mental illness where one is wild at one time and very down and out another; he tends to swing through these extremes. 33, 75, 305.

margarine - a synthetic food that is supposed to taste like butter; unfortunately it has trans fatty acids which should never be eaten. 95, 206, 210-212, 214, 217, 219-223, 254, 273, 349.

masking - the phenomenon where you really don't know you're reacting to something because your body's enzymes have revved up in response to its attempt to adapt to a stimulus; for example, the first cigarette may make one sick, but years of smoking are tolerated as cancer may be silently triggered; once you stop, the chest may be worse as it clears out and restarting could make one sick again. 5, 8, 10, 86, 98, 105, 290, 304, 305, 310.

membrane - covering, usually of a cell. 23, 40, 44, 59, 61-64, 67, 80, 93, 99, 129, 140, 142, 163, 165, 175, 184, 186, 205, 206, 210, 217, 219, 231-234, 253, 261, 270, 354, 356, 379.

mercapturic acid - a urinary metabolite of foreign chemicals, therefore a good indicator of poisoning. 54, 140, 143.

mercury - a dangerously toxic metal that can permanently poison many body enzymes; can come from inhaling industrial (city smog) exhausts, eating fish (the limit from many "pristine" New York State lakes is one a month, since we have allowed industry to pollute our waterways), dental amalgams, etc. 19, 60, 62, 65, 116, 190.

metabolism - a process of making energy or getting rid of something or changing it to another form. 25, 30, 31, 35, 36, 84, 85, 89, 92, 99, 102-105, 111, 114, 124, 125, 128, 131, 137, 142, 153, 161, 171, 172, 176, 180,

181, 184, 186, 187, 190, 191, 209, 228, 230-233, 235, 237, 254, 312, 323, 329, 353.

methacrylate - a chemical that outgasses from plastics, adhesives (often used in dentistry). 17, 18, 125, 279.

methylnaphthalene - a potent hydrocarbon that outgasses from household products and can cause cancer. 17, 18.

methylene chloride - dichloromethane; a solvent in paints, paint strippers, aerosol propellant, can rapidly metabolize in the body to a lethal level of carbon monoxide. 17, 19.

Mickey Finn - the old "knock-out drops", chloral hydrate; also forms in the brain when detox pathways are over- loaded. 32, 48, 56, 102, 167.

mitochondria - cylindrical structures within a cell (encased in a membrane) where all the energy is manufactured. 40, 44, 59, 61, 63, 64, 160, 163, 205, 310, 354.

molecular - having to do with molecules which are composed of atoms (which are composed of negatively changed electrons and positively charged protons). 41, 68, 78, 95, 169, 244, 332, 344, 364, 367, 375.

molybdenum - an mineral essential to the body, in sulfite oxidase and aldehyde oxidase enzymes, for example. 48, 49, 51, 57, 101, 156, 167, 168, 170, 171, 173, 192, 212, 319, 324.

monoamine oxidase - MAO, the enzyme that metabolizes many brain hormones. 233, 325.

monooxygenase - the cytochrome P450 enzymes in the endo- plasmic reticulum where Phase I detox begins. 52, 246, 253, 321.

multiple sclerosis - a severely progressive disease of the nervous system where the victims can end up unable to care for themselves. 33.

mutagenesis – the process that creates mutation or serious genetic change, usually for the worse; often goes on to cause cancer in the person and/or birth defects in his offspring. 55.

mycotoxins – toxins made by molds, many are potent carcinogens. 36, 38, 225.

neuropathy – pathology or disease of nervous tissue, often manifesting as numbness and tingling. 21, 88, 115, 237.

neurotic – mentally abnormal or strange but not overtly crazy or out of touch with reality. 103, 158, 163, 167.

neurotransmitter – chemicals that make nervous tissue work; in the brain they can be thought of as brain hormones that create our moods and memory; in peripheral nervous tissue (the long nerves outside of the brain that came from the spinal column) it refers to the chemicals that transmit the electricity from nerves to muscles. 81, 99, 102, 103, 111, 115, 142, 148, 161, 163, 165, 168, 169, 171, 172, 184, 191, 196, 209, 233, 235, 249, 266, 298, 307, 313, 321, 323-325, 369.

niacin – vitamin B3, very important in electron transfer in phase I detox, also used to lower cholesterol; causes flushing if dose not carefully raised. 52, 131, 175, 232.

noradrenalin – a neurotransmitter cousin to adrenalin. 102, 111, 325.

normal – (1) has taken a new meaning in this century, for example, normal levels of chemicals in the blood should be zero, but now there are "normal" ranges that represent an average or mean of what is found among the "asymptomatic" populace of the 20th century; (2) normal levels for nutrients in the blood assume there is no individual biochemical variation. 20, 48, 52, 65, 84, 112, 116, 137, 139, 142, 152, 229, 231, 248, 255, 316, 330, 333, 363, 372.

nucleic acids - the building blocks of DNA and RNA. 332.

nucleus - area within the cell, enclosed by a membrane that houses genetic material, DNA. 40, 61.

nutrient - can be a vitamin, mineral, amino acid or essential fatty acid. 48-50, 66, 84, 86, 90-96, 104, 106, 108, 131, 137, 143, 145, 148, 152-156, 160, 161, 166, 172, 175, 176, 179-181, 185-189, 194, 195, 203, 261, 265, 268, 269, 274, 275, 284, 288, 298, 303-307, 310, 312, 314, 320-324, 328, 331, 333, 339, 352, 353, 356, 368-370, 379.

nystagmus - a spasm of the eye muscles (seen best if one looks far to the side; the observer will note the eye seems to bounce back and forth ever so slightly). Magnesium deficiency can be a cause. 138, 159.

Omega-3 - one of two EFA's; from fish oils and flax (linseed) oils. 9, 207-210, 213, 216, 220-222, 229, 230, 254.

Omega-6 - one of two EFA's; from vegetable and seed oils. 194, 207-209, 216, 220, 223, 225, 254.

optimal - best for that individual, disregarding what is best for the average person. 25-28, 65, 106, 107, 150, 160, 190, 206, 214, 219, 261, 321.

organophosphorous compounds - a commonly used class of pesticides; works by inhibiting nerve transmission (via inhibition of plasma cholinesturase and rbc acetycholinesturase) much of the damage is cummulative and irreversible (Zenz). 85, 88, 123, 134, 135, 139, 140, 326.

osteoporosis - a condition of weak bones because the minerals and vitamins needed to fix calcium in the bones are missing. 95, 153, 190, 232, 234, 236-240, 252, 329, 378.

oxidation - removal or "burning off" of electrons, breakdown, metabolism, aging, burning up. 37, 39, 164, 165, 226.

palpitations - irregular heartbeat, often because of lack of minerals for normal nerve conduction and muscle relaxation and/or excess stimulation as from caffeine (and other food and chemical sensitivities); hearts with compromised blood supply as in arteriosclerosis are more vulnerable. 12, 14, 51.

Pangborn, Dr., Jon - 157, 395.

PAPS - a Phase II conjugator. 44, 52, 54, 56, 116, 153, 165, 173, 184, 185.

paresthesia - a form of neuropathy usually characterized by numbness and tingling of an extremity; a common symptom of pesticide poisoning. 126.

Parkinsonism - a degenerative nervous disease with uncontrollable tremor. 33, 148, 161, 270, 363.

PCP - pentachlorophenol, a common and toxic wood preservative. 129.

peroxidation - accelerated oxidation or destruction of cell membranes by peroxides (free radicals) that result from the body's attempt to metabolize chemicals. 67, 165.

pesticide - a chemical meant to destroy life (insects, weeds, etc.). 18, 19, 24, 34, 38, 39, 51, 57, 62, 65, 80, 81, 85, 88, 92, 95, 103, 108, 111-144, 175, 190, 192, 216, 225, 261, 264, 267, 275, 279, 281, 296, 303, 306, 326, 328, 348-350, 363, 368-374, 378.

Phase I - usually the first stage of detox and inside the endoplasmic reticulum. 39, 40, 44, 47, 51, 55, 59,

60, 63, 64, 99, 140, 170, 173, 186, 232, 319, 330, 355.

Phase II – the second stage of detox, usually occurs in the cell substance or cytosol. 39-41, 52, 54, 56, 60, 116, 153, 160, 165, 166, 173, 186, 232, 330, 354.

phases of detox – the steps you can take at any pace that suits you to gradually get healthy. 43, 153, 259, 260, 276, 279, 282, 288, 289.

phenol – a toxic benzene derivative, the old carbolic acid, a preservative in all regular allergy injections, a known carcinogen; conjugated with glucuronic acid and sulfuric acid so extracts with phenol put additional stress on detox paths (Zenz). 16-19, 23, 30, 50, 89, 106, 107, 125, 168, 171, 280, 292, 295, 296.

phosphatidyl choline – an essential lipid in all membranes, without which serious degenerative disease like Alzheimer's occurs; see auto-cannibalism. 175, 184, 194, 219, 269, 270, 319, 354-356.

phthalate – a metabolite of plasticizers and plastics. 16, 17, 24, 273.

phytates – substances from undercooked or raw vegetables and grains that can inhibit the absorption of nutrients. 231.

placebo – a dummy or fake or control. 28, 29, 146, 354.

plaque – a deposit (usually unwanted and harmful as in arterial and dental plaques). 161, 229.

plasticizer – chemicals that give plastics their desirable physical qualities; are usually carcinogens. 24.

polyaromatic – many ring structures in the chemical. 166.

polyunsaturate – a biochemical term that is supposed to lure the public into thinking there are multiple double bonds, so it's the "good" type of oil; what it actually stands for is that it is an inferior oil that has been hydrogenated and changed to the deleterious trans form as well as bleached, purified (vitamins and minerals removed) and packaged in see through bottles (so much has been removed that light can no longer damage it). 206, 210, 213, 214, 217, 326.

polyvinyl chloride - PVC, hard plastic as for pipes. 24, 34, 129.

ppm - parts per million, a unit of measure.

presenile dementia - usually referred to as Alzheimer's where the mind goes before the person is actually old enough; really it's another medical misnomer, because it suggests that it's to be expected at some time whereas there is no reason why it should occur ever. 212, 269, 270, 354, 363, 368.

prostaglandin - hormones of the immune system, some of which have good effects, others are destructive. 208, 209, 221.

protozoa - a one-celled organism that can cause disease in the body, usually is a parasite. 251, 252.

provocation-neutralization - skin testing techniques where one dose turns on symptoms and another turns them off. 25-28, 145, 151, 306, 308, 313, 347.

psoriasis - an "incurable" scaley skin problem, often corrected by finding an essential fatty acid deficiency or other metabolic abnormality. 74, 222, 225.

psychosis - "crazy, nuts", out of touch with reality (often biochemical defects and environmental triggers can be found and corrected). 115, 159.

pyridoxal-5-phosphate - the enzyme that allows vitamin B6 to be metabolized. 176, 179, 186.

Randolph, Dr. Theron G. – 16, 23, 123, 266, 341, 347, 388, 391.

Raynaud's – a spastic condition of vessels where the finger, for example, becomes abnormally cold and white. 157, 159, 240.

Rea, Dr. William J. – 10, 27, 123, 129, 154, 157, 266, 294, 305, 348, 385, 389, 393, 395, 396, 398, 399.

redox ability – the balancing or neutralization of body chemistry to minimize dangerous free radical formation. 164.

reduction – addition of electrons to a molecule or substance. 39, 53, 164, 245.

Remington, Dr. Dennis – 350.

riboflavin – vitamin B2. 52.

RNA – ribonucleic acid, the material which governs all of our cell functions; it can be damaged by chemicals so that the instructions to make cancer are followed; it works in close harmony with the genetic nucleic acid DNA, getting its instructions from it; it is the RNA that is sort of the sub-contractor; it directs the protein and enzyme synthesis and actually sees that the genetic work is carried out. 186, 330.

Rogers' Rules – 106.

sarcoid – one of many syndromes of "unknown cause" which causes a severe arthritis, lung disease, dermatitis, and many other symptoms; sometimes goes into a long remission. 70, 73.

schizophrenia – a form of mental illness where one hallucinates, and has a zombie-type "flat" affect, and appears crazy in speech or actions. 33, 70, 71, 75, 139, 237.

senility – "old age", usually connotes not being in full mental control, as well. 20, 161, 226, 232, 234, 239, 241, 354, 356, 378, 379.

serial dilution titration – the logical approach to skin testing for allergies where the precise dose is found for each antigen rather than trying to give everyone the same dose. 313.

serotonin – a brain neurotransmitter. 9, 111, 148, 163, 166, 321, 324, 372.

Shambaugh, Dr. George – 348.

single blind – testing where the patient does not know what is being tested. 29, 30, 106, 146, 151, 306, 308.

skin brushing – to stimulate lymphatics. 200, 323.

snowball effect – whereby a condition gets worse and worse as symptoms pile on, spreading phenomenon, cascade. 29, 66, 96.

SOD – superoxide dismutase, the body's natural anti-inflammatory enzyme. 160, 169, 173, 186.

spreading phenomenon – same as snowball effect. 81, 162, 166, 186, 302–304, 309.

styrene – a carcinogenic chemical that plastics are made from, has been found in biopsies of arteriosclerotic plaques; excreted in urine as mandelic acid and phenylglyoxylic acid. 17–20, 23, 137, 138.

sulfhydryl – a sulfur and hydrogen atom which are attached to a molecule; this group is used to connect a molecule with a chemical so it can be dragged out of the body (as on the sulfhydryl group of GSH). 52, 116, 184.

sulfite – (1) can refer to a sulfur-containing food additive, or (2) the pathway in the body that metabolizes these. 171, 172, 319.

sulfo-transferase - an enzyme that moves sulfur groups from one molecule to another. 170, 171, 325.

sulfur - an essential element in the body, especially important in detox. 52, 53, 55, 116, 170, 172, 173, 324, 325.

superoxide dismutase - SOD, an antioxidant that protects against free radical destruction, especially in inflammatory reactions; can be likened to the body's own anti-arthritis substance. 140-143, 160.

synovium - tissue that lines joints; it's the area where chemicals, antigens and free radicals can go on to cause arthritis symptoms. 341.

synthesis - manufacture or creation of. 34, 48, 92, 96, 102, 108, 158, 165, 167, 168, 172-175, 184-186, 191, 218, 221, 231, 318, 320, 324, 328, 330, 332.

tachycardia - abnormally fast heart beat.

target organ - the body area predominantly affected by an environmental trigger or nutrient deficiency. 23, 32, 46, 74-76, 79-83, 88, 106, 128, 189, 237, 257, 266, 302, 309-311, 356, 363, 370.

TCE or tce - trichloroethylene, a ubiquitous solvent and xenobiotic; forms chloral hydrate in the brain if detox paths are overloaded by other chemicals of blocked by an unsuspected nutrient deficiency. 21, 152.

teratogenesis - causing harmful genetic change in the fetus. 55.

tetrachloroethylene - perchloroethylene or Perc (dry cleaning fluid), a cousin of tce. 17-19, 152.

tetrahydroisoquinolines - false neurotransmitters that are formed when aldehydes attack brain hormones. 163.

T helper cells - important cells in the immune system that direct other cells into action.

thiaminase - an enzyme made by some species of fungi like Candida in the gut, that destroys vitamin Bl before it can get absorbed. 247, 252, 320.

thiamine - vitamin Bl. 131, 175, 191, 247, 252, 318, 322.

TIA - transient ischemic attack, or mini-strokes where the person does not progress to a full stroke, but it's a good warning that one is around the corner. 159.

TIBC - total iron binding capacity, part of the measure of iron storage.

tight building syndrome - also known as sick buidling syndrome; retrofitting to conserve heat has captured the outgassings of many indoor building materials and synthetic products; this heightened level of chemicals causes disease. 16, 18, 106, 295, 348.

toluene - methyl benzene; solvent, outgasses from many products like paints; biotransformed to hippuric acid in the urine. 16-19, 23, 24, 29, 57, 88, 89, 103, 125, 138, 141, 142, 192, 279, 295, 303, 304, 383.

total load - the summation of body burden in terms of what the body has to deal with (adapt to or detoxify). 66-68, 83, 85, 88, 89, 102, 106, 124, 136, 145, 146, 166, 203, 246, 278, 302, 304, 308-310, 313, 361, 368, 369.

toxic brain syndrome - any brain symptoms caused by a toxin; can include confusion, depression, spaciness, etc. 56, 61, 63, 88, 158, 165, 170, 363, 371.

trans fatty acids - the harmful and abnormal form caused by hydrogenation. 206, 211, 222, 254, 379.

transition - a change. 259, 288, 328.

trichloroethane - methyl chloroform, metabolized to trichloroethanol and trichloroacetic acid, related to the solvent tce. 17-20, 328.

trichloroethylene - tce, metabolized to same two metabolites as trichloroethane; metabolism inhibited by alcohol, trichloroethanol is conjugated with glucuronic acid (Zenz). 16-23, 31, 50, 55, 65, 99, 103, 125, 137, 167, 280, 308, 326, 363, 372, 373.

trypsin - a chromium requiring digestive enzyme that breaks down amino acids for absorption.

T suppressor cell - important immune system cell that acts as a governor or regulator of cell activity. 114.

tyrosine - an amino acid from which adrenalin is formed. 148, 184, 324.

UDPGA - a Phase II conjugator. 44.

U.F.F.I. - urea foam formaldehyde insulation or "foam insulation" for short. 12, 14, 15, 23, 311.

unmasking - the process of becoming unadapted, loss of adaptive enzymes as a substance is avoided for a while. 271, 362.

vaginitis - chronic inflammation of vaginal tissues with burning and itching; the vagina can be the target organ for a food sensitivity, and of course, it is vulnerable to repeated infections if there are undiscovered nutrient deficiencies. 70.

vasculitis - inflammation of blood vessels. 159, 240.

vertigo - dizziness. 138, 159.

vinyl - a form of plastic. 17, 280, 295.

vinyl chloride - outgasses from plastics, can cause toxic brain symptoms. 24, 48, 65, 67, 129, 161.

VIP - vasoactive intestinal peptide, a gut neurotransmitter which has receptor sites in other parts of the body, including the brain; is one of the ways the gut talks to or communicates with the brain.

vitamin L - love and laughter. 150, 195.

VOC - volatile organic (hydrocarbon) compounds is just another name for one class of xenobiotics; volatile means it gets into the air (and brain) easily. 34.

xenobiotic - foreign chemical. 16, 34-39, 42, 43, 46, 56, 60, 64, 81-84, 89, 91, 98, 130, 131, 140-145, 153, 161, 166, 170, 171, 253, 279, 302, 303, 306, 308, 310, 313, 322-328, 356, 369.

xylene - a relative of benzene (dimethyl benzene), can be carcinogenic, outgasses from many products; eliminated as urinary methyl hippuric acid. 16-20, 23, 29, 50, 82, 125, 151, 279, 295, 296, 303, 383.

zinc - an essential mineral in over 90 enzymes. 48-52, 56, 57, 84, 94, 101, 152, 156, 165, 167-173, 184-187, 191-193, 209, 211-214, 228, 231-239, 253, 254, 303, 307, 314, 316, 320, 336, 378.

438

My special thanks to Jack and Carol Roshia of Liverpool, NY. For 22 years ago they had a dream of bringing a gift to the world. And that gift has typed and edited, and retyped, and re-edited this book. Thank you, Jackie.